Clinical Electrocardiography

PreTest® Self-Assessment and Review

Clinical Electrocardiography

PreTest® Self-Assessment and Review

Franklin H. Zimmerman, M.D.
Assistant Clinical Professor of Medicine (Cardiology)
Columbia University College of Physicians and Surgeons
New York, New York
Attending Cardiologist
Phelps Memorial Hospital Center
North Tarrytown, New York
Westchester County Medical Center
Valhalla, New York
St. Luke's–Roosevelt Hospital Center
New York, New York

McGraw-Hill, Inc.
Health Professions Division/PreTest Series

New York St. Louis San Francisco Auckland
Bogotá Caracas Lisbon London Madrid
Mexico City Milan Montreal New Delhi Paris
San Juan Singapore Sydney Tokyo Toronto

Clinical Electrocardiography: PreTest Self-Assessment and Review
International Editions 1994

2 3 4 5 6 7 8 9 0 SLP PMP 9 8 7 6 5

Library of Congress Cataloging-in-Publication Data

Zimmerman, Franklin H.
Clinical electrocardiography : PreTest self-assessment and review / Franklin H. Zimmerman.
p. cm.
Includes bibliographical references.
ISBN 0-07-052008-9
1. Electrocardiography-Examinations, questions, etc.
2. Electrocardiography-Problems, exercises, etc. I. Title.
[DNLM: 1. Electrocardiography-examination questions. WG 18 Z72c 1994]
RC683.5.E5Z538 1994
616.1'207547'076-dc20
DNLM/DLC
for Library of Congress 93-13548
CIP

The editors were Gail Gavert and Bruce MacGregor.
The production supervisor was Gyl A. Favours.
This book was set in Times Roman by Compset, Inc.

When ordering this title, use ISBN 0-07-113587-1

Printed in Singapore

To

Laurie, Stacey and Ricky

for their support, sacrifice, and encouragement

Contents

Introduction

Clinical Electrocardiography: PreTest Self-Assessment and Review has been designed to provide physicians with a clinically relevant, academic approach to the interpretation of electrocardiograms. This text should be useful to any physician who interprets electrocardiograms, including cardiologists, internists, family practitioners, anesthesiologists, medical students, or any health care provider who wishes to maintain a high competency in the interpretation of electrocardiograms. The board review format should provide a particularly useful instrument for candidates taking the cardiology board examination. Use of this review text should help the reader to (1) recognize common and uncommon electrocardiographic diagnoses, (2) learn the principles of interpreting cardiac arrhythmias, (3) identify areas of weakness, and (4) correlate electrocardiographic data with clinically relevant information.

This text contains a total of 200 electrocardiograms. All use a three-channel format with a concomitant lead II rhythm strip. Both a narrative and a board-examination type of format are used for interpretation. The narrative interpretation is designed to simulate that used in a hospital's electrocardiographic laboratory. The board review format is designed to resemble that which appears on the electrocardiographic portion of the cardiology board examination.

The 200 electrocardiograms are divided into 5 tests of 40 tracings each. The reader may wish to practice using a time limit of 4 hours for each in order to simulate the format of the actual board examination. A brief clinical history appears with each electrocardiogram. Answers, explanations, and references are given after each electrocardiogram. The references may indicate specific citations for the commentary or offer opportunities for further reading. Book references appear with the author's name and the appropriate page number. Journal references appear with the author's name only; if more than one article by an author is listed in the bibliography, articles are differentiated by parenthetical notations. A section of diagnostic criteria for standard electrocardiographic diagnoses precedes the first test.

Acknowledgments

Special appreciation is given to Dr. Arthur E. Fass, Assistant Clinical Professor of Medicine (Cardiology) at New York Medical College and Chief of Cardiology at Phelps Memorial Hospital Center. Dr. Fass reviewed and interpreted each ECG and was the major contributor to and editor of the section on diagnostic criteria that opens this text.

I wish to thank Dr. James Levy, Director of the Electrocardiography Laboratory, Westchester County Medical Center; Dr. Carmine Sorbera, Associate Director of the Electrophysiology Laboratory, Westchester County Medical Center; and Dr. Julian Frieden, Chief of Cardiology, New Rochelle Hospital for their review of the electrocardiograms.

The clerical and nursing staffs of Phelps Memorial Hospital Center, Westchester County Medical Center, and New Rochelle Hospital were instrumental in collecting the electrocardiographic tracings.

I also wish to thank Gail Gavert at McGraw-Hill, whose efforts and confidence are in large part responsible for the successful completion of this project.

Test Instructions

The reader should first interpret the electrocardiograms in a narrative format. The tracing should be analyzed in terms of the cardiac rhythm with identification of the atrial and ventricular rates. The PR, QRS, and QT intervals should be measured, and the electrical axis determined within 15 degrees. Electrocardiographic abnormalities should be identified. The data should then be synthesized into an integrated interpretation.

A board-review format may also be used for practice. The following section provides a table of electrocardiographic diagnoses that should be used with the sample tracings. The reader should select the diagnoses that apply to each electrocardiogram. Multiple diagnoses are likely for each example. There may not be an exact diagnosis to conform with the narrative interpretation; however, the reader should choose those diagnoses which best apply. The author has listed the preferred selections in the answer section. Potential, unconfirmed, or alternative diagnoses appear in parentheses.

The selection of test answers is derived from standard electrocardiographic diagnoses. The test is similar but not identical to the cardiology board examination. The author makes no claim that the American Board of Internal Medicine or the American College of Cardiology would interpret the enclosed tracings exactly as the author has done.

Abbreviations

AFIB *Atrial fibrillation*
APC *Atrial premature complex*
AV *Atrioventricular*
CCU *Coronary care unit*
CHF *Congestive heart failure*
COPD *Chronic obstructive pulmonary disease*
ECG *Electrocardiogram*
ER *Emergency room*
ICU *Intensive care unit*
JPC *Junctional premature complex*
LBBB *Left bundle branch block*
LVH *Left ventricular hypertrophy*
MAT *Multifocal atrial tachycardia*
MI *Myocardial infarction*
PAT *Paroxysmal atrial tachycardia*
RBBB *Right bundle branch block*
RVH *Right ventricular hypertrophy*
SA *Sinoatrial*
SVT *Supraventricular tachycardia*
VA *Ventriculoatrial*
VPC *Ventricular premature complex*
VT *Ventricular tachycardia*
WPW *Wolff-Parkinson-White pattern (or syndrome)*

Table of Electrocardiographic Diagnoses

I. RHYTHM ABNORMALITIES

A. Supraventricular Rhythms and Complexes

- □ 1. Sinus rhythm
- □ 2. Sinus arrhythmia
- □ 3. Sinus bradycardia
- □ 4. Sinus tachycardia
- □ 5. Wandering atrial pacemaker within the sinus node
- □ 6. Wandering atrial pacemaker to the AV junction
- □ 7. Sinus arrest or pause
- □ 8. Sinoatrial exit block
- □ 9. Ectopic atrial rhythm
- □ 10. Atrial premature complexes, normally conducted
- □ 11. Atrial premature complexes, aberrantly conducted
- □ 12. Atrial premature complexes, nonconducted
- □ 13. Multifocal atrial rhythm
- □ 14. Multifocal atrial tachycardia
- □ 15. Atrial tachycardia, regular 1:1 conduction, sustained
- □ 16. Atrial tachycardia, regular 1:1 conduction, short paroxysms
- □ 17. Atrial tachycardia, with non-1:1 conduction (with block)
- □ 18. Supraventricular tachycardia, unspecified
- □ 19. Atrial flutter
- □ 20. Atrial fibrillation

B. AV Junctional Rhythms and Complexes

- □ 21. AV junctional rhythm
- □ 22. AV junctional escape rhythm
- □ 23. AV junctional rhythm, accelerated
- □ 24. AV junctional escape complexes
- □ 25. AV junctional premature complexes

C. Ventricular Rhythms and Complexes

- □ 26. Ventricular premature complex(es), uniform
- □ 27. Ventricular premature complex(es), multiform
- □ 28. Ventricular premature complexes, paired
- □ 29. Ventricular parasystole
- □ 30. Ventricular tachycardia
- □ 31. Accelerated idioventricular rhythm
- □ 32. Ventricular fibrillation
- □ 33. Torsades de pointes

D. Pacemaker Function, Rhythms, and Complexes

- □ 34. Single-chamber pacemaker, atrial pacing
- □ 35. Single-chamber pacemaker, ventricular pacing on demand
- □ 36. Single-chamber pacemaker, ventricular pacing with complete control
- □ 37. Dual-chamber pacemaker, atrial sensing with ventricular pacing
- □ 38. Dual-chamber pacemaker, atrial and ventricular sensing and pacing
- □ 39. Pacemaker malfunction, failure to capture atrium or ventricle appropriately
- □ 40. Pacemaker malfunction, failure to sense atrial or ventricular complexes appropriately
- □ 41. Pacemaker malfunction, failure to fire appropriately on demand (inappropriate sensing of stimuli or complex)

II. AV CONDUCTION ABNORMALITIES

- □ 42. AV block, first-degree
- □ 43. AV block, second-degree, Mobitz I (Wenckebach)
- □ 44. AV block, second-degree, Mobitz II
- □ 45. AV block, second-degree, 2:1
- □ 46. AV block, high-grade
- □ 47. AV block, third-degree or complete
- □ 48. Accelerated AV conduction (short PR interval pattern with normal QRS duration in sinus rhythm)
- □ 49. Ventricular preexcitation (WPW pattern)
- □ 50. Physiologic AV conduction delay associated with supraventricular tachyarrhythmias
- □ 51. Nonphysiologic AV conduction delay associated with supraventricular tachyarrhythmias

III. MISCELLANEOUS AV RELATIONSHIPS

- □ 52. Ventriculophasic sinus arrhythmia
- □ 53. AV dissociation
- □ 54. Reciprocal (echo) complexes
- □ 55. Retrograde atrial activation from a ventricular focus
- □ 56. Fusion complexes
- □ 57. Ventricular capture complexes
- □ 58. Interpolation of ventricular premature complexes

IV. P-WAVE ABNORMALITIES

- □ 59. Right atrial abnormality
- □ 60. Left atrial abnormality
- □ 61. Biatrial abnormality
- □ 62. Nonspecific atrial abnormality
- □ 63. PR depression

V. ABNORMALITIES OF QRS AXIS OR VOLTAGE

- □ 64. Left axis deviation
- □ 65. Right axis deviation
- □ 66. Poor R-wave progression
- □ 67. Low voltage, limb leads
- □ 68. Low voltage, precordial leads
- □ 69. Electrical alternans

VI. INTRAVENTRICULAR CONDUCTION ABNORMALITIES

- □ 70. Right bundle branch block, complete
- □ 71. Right bundle branch block, incomplete
- □ 72. Left anterior fascicular block
- □ 73. Left posterior fascicular block
- □ 74. Left bundle branch block, complete
- □ 75. Left bundle branch block, incomplete
- □ 76. Intraventricular conduction delay, nonspecific (includes IVCD associated with chamber enlargement)
- □ 77. Probable aberrant intraventricular conduction associated with supraventricular arrhythmia

VII. VENTRICULAR HYPERTROPHY OR ENLARGEMENT

- □ 78. Left ventricular hypertrophy by voltage criteria, with or without associated ST-T-wave abnormalities
- □ 79. Right ventricular hypertrophy
- □ 80. Combined ventricular hypertrophy

VIII. Q-WAVE MYOCARDIAL INFARCTION

- □ 81. Anteroseptal, acute or recent
- □ 82. Anteroseptal, old or of indeterminate age
- □ 83. Anterior, acute or recent
- □ 84. Anterior, old or of indeterminate age
- □ 85. Anterolateral, acute or recent
- □ 86. Anterolateral, old or of indeterminate age
- □ 87. Extensive anterior, acute or recent
- □ 88. Extensive anterior, old or of indeterminate age
- □ 89. Lateral or high lateral, acute or recent
- □ 90. Lateral, old or of indeterminate age
- □ 91. Inferior or diaphragmatic, acute or recent
- □ 92. Inferior or diaphragmatic, old or of indeterminate age
- □ 93. Posterior, acute or recent
- □ 94. Posterior, old or of indeterminate age
- □ 95. Suggestive of ventricular aneurysm

IX. ST-, T-, U-WAVE ABNORMALITIES

- □ 96. Normal variant, isolated J-point elevation (early repolarization pattern)
- □ 97. Isolated J-point depression
- □ 98. Normal variant, RSR′ pattern lead V1
- □ 99. Normal variant, persistent juvenile T-wave pattern
- □ 100. ST- and/or T-wave abnormalities suggesting acute or recent myocardial injury
- □ 101. ST- and/or T-wave abnormalities in the setting of acute myocardial injury suggesting either reciprocal change or myocardial ischemia
- □ 102. ST- and/or T-wave abnormalities in the absence of acute myocardial injury suggesting myocardial ischemia
- □ 103. ST- and/or T-wave abnormalities associated with ventricular hypertrophy
- □ 104. ST- and/or T-wave abnormalities associated with ventricular conduction abnormality
- □ 105. ST- and/or T-wave abnormalities suggesting early, acute pericarditis
- □ 106. Nonspecific ST- and/or T-wave abnormalities
- □ 107. Post extrasystolic T-wave abnormality
- □ 108. Peaked T waves
- □ 109. Prolonged QT interval for heart rate (QTc)
- □ 110. Prominent U waves
- □ 111. Inverted U waves

X. GENERAL FEATURES

- □ 112. Incorrect electrode placement
- □ 113. Artifact secondary to tremor

Clinical Electrocardiography

PreTest®
Self-Assessment and Review

Diagnostic Criteria

Arthur E. Fass, M.D., Editor

The following are suggested diagnostic criteria for the items listed in the test section. These are not intended to be comprehensive, and minor variations of these criteria exist in textbooks of electrocardiography. The suggested test answers in this text, however, use the following basic criteria.

OUTLINE

I. **Rhythm Abnormalities**
   A. Supraventricular rhythms and complexes
   B. AV junctional rhythms and complexes
   C. Ventricular rhythms and complexes
   D. Pacemaker function, rhythms, and complexes

II. **AV Conduction Abnormalities**

III. **Miscellaneous AV Relationships**

IV. **P-Wave Abnormalities**

V. **Abnormalities of QRS Axis or Voltage**

VI. **Intraventricular Conduction Abnormalities**

VII. **Ventricular Hypertrophy (or Enlargement)**

VIII. **Q-Wave Myocardial Infarction**

IX. **ST-, T-, U-Wave Abnormalities**

X. **General Features**

ELECTROCARDIOGRAPHIC DIAGNOSES

I. **Rhythm Abnormalities**

A. Supraventricular Rhythms and Complexes

1. *Sinus rhythm*
   A physiologic rhythm initiated in the sinus node and characterized by a heart rate of 60 to 100 beats per minute. The configuration of the P wave is upright in leads I, II, and aVF and inverted in lead aVR.
2. *Sinus arrhythmia*
   Sinus rhythm in which the PP interval varies by 0.16 s or more.
3. *Sinus bradycardia*
   Sinus rhythm with a heart rate less than 60 beats per minute.
4. *Sinus tachycardia*
   Sinus rhythm with a heart rate greater than 100 beats per minute.
5. *Wandering atrial pacemaker within the sinus node*
   Sinus rhythm with minor variations in P-wave morphology remaining upright in leads I and II and inverted in aVR. The PR interval is variable but remains 0.12 s or greater.
6. *Wandering atrial pacemaker to the AV junction*
   Sinus rhythm with progressive alteration in P-wave configuration becoming inverted and retrograde. The PR interval of the AV junctional focus characteristically becomes less than 0.12 s.
7. *Sinus arrest or pause*
   A failure of the SA node to initiate an impulse, which results in absence of P waves or QRS complexes. The pause is not a multiple of the intrinsic PP interval.
8. *Sinoatrial exit block*
   An abnormality of transmission of the sinus impulse, which results in a delay or failure of production of a P wave. Only second-degree SA block can be identified on the surface electrocardiogram. It may manifest in two patterns. Type I second-degree SA block is characterized by progressive shortening of the PP interval prior to an absent P wave. Type II is characterized by a pause in the PP cycle that is an exact multiple of the intrinsic sinus rate.
9. *Ectopic atrial rhythm*
   A rhythm initiated by an atrial pacemaker other than the sinus node. It is characterized by a rate less than 100 beats per minute with a P-wave morphology different from that of the sinus node. The PR interval is within normal limits.

10. *Atrial premature complexes, normally conducted*
A premature complex originating in the atrium and characterized by a P-wave morphology different from the normal sinus complex. The PR interval of the premature beat may be shorter, longer, or no different from the sinus complex. The PR interval characteristically is ≥ 0.12 s, which helps distinguish it from a premature complex of AV junctional origin.

11. *Atrial premature complexes, aberrantly conducted*
An atrial premature complex that, because of partial refractoriness of the conduction system, is conducted to the ventricles in an abnormal fashion and results in an alteration in the normal morphology of the QRS complex.

12. *Atrial premature complexes, nonconducted*
An atrial premature complex that, because of complete refractoriness of the conduction system, fails to conduct to the ventricles and is therefore not followed by a QRS complex.

13. *Multifocal atrial rhythm*
An atrial rhythm at a rate less than 100 beats per minute and characterized by absence of one dominant pacemaker and P waves of at least three different morphologies.

14. *Multifocal atrial tachycardia*
An atrial rhythm at a rate 100 beats per minute or greater characterized by absence of one dominant pacemaker and P waves of at least three different morphologies.

15. *Atrial tachycardia, regular 1:1 conduction, sustained*
A supraventricular arrhythmia characterized by abnormal P waves and an atrial rate of 100 to 200 beats per minute. The term *sustained* indicates a rhythm that lasts 30 s or more, or for standard electrocardiographic interpretive purposes, the entire tracing.

16. *Atrial tachycardia, regular 1:1 conduction, short paroxysms*
An atrial tachycardia that is at least three complexes or more but is not sustained.

17. *Atrial tachycardia, with non-1:1 AV conduction (with block)*
Atrial tachycardia characterized by an atrial rate of 150 to 250 beats per minute with lack of 1:1 conduction. An isoelectric interval is characteristically present between the abnormal P waves in contrast to the "sawtooth" baseline of atrial flutter.

18. *Supraventricular tachycardia, unspecified*
A supraventricular tachyarrhythmia in which the mechanism cannot be determined.

19. *Atrial flutter*
An atrial rhythm characterized (classically) by an atrial rate of 250 to 350 beats per minute with flutter waves exhibiting a "sawtooth" appearance in leads II, III, aVF, and V1.

20. *Atrial fibrillation*
An absence of organized P waves with replacement by irregular atrial fibrillatory waves.

B. AV Junctional Rhythms and Complexes

21. *AV junctional rhythm*
A regular rhythm characteristically at a rate of 35 to 60 beats per minute that originates in the AV junction, with inverted, retrograde P waves in leads II, III, and aVF. The P waves may occur prior to, within, or after the QRS complex. In the absence of retrograde block, the PR interval is characteristically less than 0.12 s.

22. *AV junctional escape rhythm*
An AV junctional rhythm that emerges as a result of a failure of conduction or slowing of a normally faster physiologic pacemaker (e.g., sinus node).

23. *AV junctional rhythm, accelerated*
An AV junctional rhythm that is more rapid (generally between 70 and 130 beats per minute) than the usual rate of the AV junction. It is secondary to enhanced automaticity of the AV junction and lacks a paroxysmal onset and termination. An equivalent term for this rhythm is *nonparoxysmal junctional tachycardia*.

24. *AV junctional escape complexes*
Isolated AV junctional complexes that emerge as a result of a failure of conduction or slowing of a normally faster physiologic pacemaker.

25. *AV junctional premature complexes*
Isolated AV junctional complexes that occur prematurely relative to the basic sinus cycle.

C. Ventricular Rhythms and Complexes

26. *Ventricular premature complex(es), uniform*
Premature depolarizations relative to the intrinsic cycle that originate in the ventricles. They are characterized by a wide, abnormal QRST morphology.

27. *Ventricular premature complex(es), multiform*
Ventricular premature complexes that demonstrate more than one morphology.

28. *Ventricular premature complexes, paired*
Two ventricular premature complexes in a row.

29. *Ventricular parasystole*
Ventricular complexes that are independent of the intrinsic rhythm. These complexes are characterized by varying coupling intervals and fusion beats. The interectopic intervals are constant or are multiples of a common denominator.

30. *Ventricular tachycardia*
Three or more ventricular complexes in succession at a rate greater than 100 beats per minute.

31. *Accelerated idioventricular rhythm*
Three or more ventricular complexes in succession at a rate of 100 beats per minute or less.

32. *Ventricular fibrillation*
A disorganized rhythm originating in the ventricles characterized by absence of discernible QRS complexes and by fibrillatory waves of variable rate and amplitude.

33. *Torsades de pointes*
A polymorphous ventricular tachycardia with an alternating amplitude and polarity.

D. Pacemaker Function, Rhythms, and Complexes

34. *Single-chamber pacemaker, atrial pacing*
A pacemaker stimulus captures the atrium. In the absence of conduction abnormality, a QRS complex follows.

35. *Single-chamber pacemaker, ventricular pacing on demand*
A pacemaker stimulus captures the ventricles after a pause in the native rhythm.

36. *Single-chamber pacemaker, ventricular pacing with complete control*
A ventricular pacemaker captures the ventricles without evidence of intrinsic ventricular depolarization.

37. *Dual-chamber pacemaker, atrial sensing with ventricular pacing*
A ventricular pacemaker captures the ventricles following a normal P wave. There should be evidence of atrial sensing and not fortuitous ventricular pacing at a rate similar to the intrinsic atrial rate.

38. *Dual-chamber pacemaker, atrial sensing with ventricular pacing*
A pacemaker rhythm characterized by atrial and ventricular sensing and pacing.

39. *Pacemaker malfunction, failure to capture atrium or ventricle appropriately*
A pacemaker stimulus that fails to capture the appropriate chamber when nonrefractory.

40. *Pacemaker malfunction, failure to sense atrial or ventricular complexes appropriately*
A pacemaker stimulus that fails to be appropriately inhibited by an intrinsic depolarization of either the ventricles or atria.

41. *Pacemaker malfunction, failure to fire appropriately on demand*
A pacemaker stimulus that does not appear when it would normally be expected.

II. AV Conduction Abnormalities

42. *AV block, first-degree*
In sinus rhythm, a consistent PR interval of greater than 0.20 s.

43. *AV block, second-degree, Mobitz I (Wenckebach)*
In sinus rhythm, classic Wenckebach is characterized by progressive lengthening of the PR interval until a P wave fails to conduct to the ventricles. There is associated progressive shortening of the RR interval until a beat is dropped. The resulting pause is the sum of two PP intervals. Mobitz type I second-degree AV block may also be present without the Wenckebach phenomenon. In this instance, there is prolongation of the PR interval prior to the dropped beat but without a gradual progressive increase in the PR interval and shortening of the RR interval.

44. *AV block, second-degree, Mobitz II*
In sinus rhythm, a constant PR interval is identified in consecutively conducted beats with intermittent failure of the P wave to conduct to the ventricles.

45. *AV block, second-degree, 2:1*
In sinus rhythm, there is a 2:1 relationship of the P waves to QRS complexes. Mobitz type I and type II cannot be differentiated.

46. *AV block, high-grade*
In sinus rhythm, conduction of the P waves to the ventricles in a ratio of 3:1 or more. The atrial rate must be greater than the ventricular rate. This is also applicable when the majority (but not all) of the P waves fail to conduct to the ventricles and the rhythm is maintained by a subsidiary pacemaker. Conduction must be expected and not interfered with by the subsidiary pacemaker. The identification of occasional conduction to the ventricles defines the conduction abnormality as high-grade rather than complete AV block.

47. *AV block, third-degree or complete*
Absence of AV conduction. The atrial rate must be greater than the ventricular rate.

48. *Accelerated AV conduction (short PR interval pattern with normal QRS duration in sinus rhythm)*
Characterized by a PR interval of less than 0.12 s, a normal P-wave morphology, and normal QRS duration.

49. *Ventricular preexcitation (WPW pattern)*
Characterized by a PR interval of less than 0.12 s, a normal P-wave morphology, an initial slurring (delta wave) prior to a wide QRS complex of 0.11 s or more, and secondary ST-T wave changes.

50. *Physiologic AV conduction delay associated with supraventricular tachyarrhythmias*
A manifestation of physiologic delay in AV conduction associated with a supraventricular tachyarrhythmia (responses at heart rates listed are approximations and are dependent on autonomic tone). Included are
a. Prolongation of the PR interval with 1:1 conduction at atrial rates of 150 beats per minute or more.
b. The Wenckebach phenomenon at atrial rates of 130 to 200 beats per minute.
c. Uniform, 2:1 AV conduction at atrial rates greater than 200 beats per minute in atrial tachycardia and atrial flutter.
d. Atrial fibrillation with an average ventricular response of 100 to 180 beats per minute.

51. *Nonphysiologic AV conduction delay associated with supraventricular tachyarrhythmias*
A nonphysiologic impairment of AV conduction secondary to either intrinsic disease or pharmacologic agents (responses at heart rates listed are approximations and are dependent on autonomic tone). Included are
a. PR interval prolongation with 1:1 conduction at atrial rates between 100 and 150 beats per minute.
b. The Wenckebach phenomenon at atrial rates between 100 and 130 beats per minute.
c. A greater than 2:1 AV conduction ratio (either uniform or variable) at atrial rates greater than 200 beats per minute in atrial tachycardia and atrial flutter.
d. Atrial fibrillation with an average ventricular response of less than 100 beats per minute.

III. Miscellaneous AV Relationships

52. *Ventriculophasic sinus arrhythmia*
A form of sinus arrhythmia in which the sinus cycles that contain ventricular depolarizations are shorter than those cycles which do not.

53. *AV dissociation*
Independent and unrelated atrial and ventricular rhythm mechanisms.

54. *Reciprocal (echo) complexes*
A reentry complex that results from an impulse depolarizing the chamber of its origin and returning to depolarize the same chamber. The impulse may arise from the SA node, atria, AV junction, or ventricles.

55. *Retrograde atrial activation from a ventricular focus*
Activation of the atria in a retrograde fashion from an independent depolarization in the ventricles.

56. *Fusion complexes*
A complex or complexes arising from the simultaneous transmission of impulses from more than one focus. The resulting hybrid complex demonstrates a morphology intermediate between the usual, undisturbed pattern of the two depolarizations.

57. *Ventricular capture complexes*
The presence of conducted beats from supraventricular impulses during a period of AV dissociation. This generally refers to capture during a period of ventricular tachycardia.

58. *Interpolation of ventricular premature complexes*
Ventricular extrasystoles that are interposed between two sinus beats and do not disturb the sinus rhythm. A prolongation of the subsequent PR interval is characteristic secondary to concealed retrograde conduction to the AV junction.

IV. P-Wave Abnormalities

59. *Right atrial abnormality*
—The P-wave amplitude is 2.5 mm or more in leads II, III, and aVF. The P-wave duration is less than 0.12 s.
—The initial positive component of the P wave in lead V1 is 1.5 mm or more.
Supporting criteria: The P-wave axis in the frontal plane is +75 degrees or more.

60. *Left atrial abnormality*
—The P-wave duration is prolonged (0.12 s or more) and notched in leads I, II, and aVL.
—There is an abnormal P terminal force in lead V1 with the product of the depth and duration equal to or greater than 0.04.
Supporting criteria: The P-wave axis in the frontal plane is leftward of +15 degrees.

61. *Biatrial abnormality*
—An abnormal P terminal force combined with an initial positive P-wave component of 1.5 mm or more in lead V1.
—Combined wide (greater than 0.12 s) and tall (greater than 2.5 mm) P waves in the limb leads.

62. *Nonspecific atrial abnormality*
A wide P wave (duration 0.12 s or more) without other criteria for abnormality.

63. *PR depression*
A depressed PR segment below the baseline of more than 0.8 mm.

V. Abnormalities of QRS Axis or Voltage

64. *Left axis deviation*
A frontal plane QRS axis between −30 and −90 degrees.

65. *Right axis deviation*
A frontal plane QRS axis between +90 and +270 degrees.

66. *Poor R-wave progression*
R waves are present in leads V1–V3, but the R-wave magnitude is 3.0 mm or less in V3, and the R wave in V2 is equal to or smaller than the R wave in V3. Reverse R-wave progression is as above except that R-wave voltage decreases from V1–V3. Patients with low voltage in the precordial leads (see below), left bundle branch block, or preexcitation (WPW) are excluded.

67. *Low voltage, limb leads*
The sum of the R and S waves in all limb leads is 5 mm or less.

68. *Low voltage, precordial leads*
The sum of the R and S waves in all precordial leads is 10 mm or less.

69. *Electrical alternans*
A regular alternation of the amplitude of the P, QRS, or T waves, either alone or in combination. The complexes must originate from a single pacemaker.

VI. Intraventricular Conduction Abnormalities

70. *Right bundle branch block, complete*
—A QRS duration of 0.12 s or greater.
—A secondary R′ wave in the right precordial leads with the terminal R′ greater than the initial R wave.
—Secondary ST-T wave abnormalities in the right precordial leads.
Additional supporting findings: Slurred S waves in leads I and aVL and in the left precordial leads.

71. *Right bundle branch block, incomplete*
Criteria for right bundle branch block, but with a QRS duration of 0.09 to 0.11 s.

72. *Left anterior fascicular block*
—Left axis deviation between −30 and −90 degrees.
—A positive terminal deflection in aVL and aVR with the peak of the terminal R wave in aVR occurring later than in aVL.
—Normal or slightly prolonged QRS duration (less than 0.12 s)
—No other cause of left axis deviation.
Additional supporting findings: A qR complex in leads I and aVL; an rS complex in leads II, III, and aVF; and an S wave in lead III larger than that in lead II.

73. *Left posterior fascicular block*
—Right axis deviation between +90 and +180 degrees.
—An rS pattern in lead I and aVL and a qR pattern in leads II, III, and aVF. (Q waves less than 0.04 s in duration.)
—Normal, or slightly prolonged QRS duration (less than 0.12 s).
—No other cause of right axis deviation.
Additional findings: The R wave in lead III should equal or exceed that in lead II.

74. *Left bundle branch block, complete*
—QRS duration of 0.12 s or more.
—Broad, notched, or slurred R waves in leads I, aVL, and V5–V6.
—Secondary ST-T wave abnormalities in leads I, aVL, and V5–V6.
—Absence of Q waves in leads I and V5–V6.

75. *Left bundle branch block, incomplete*
Three of four criteria are required:
—QRS duration of 0.10 to 0.11 s.
—Absence of Q waves in leads I and V5–V6.
—Broad, notched, or slurred R waves in leads I, aVL, and V5–V6.
—R peak time (intrinsicoid deflection) prolonged to 0.06 s or greater measured in leads V5–V6.

76. *Intraventricular conduction delay (IVCD), nonspecific (includes IVCD associated with chamber enlargement)*
Prolongation of the QRS duration to 0.11 s or more in the absence of criteria for either left bundle branch block or right bundle branch block.

77. *Probable aberrant intraventricular conduction associated with a supraventricular arrhythmia*
Transient abnormal intraventricular conduction secondary to partial refractoriness of the intraventricular conduction system.

VII. Ventricular Hypertrophy (or Enlargement)

78. *Left ventricular hypertrophy by voltage criteria with or without associated ST-T wave abnormalities (acceptable in patients over 40 years of age)*
—Sum of S wave in leads V1 or V2 and R wave in leads V5 or V6 is greater than 35 mm, or
—R wave in lead aVL is greater than 11 mm, or
—Sum of R wave in lead I and S wave in lead III is greater than 25 mm, or
—The Lewis index is 17 or more.
(R lead I − S lead I) + (S lead III − R lead III)
Supporting findings: Left ventricular "strain" pattern; prolongation of the R peak time (intrinsicoid deflection) to 0.05 s or more in the left precordial leads; left atrial abnormality.

79. *Right ventricular hypertrophy*
—Right axis deviation (in the absence of other causes).
—R-wave voltage greater than S wave in lead V1.
—R wave in lead V1 is greater than or equal to 7 mm.
—qR pattern in lead V1.

—rSR′ pattern (with normal QRS duration), with R′ greater than or equal to 10 mm.
—The R/S ratio in lead V5 or V6 is less than or equal to 1.
Additional or supporting findings: Delay in the R peak time (intrinsicoid deflection) measured in lead V1 to greater than or equal to 0.035 s; ST depression and T-wave inversion in the right precordial leads; and S wave in lead V1 is less than 2 mm.

80. *Combined ventricular hypertrophy*
The criteria for left and right ventricular hypertrophy are simultaneously present.

VIII. Q-Wave Myocardial Infarction

Old or of Indeterminate Age

Old or indeterminate infarction should be identified when there are diagnostic Q waves on the electrocardiogram without associated ST-segment or T-wave abnormalities to suggest acute or recent injury. Q (or QS) waves are considered diagnostic when they have a width of 0.04 s or more and a depth equal to or greater than 25 percent of the R wave in that lead.

Acute or Recent

Acute infarction is characterized by diagnostic Q waves (or developing Q waves) in conjunction with ST abnormalities of acute myocardial injury. The abnormality is horizontal or concave down (coved) ST elevation in the affected leads (ST depression in leads V1–V2 for posterior infarction). Recent or subacute infarction is characterized by resolving ST-segment abnormalities associated with T-wave inversion in the infarction leads (upright T wave for posterior infarction). It is often impossible to definitively assess the duration of the infarction without clinical correlation or serial tracings. Multiple patterns as well as those which do not conform exactly to the following diagnoses may be seen.

81–82. Anteroseptal
Leads V1–V3.

83–84. Anterior
Leads V2–V4.

85–86. Anterolateral
Leads I, aVL, V4–V6.

87–88. Extensive anterior
Leads V1–V5 (V6).

89–90. Lateral or high lateral
Leads I, aVL.

91–92. Inferior or diaphragmatic
Leads II, III, aVF.

93–94. Posterior
Tall R waves of 0.04 s or more with R > S leads V1–V2.

95. *Suggestive of ventricular aneurysm*
ST elevation in leads containing Q waves that persists for at least 2 weeks following myocardial infarction.

IX. ST-, T-, U-Wave Abnormalities

96. *Normal variant, isolated J-point elevation (early repolarization pattern)*
Upward displacement of the ST segment at the J junction from 1–4 mm above the isoelectric line. The ST segment demonstrates upward concavity associated with tall, broad, symmetric T waves.

97. *Isolated J-point depression*
Upsloping ST depression at the J junction found in an otherwise normal person.

98. *Normal variant, RSR′ pattern lead V1*
—The RSR′ complex is of normal duration.
—A primary R wave in lead V1 less than 8 mm.
—An R′ less than 6 mm.
—An R′/S ratio less than 1 in any right precordial lead.

99. *Normal variant, persistent juvenile T-wave pattern*
Characterized by T-wave inversion in V1 and V2 in an otherwise normal adult.

100. *ST or T-wave abnormality or both suggesting acute or recent myocardial injury*
Horizontal or concave downward (coved) elevation with or without associated T-wave inversion. (Horizontal ST depression with an upright T wave in leads V1–V2 for posterior wall injury.)

101. *ST or T-wave abnormality or both in the setting of acute myocardial injury suggesting either reciprocal change or myocardial ischemia*
Horizontal or downsloping ST depression with or without T-wave abnormalities in leads opposite to those with ST elevation.

102. ST or T-wave abnormality or both in the absence of acute myocardial injury suggesting myocardial ischemia
Horizontal or downsloping ST depression with or without T-wave inversion in the absence of concomitant ST elevation in additional leads.

103. ST or T-wave abnormality or both associated with ventricular hypertrophy
—In left ventricular hypertrophy: ST depression with downward concavity and T-wave inversion in the left precordial leads; also often in leads I and aVL with a horizontal QRS axis and in leads II, III, and aVF with a vertical axis.
—In right ventricular hypertrophy: ST depression with downward concavity and T-wave inversion in the right precordial leads.

104. ST or T-wave abnormality or both associated with ventricular conduction abnormality
—In left bundle branch block: ST depression and T-wave inversion in the left precordial leads.
—In right bundle branch block: ST depression and T-wave inversion in the right precordial leads.

105. ST or T-wave abnormality or both suggesting early, acute pericarditis
Characterized by diffuse ST elevation that is concave upward. The findings are often in multiple leads but are most common in leads I, II, and V5–V6. The absence of reciprocal changes and concomitant T-wave inversion helps to distinguish this from acute myocardial injury. The T wave remains concordant with the direction of the ST segment in early pericarditis.

106. Nonspecific ST or T-wave abnormality or both
Slight ST depression or elevation or isolated T-wave inversion or other abnormality that cannot be characterized as secondary to a specific abnormality.

107. Post extrasystolic T-wave abnormality
An alteration in the T-wave morphology in the complex following a ventricular premature depolarization.

108. Peaked T waves
The T-wave amplitude is greater than 6 mm in the limb leads or 10 mm in any precordial lead.

109. Prolonged QT interval for heart rate (QTc)
—The QT interval varies inversely with the heart rate. A number of formulas have been proposed for correcting the QT interval for heart rate variability. All have been called into question. The most commonly used formula for correcting the QT interval for the heart rate (QTc) is Bazett's formula:

QTc = QT interval (s)/square root of RR interval (s)

The upper limit of normal for the QTc that has been used for clinical studies is 0.44 s.
—The use of Bazett's formula is not always feasible in routine interpretation. A brief approximation for determining the normal limits for the QT interval (uncorrected) has been suggested. This method is to assign an upper limit of 0.40 s for a heart rate of 70 beats per minute. For every increase or decrease in the heart rate of 10 beats per minute, subtract 0.02 s from or add 0.02 s to the QT interval, respectively. Measurements that fall outside these values should suggest a prolonged QT interval.

110. Prominent U waves
The maximum amplitude of the U wave is usually 1.0 mm, but it may rarely reach 2.0 mm. The amplitude of the U wave is proportional to that of the T wave but should be no greater than 25 percent of the height of the T wave.

111. Inverted U waves
The U wave generally follows the vector of the T wave. U-wave inversion in leads with a normally upright T wave should be considered abnormal.

X. General Features

112. Incorrect electrode placement

113. Artifact due to tremor

TEST A

A-1

Clinical History

A 79-year-old man with chronic dyspnea. He is a heavy smoker.

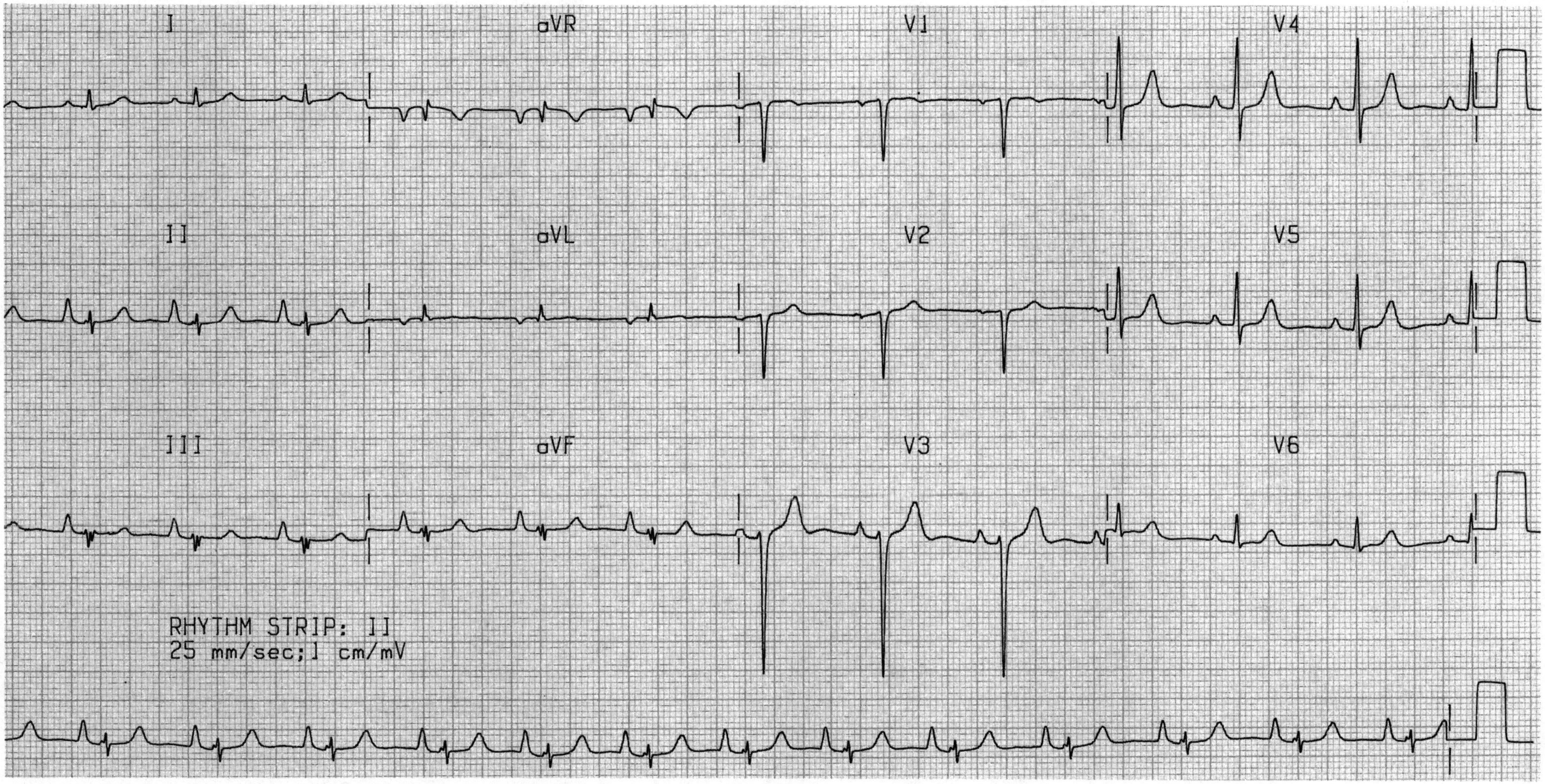

A-1

NARRATIVE INTERPRETATION

Rhythm:	**Sinus**
Rate:	**82**
Intervals:	**PR 0.16, QRS 0.08, QT 0.36**
Axis:	**−30 degrees**

Abnormalities

P-wave voltage greater than 2.5 mm, leads II, III, aVF. Limb-lead voltage less than 6 mm. R-wave voltage V1–V3 less than 3 mm.

Synthesis

Sinus rhythm. Low voltage limb leads. Right atrial abnormality. Poor R-wave progression.

TEST ANSWERS: 1, 59, 66, 67.

Comment: Low voltage (the total amplitude of the R and S waves is less than 6 mV in any limb lead) is present in this tracing. Low voltage may be seen in patients with pericardial effusion, myxedema, amyloidosis, profound obesity, chronic obstructive pulmonary disease, and extensive loss of functioning myocardial tissue as might occur after multiple myocardial infarctions. Poor R-wave progression is identified when R waves are present in the anterior precordial leads, but R-wave magnitude is <3.0 mm in lead V3. Causes include anterior wall myocardial infarction (MI), left ventricular hypertrophy (LVH), right ventricular hypertrophy (RVH), left anterior fascicular block, chronic obstructive pulmonary disease (COPD), or normal variants. In this case, the most likely cause of both low voltage and poor R-wave progression is COPD. The tall peaked P waves represent right atrial hypertrophy secondary to elevated right heart pressures.

REFERENCES: Zema (1982). Kilcoyne. Selvester.

A-2

Clinical History

A 60-year-old man with long-standing hypertension.

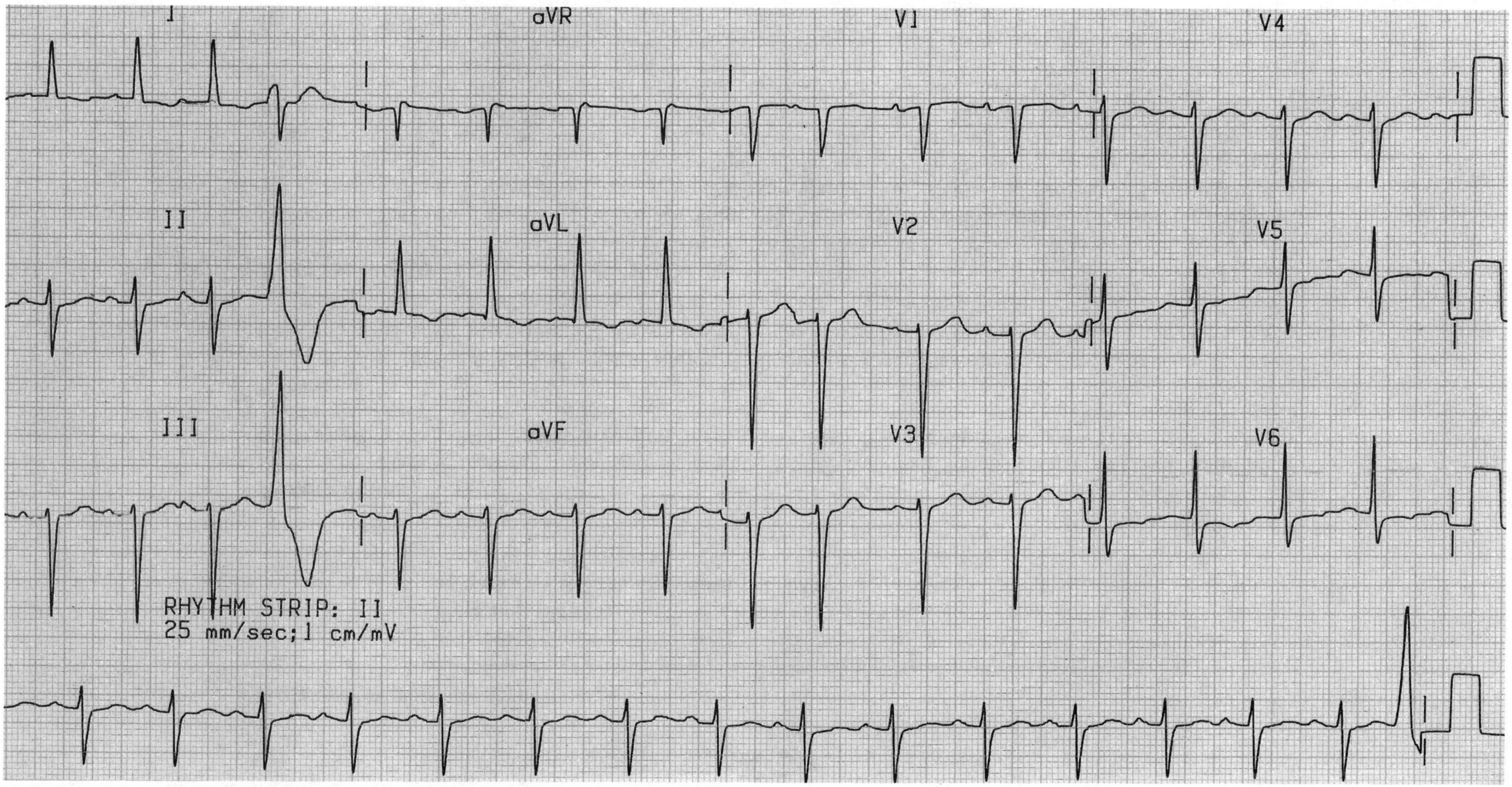

A-2

NARRATIVE INTERPRETATION

Rhythm: **Sinus**
Rate: **94**
Intervals: **PR 0.20, QRS 0.08, QT 0.36**
Axis: **−45 degrees**

Abnormalities

APC. VPC. Axis leftward of −30 degrees. R wave V1–V3 less than 3 mm. R wave aVL is 15 mm. ST depression, leads I, V6. T-wave inversion, leads I, aVL, V6. T wave biphasic lead V5.

Synthesis

Sinus rhythm. VPC. APC. Left axis deviation. Left anterior fascicular block. LVH. Poor R-wave progression. ST-T-wave abnormalities associated with ventricular hypertrophy.

TEST ANSWERS: 1, 10, 26, 64, 66, 72, 103 (106).

Comment: Note that "classic" precordial voltage criteria for LVH are absent in this tracing. However, the presence of an R wave in aVL $\geq$ 13 mm is very specific for LVH. The presence of left anterior fascicular block (LAFB) tends to mask precordial voltage for LVH in the chest leads while it increases voltage in the limb leads. Nevertheless, additional criteria for LVH in the presence of LAFB are met in this tracing (S wave lead III $\geq$ 15 mm, R wave lead aVL $\geq$ 13 mm). The ST-T-wave abnormalities are likely secondary to ventricular hypertrophy but may also be considered nonspecific.

REFERENCES: Milliken. Gertsch.

A-3

Clinical History

A 52-year-old man with chest pain and hypotension.

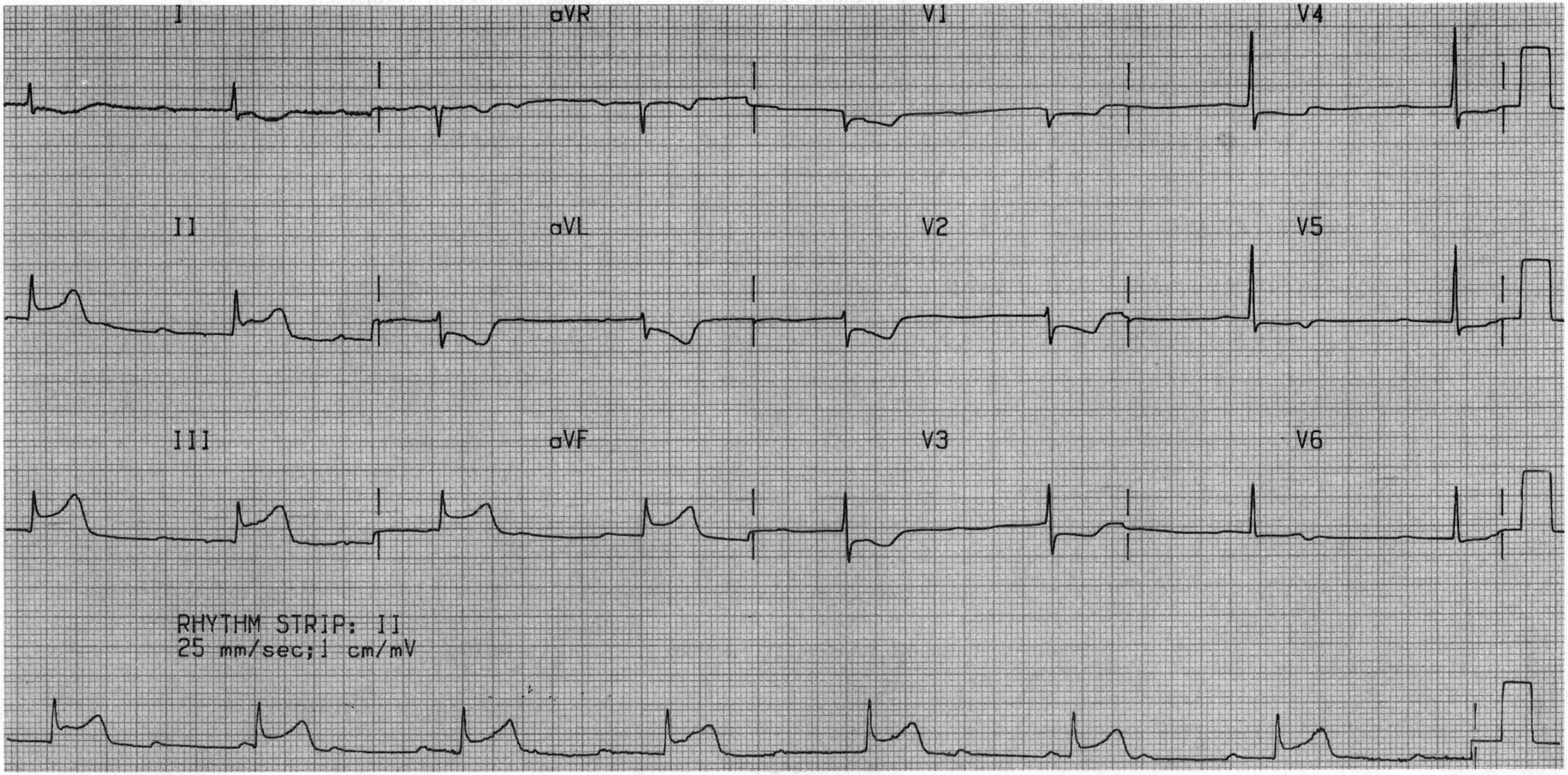

A-3

NARRATIVE INTERPRETATION

Rhythm:	**Sinus with complete AV block; AV junctional escape rhythm**
Rate:	**Sinus rate 98; AV junctional escape rate 43**
Intervals:	**PR –, QRS 0.08, QT 0.44**
Axis:	**+75 degrees**

Abnormalities

P waves nonconducted. AV dissociation. ST elevation leads II, III, aVF. ST depression leads I, aVL, V1–V6. T-wave inversion leads I, aVL, V2–V3. Biphasic T waves leads V4–V6..

Synthesis

Sinus rhythm with complete AV block. Junctional escape rhythm. AV dissociation. Inferior wall myocardial infarction with ST elevation suggestive of acute myocardial injury. ST depression with T-wave inversion in leads I, aVL, and precordial leads compatible with either reciprocal change, myocardial ischemia, or possible posterior myocardial injury.

TEST ANSWERS: 1, 22, 47, 53, 91, (93), 100, 101.

Comment: It is important to note that AV dissociation is not synonymous with complete heart block. In this example, heart block and AV dissociation are both present. In contrast, ventricular tachycardia demonstrates AV dissociation without heart block. Patients with acute inferior wall myocardial infarction may develop complete AV block as a result of profound vagal influences. In contrast to patients with anterior wall myocardial infarction, this is not a sign of extensive necrosis to the cardiac conduction system. Unless there is hemodynamic compromise, temporary pacemaker therapy is usually not required. Complete AV block in the setting of acute inferior myocardial infarction is usually transient and resolves within several days.

REFERENCES: Berger. Nicod.

A-4

Clinical History

A 21-year-old man with end-stage renal disease.

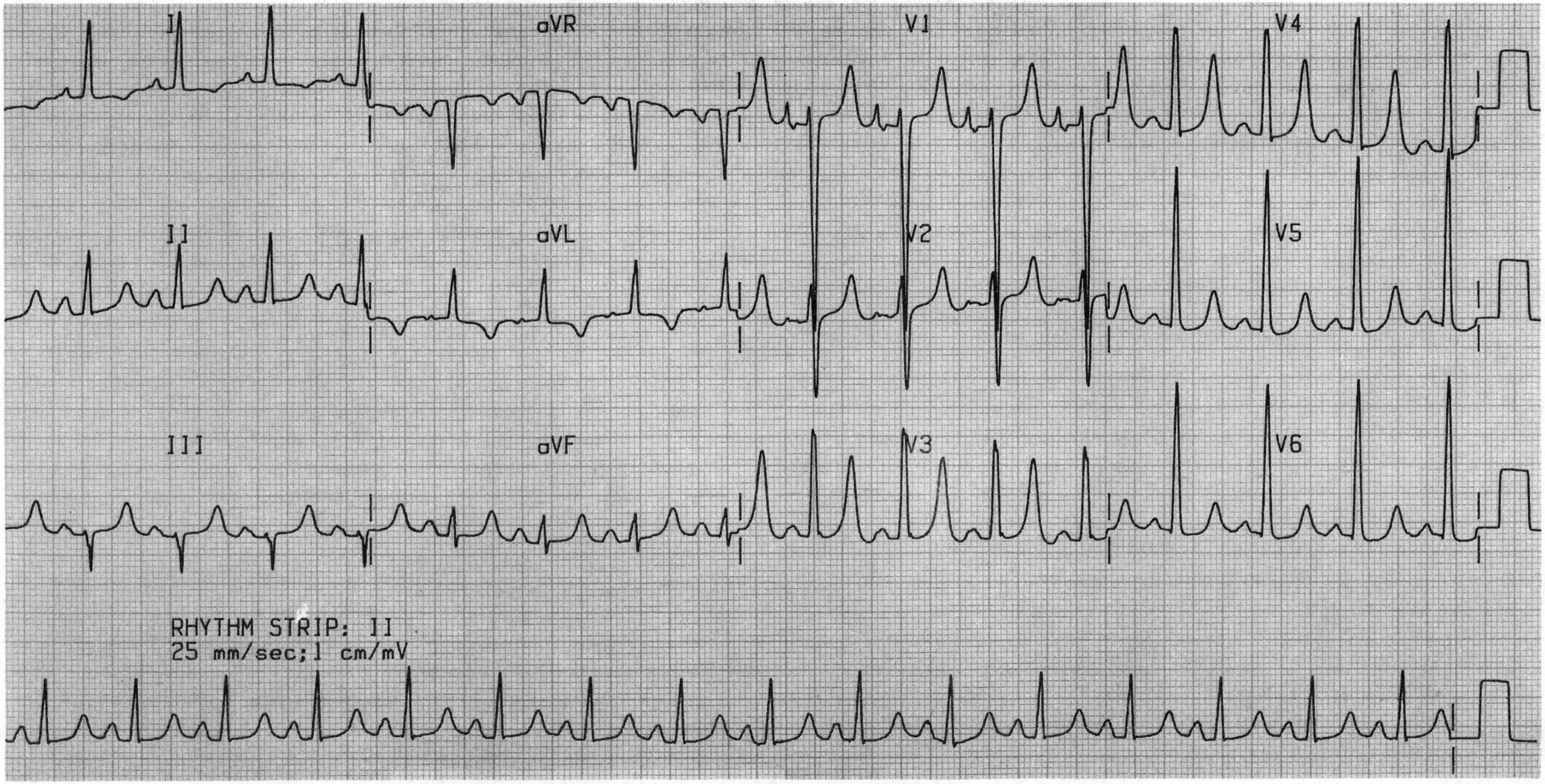

A-4

NARRATIVE INTERPRETATION

Rhythm: **Sinus**
Rate: **98**
Intervals: **PR 0.18, QRS 0.08, QT 0.36**
Axis: **+15 degrees**

Abnormalities

Increased P-wave voltage leads II, III, aVF, V1. R wave V5 + S wave V1 equals 63 mm. ST depression I, aVL, V4–V6. T-wave inversion I, aVL. Peaked, "tent-shaped" T waves most prominent in precordial leads. QT interval prolonged for heart rate.

Synthesis

Sinus rhythm. Right atrial abnormality. LVH by voltage criterion. Nonspecific ST-T-wave abnormalities. Peaked T waves suggestive of hyperkalemia. Prolonged QTc interval.

TEST ANSWERS: 1, 59, 78, 106, 108, 109.

Comment: The tall, narrow, peaked T waves noted in this example are characteristic of hyperkalemia. This patient had a serum potassium of 7.6 meq/dL. Other electrocardiographic abnormalities, including prolongation of QRS duration and decrease in P-wave amplitude, may be observed in patients with moderate hyperkalemia. This patient had a P pulmonale pattern despite hyperkalemia. Interestingly, the P pulmonale pattern may occasionally represent left atrial enlargement. Such was the case in this patient. Note that in young patients different precordial voltage criteria for LVH must be used. In patients 20 to 30 years of age, precordial voltage up to 60 mm may be seen. This patient had values exceeding this and is diagnosed with LVH. The slightly prolonged QT interval may have been secondary to hypocalcemia.

REFERENCES: Chou p 487. Friedman pp 68, 130. Manning. Walker.

A-5

Clinical History

An 83-year-old man with a recently implanted pacemaker. He has a history of heavy smoking.

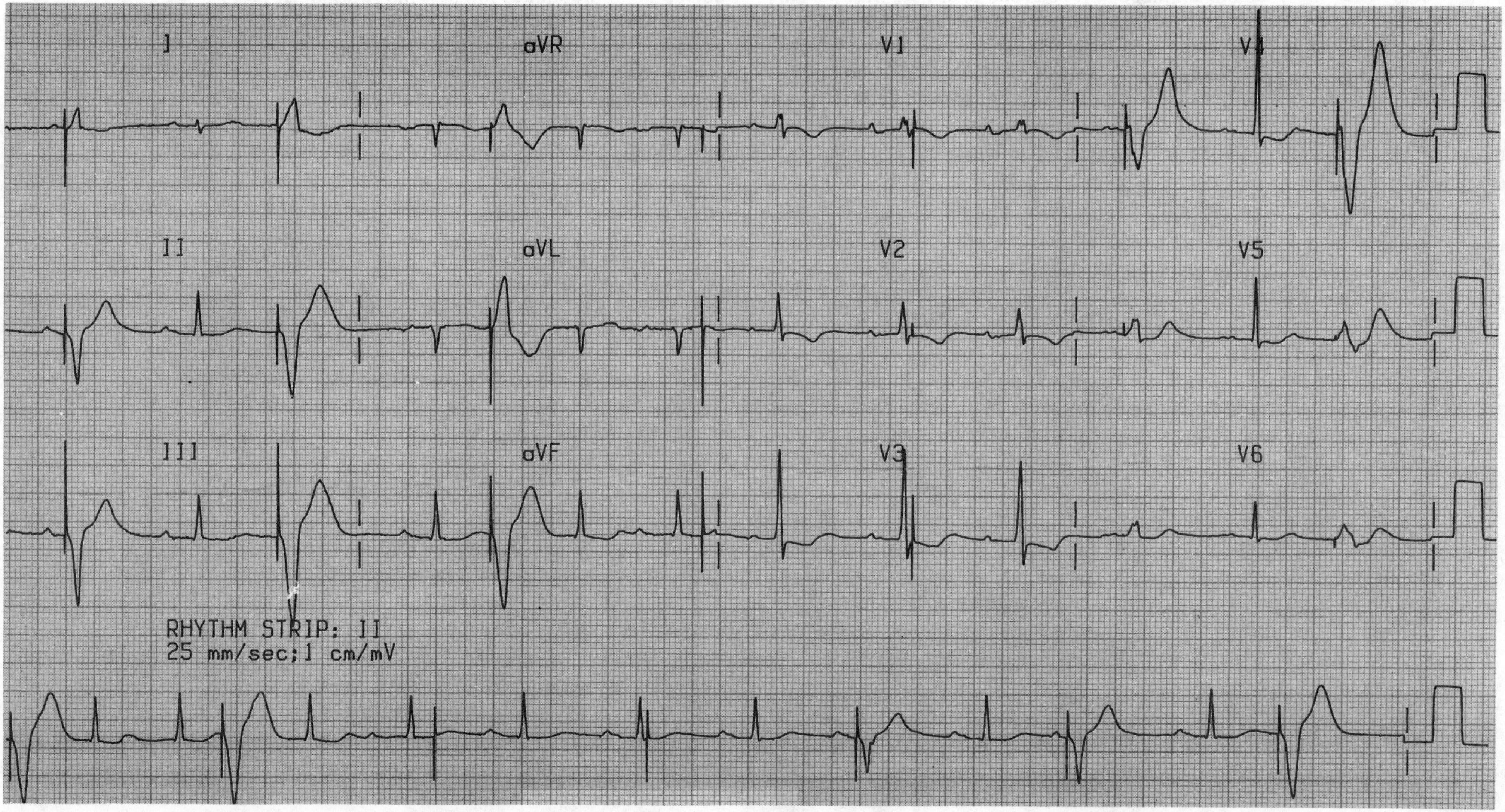

A-5

NARRATIVE INTERPRETATION

Rhythm: **Sinus with first-degree AV block**
Rate: **75**
Intervals: **PR 0.26, QRS 0.06, QT 0.40**
Axis: **+105 degrees**

Abnormalities

Prolonged PR interval. Axis rightward of +90. R wave greater than S wave leads V1–V3. ST depression leads II, III, aVF, V3–V6. Biphasic T wave leads V4–V5. T-wave inversion leads V2–V3. Ventricular pacemaker complexes, rate 60, with occasional capture. Ventricular pacemaker malfunction with failure to sense. Pacemaker fusion complexes.

Synthesis

Sinus rhythm with first-degree AV block. Right axis deviation. RVH. Nonspecific ST-T-wave abnormalities. Ventricular pacemaker complexes with intermittent capture. Pacemaker fusion complexes. Pacemaker malfunction, failure to sense.

TEST ANSWERS: 1, 40, 42, 56, 65, 79, (103), 106.

Comment: This tracing is suggestive of cor pulmonale secondary to obstructive airway disease. An axis rightward of +90 degrees is unusual in patients over the age of 40 and is suggestive of RVH, particularly in view of the tall R waves in the right precordial leads. There are nonspecific ST-T-wave abnormalities present although the ST depression and T-wave inversion in the right precordial leads may be associated with RVH. The pacemaker demonstrates complete sensing failure and is functioning independently of the native rhythm. It is seen to capture the ventricle when it does not fall within the ventricular refractory period, but it is not functioning "on demand." This activity results in occasional pacemaker fusion complexes, which are seen best in the rhythm strip. The pacemaker capture will occasionally become interpolated between two sinus complexes. The next two beats show a prolonged PR interval probably secondary to concealed retrograde conduction into the AV junction.

REFERENCES: Chou pp 55, 263. Kilcoyne. Selvester. Schaeffer. Schmock (pp 328–334). Schmock (pp 335–340).

A-6

Clinical History

A 68-year-old woman with a history of palpitations.

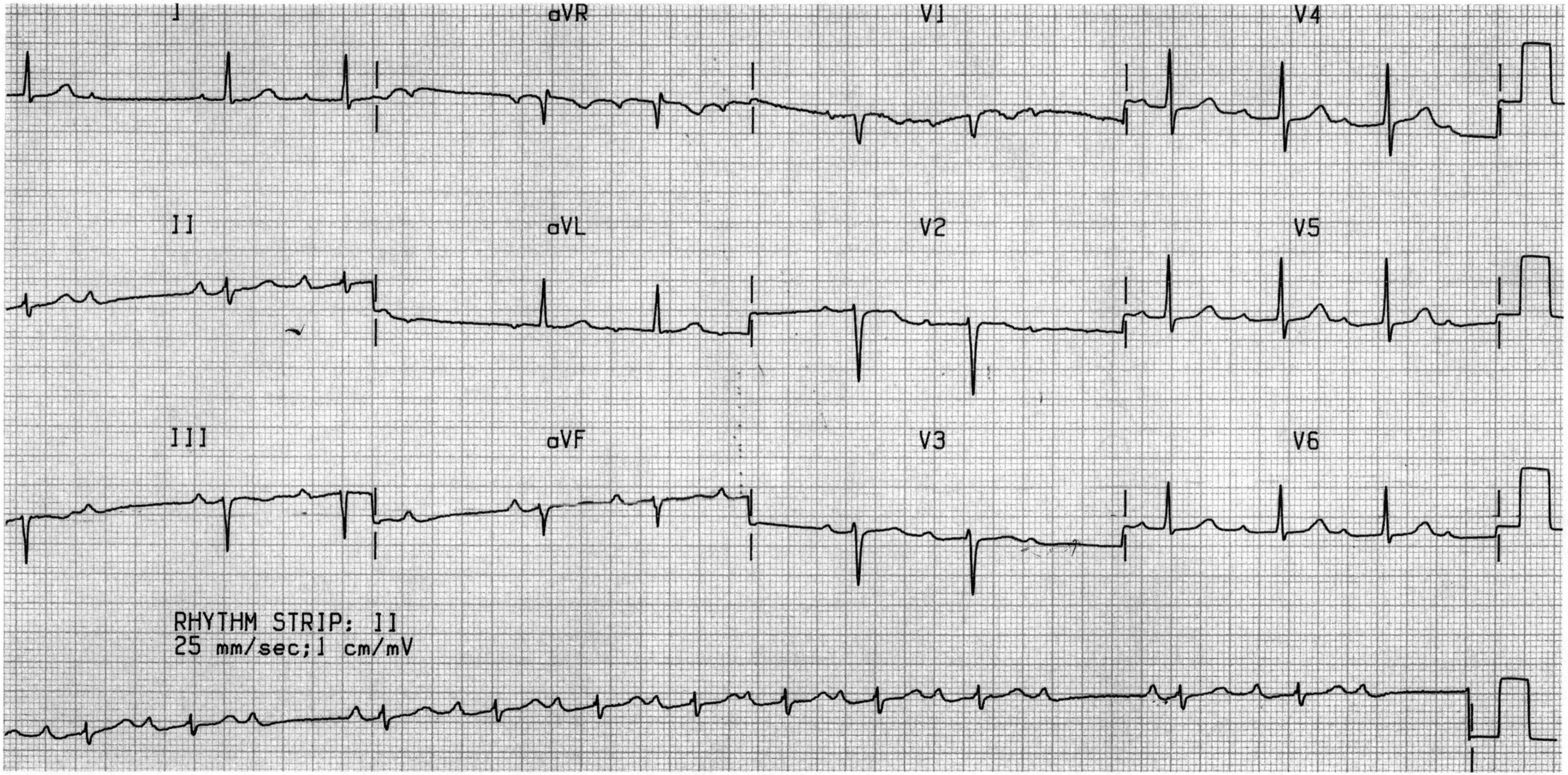

A-6

NARRATIVE INTERPRETATION

Rhythm:	**Sinus with second-degree AV block, Mobitz I**
Rate:	**90**
Intervals:	**PR 0.20, QRS 0.07, QT 0.34**
Axis:	**−30 degrees**

Abnormalities
Progressive increase in PR interval with eventual failure to conduct P wave. R wave less than 3 mm leads V1–V3.

Synthesis
Sinus rhythm with second-degree AV block, Mobitz I. Poor R-wave progression.

TEST ANSWERS: 1, 43, 66.

Comment: This patient demonstrates second-degree AV block of Mobitz type I (Wenckebach). As seen in this example, the Wenckebach phenomenon may not always be present in second-degree AV block, Mobitz type I. In classic Wenckebach, there is progressive lengthening of the PR interval until there is failure of the P wave to conduct to the ventricles. Additional features include a shortening of the RR interval until a blocked P wave occurs and the fact that the RR interval that contains the blocked P wave is less than twice the sum of two PP intervals. In the present example, the RR intervals at first shorten but then lengthen prior to the blocked P wave. The PR interval is also seen to increase most in the second complex after the pause and does not progressively lengthen. The site of origin of the conduction abnormality in patients with second-degree AV block, type I, with a narrow QRS complex is usually the AV node.

REFERENCES: Chou pp 413–416. Hecht. Zipes.

A-7

Clinical History

An asymptomatic 70-year-old man who has been treated with a calcium channel blocking agent for a history of angina.

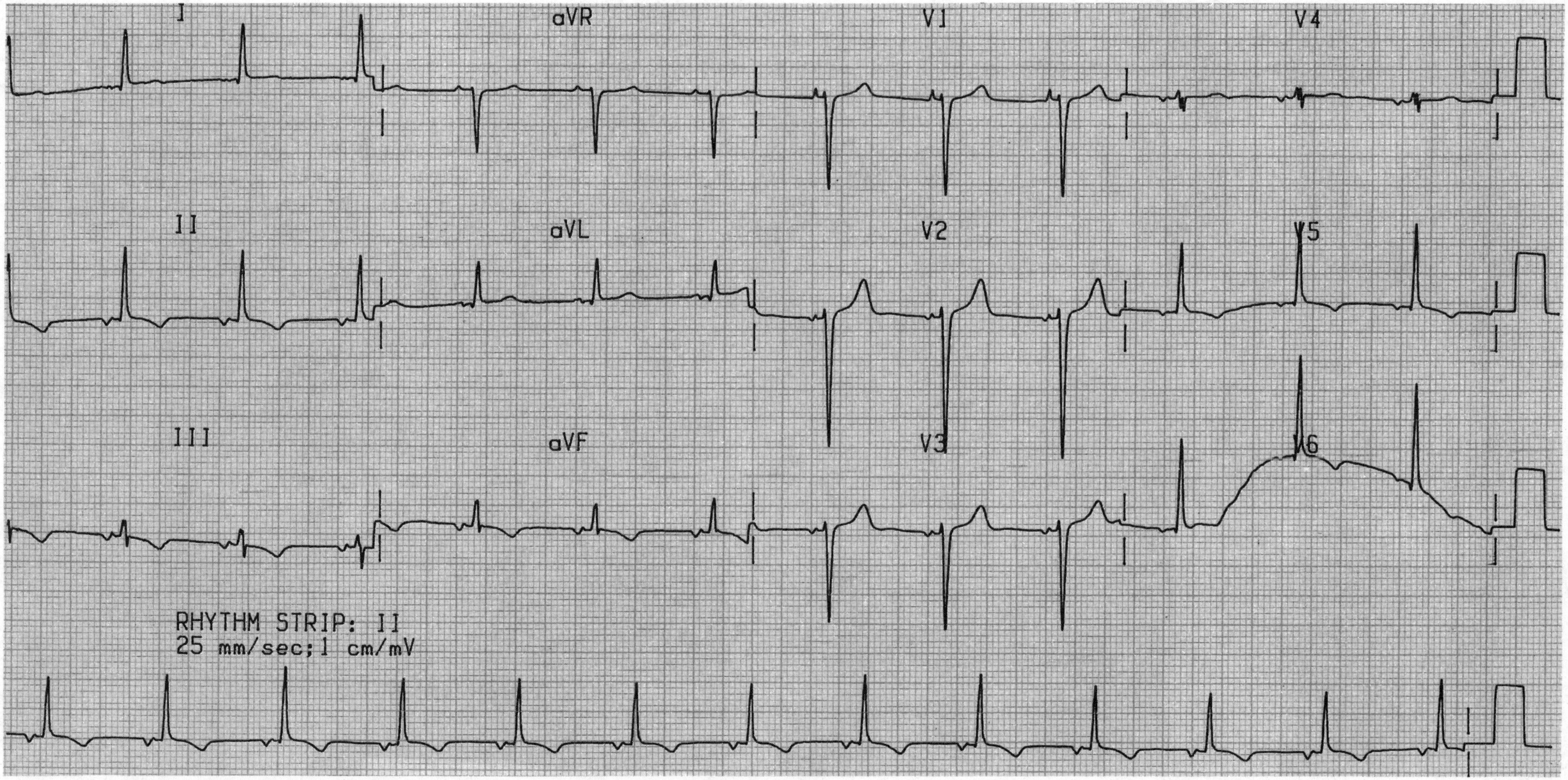

A-7

NARRATIVE INTERPRETATION

Rhythm: **Accelerated AV junctional rhythm**
Rate: **77**
Intervals: **PR 0.10, QRS 0.07, QT 0.34**
Axis: **+30 degrees**

Abnormalities

Inverted P waves leads II, III, aVF with short PR interval. R wave less than 3 mm leads V1–V4. T-wave inversion leads II, III, aVF, V5–V6.

Synthesis

Accelerated AV junctional rhythm. Poor R-wave progression. Nonspecific T-wave abnormalities.

TEST ANSWERS: 23, 66, (82), 106.

Comment: The cause of the poor R-wave progression in this patient is most likely a prior anteroseptal wall MI. This diagnosis is supported in this patient by a history of coronary artery disease and the absence of significant R-wave voltage in the anterior precordium. It is the author's practice to add "probable" when making this diagnosis on the basis of poor R-wave progression alone in the absence of Q waves. The additional ST-T-wave abnormalities suggest potential coronary artery disease; however, they are nonspecific and not diagnostic. This patient was known to have sustained an anterior wall MI in the past and was treated with verapamil. Remember that in an AV junctional rhythm, the inverted P wave can occur either before, after, or within the QRS complex. By definition, the rate of the AV junctional rhythm qualifies as accelerated.

REFERENCES: Zema (*J Electrocardiol* 23:147–156, 1990). Zema (*J Electrocardiol* 17:129–138, 1984). DePace. Warner (*Am J Cardiol* 52:690–692, 1983).

A-8

Clinical History

A 16-year-old healthy female with atypical chest pain.

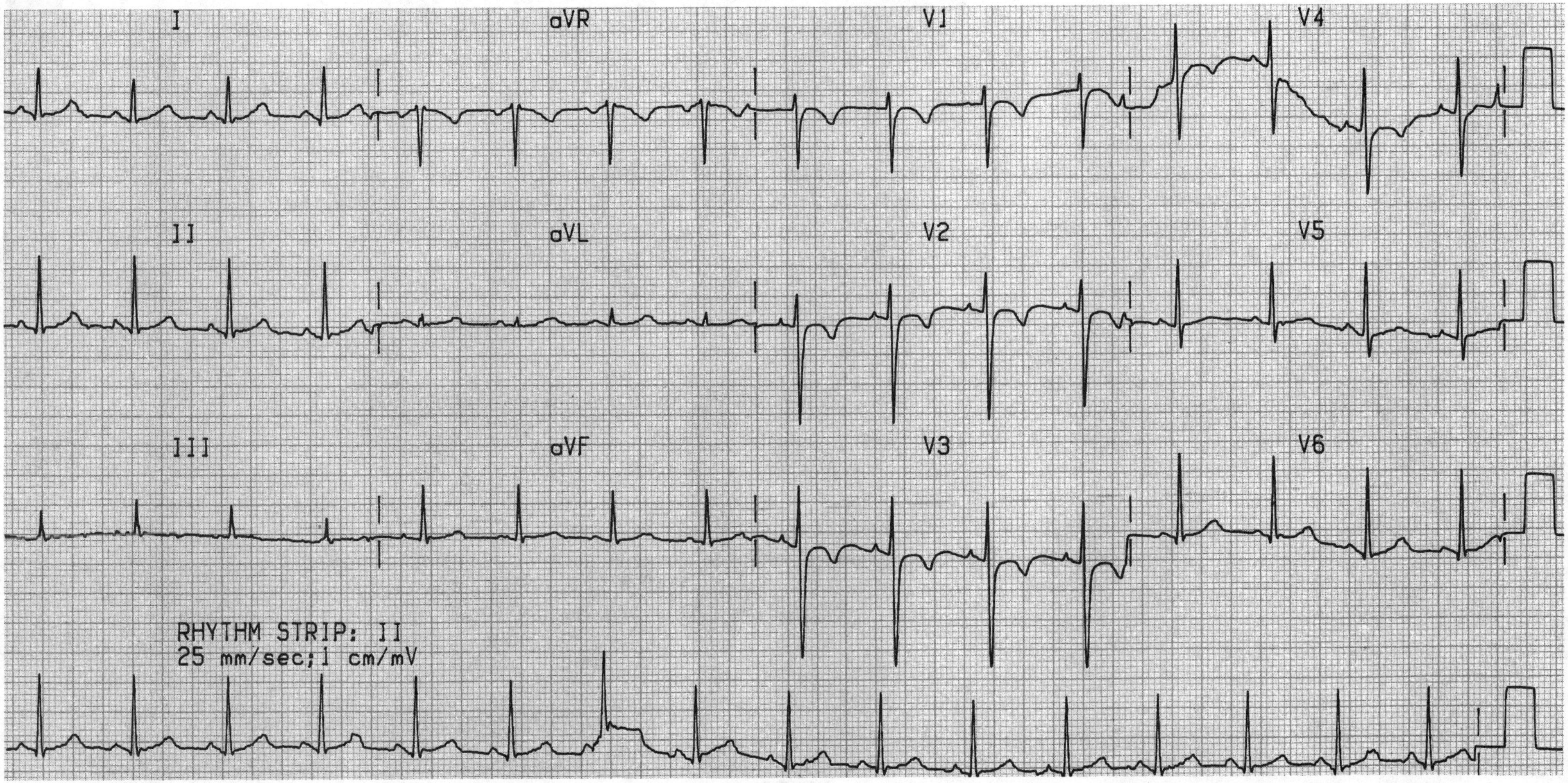

A-8

NARRATIVE INTERPRETATION

Rhythm: **Sinus**
Rate: **98**
Intervals: **PR 0.14, QRS 0.08, QT 0.32**
Axis: **+45 degrees**

Abnormalities

T waves inverted V1–V4.

Synthesis

Sinus rhythm. Normal variant, persistent juvenile T-wave pattern.

TEST ANSWERS: 1, 99.

Comment: In infants and children, the T-wave vector in the horizontal plane is oriented leftward and posterior; hence, T-wave inversion is normally seen in the right and mid precordial leads. With increasing age, the T-wave vector becomes anterior. With the exception of V1, which may normally remain inverted, the T wave in the adult is upright in the precordial leads. Normal persons who continue to demonstrate T-wave inversion in the right and mid precordial leads are described as having a persistent juvenile pattern.

REFERENCES: Chou pp 14, 519. Blackman.

A-9

Clinical History

A 75-year-old man with a history of palpitations.

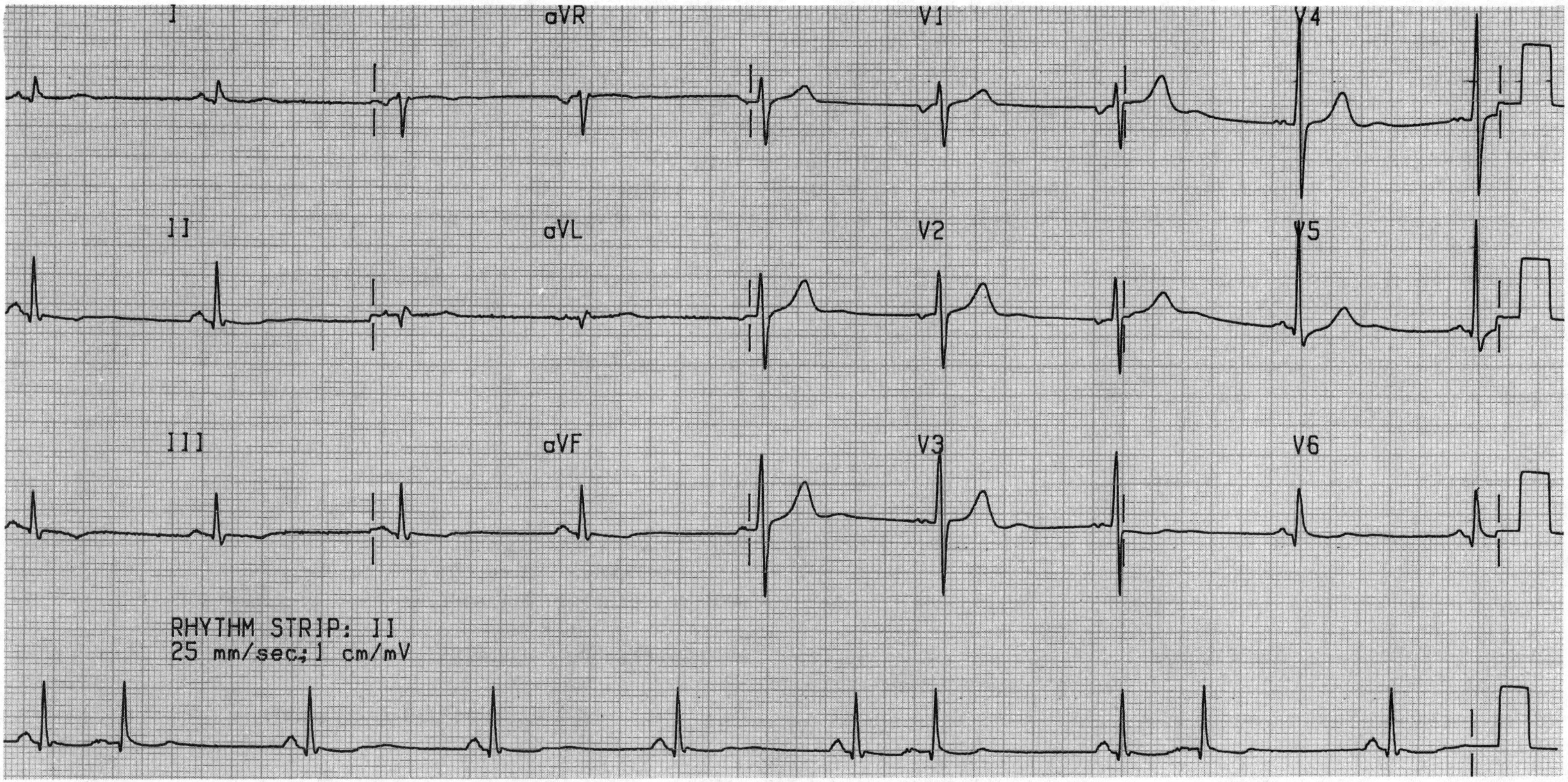

A-9

NARRATIVE INTERPRETATION

Rhythm: **Sinus bradycardia**
Rate: **50**
Intervals: **PR 0.16, QRS 0.08, QT 0.42**
Axis: **+60 degrees**

Abnormalities
Slow heart rate. APCs. Abnormal P terminal force V1. ST depression leads II, III, aVF, V5–V6. T-wave inversion leads II, III, aVF.

Synthesis
Sinus bradycardia. APCs normally conducted. Left atrial abnormality. Nonspecific ST-T-wave abnormalities.

TEST ANSWERS: 3, 10, 60, 106.

Comment: It is not unreasonable to use a descriptive term such as "sag" in the narrative comments. Technically, there is ST depression. Note the U waves in the precordial leads. The U wave is a low-amplitude deflection that follows the T wave. Its amplitude is normally 5 to 25 percent that of the preceding T wave. It is considered abnormal if the amplitude of the U wave is 1.5 mm in any lead. The U waves in this example are within normal limits. Common causes of prominent U waves include bradycardia, hypokalemia, LVH, central nervous system abnormalities, and mitral valve prolapse.

REFERENCES: Chou pp 14, 519–521. Lepeschkin.

Date : 12/09/2026

Location Slip

Time : 4:47 pm

Reference : **EDUCATIONAL TRSPL 110926** Local Slip

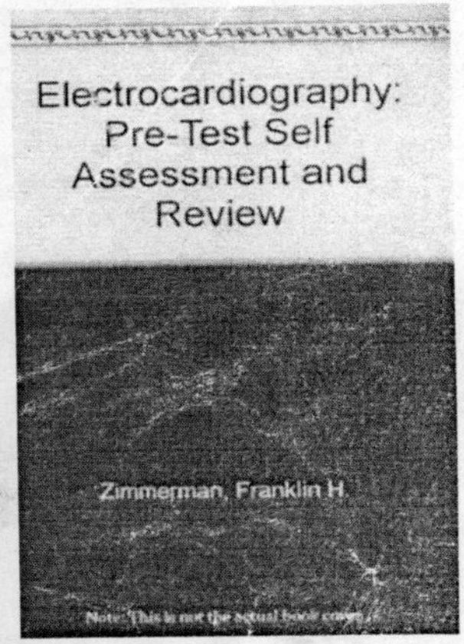

0071135871 **Qty : 1**

Title : **Electrocardiography**

Author : Franklin H. Zimmerman,

Publisher : McGraw-Hill Professional

Yr : 1993

Edn No. : 1st

Cover. : Paperback

SKU Scan Location

Skucode	Godown	Floor	Location	Transaction Date
53A1060179	0	0	AL080	10/04/2007 14:10:24
53A1100408	4	0	AL088	10/04/2007 13:11:45
53A1150231	4	0	AL096	03/04/2007 13:42:56
51A0650426	6	0	AL071	03/02/2007 19:00:26
51A0650357	6	0	AL114	03/02/2007 19:00:26

ISBN Location

ISBN	GodownNo	Floor	BoxNo	Qty	FileID
0071135871	0	0	UNKNOWN	1	Stock Sync
071135871	4	0	Unknown	2	Dashboard Transfe
1135871	6	0	Unknown	1	Dashboard Transfe
35871	6	0	Unknown	1	Dashboard Transfe

d History

Floor No	Box No	Qty	scandate

A-10

Clinical History

A 78-year-old asymptomatic woman.

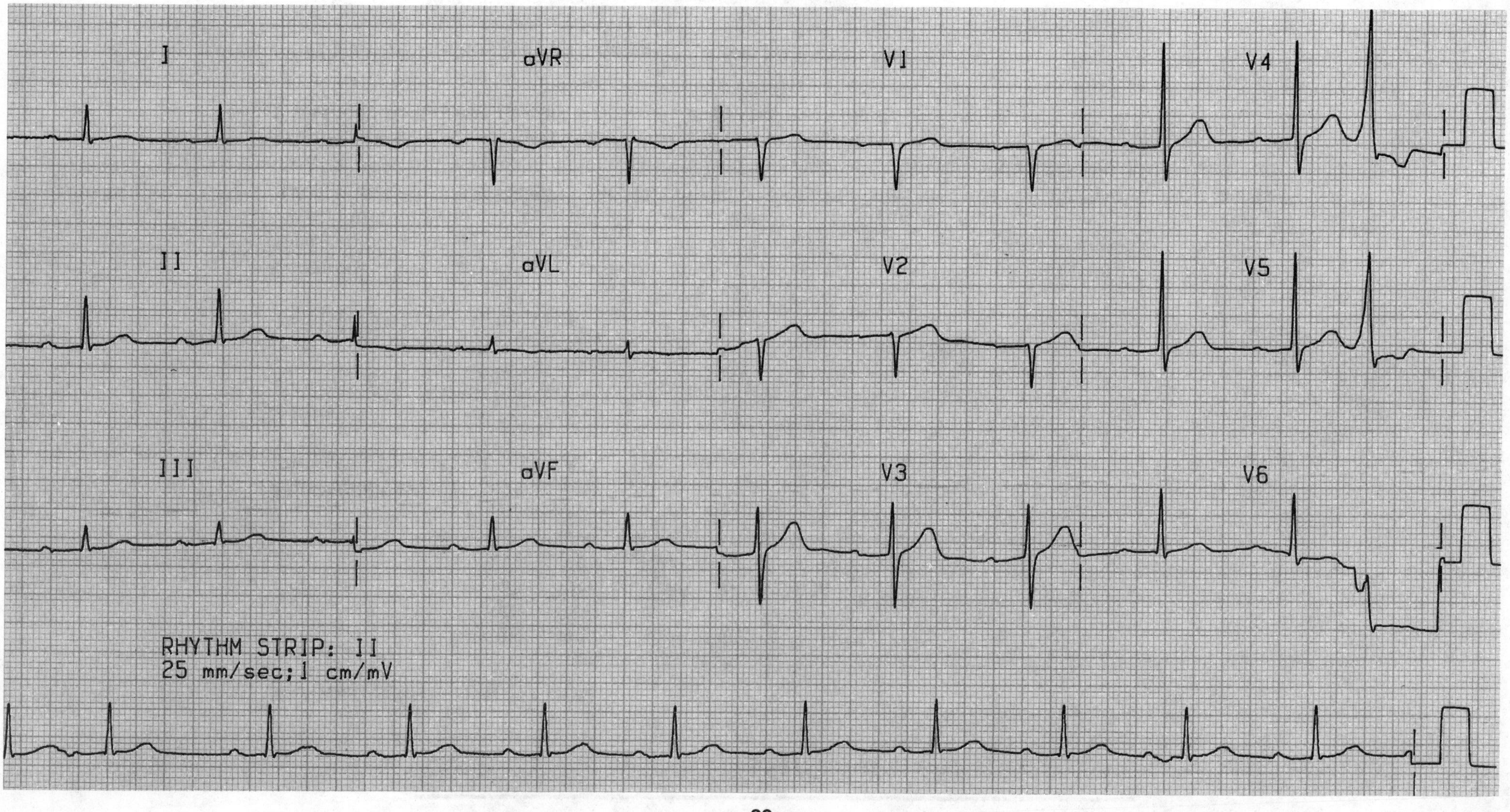

A-10

NARRATIVE INTERPRETATION

Rhythm:	**Sinus, with first-degree AV block**
Rate:	**65**
Intervals:	**PR 0.26, QRS 0.08, QT 0.38**
Axis:	**+75 degrees**

Abnormalities

Prolonged PR interval. VPC. APC.

Synthesis

Sinus rhythm with first-degree AV block. VPC. APC.

TEST ANSWERS: 1, 10, 26, 42.

Comment: First-degree AV block is the most common cardiac conduction abnormality. It is frequently seen in older patients in the absence of clinical cardiac disease. In patients with a narrow QRS complex, the conduction abnormality usually lies within the AV node. In most patients, asymptomatic first-degree AV block is clinically insignificant. The clinician should be alerted, however, that conduction disease may be present and pharmacologic agents that may worsen cardiac conduction should be used with caution. Finally, do not forget to carefully review the rhythm strip of each tracing. The APC present in the second beat of the rhythm strip could easily be overlooked.

REFERENCES: Chou p 412. Chung pp 275–281. Myrin.

A-11

Clinical History

A 65-year-old woman taking digoxin for congestive heart failure.

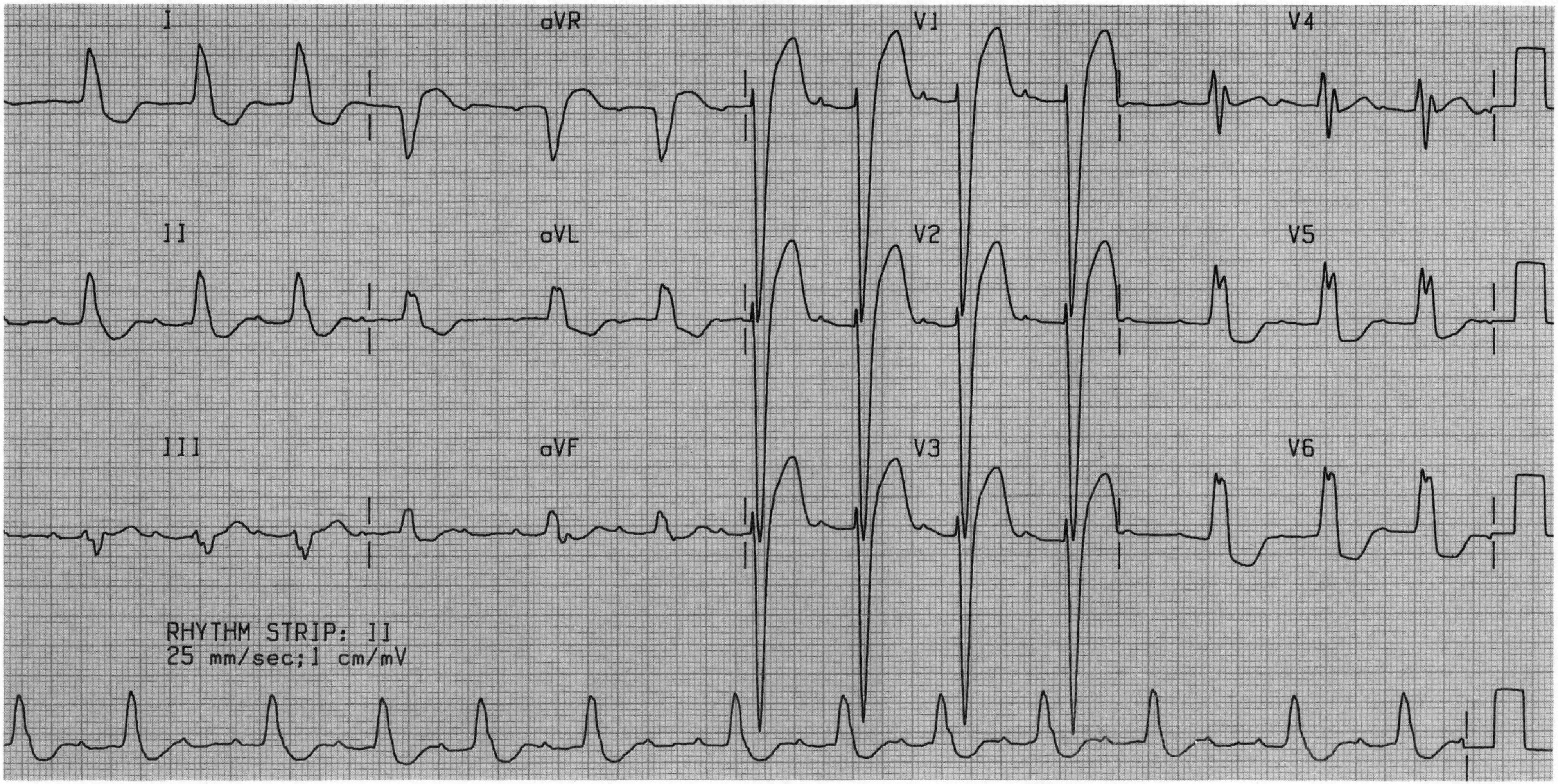

A-11

NARRATIVE INTERPRETATION

Rhythm:	**Atrial tachycardia with variable conduction**
Rate:	**Atrial rate 175, average ventricular rate 75**
Intervals:	**PR variable, QRS 0.16, QT 0.40**
Axis:	**+15 degrees**

Abnormalities

Progressive prolongation of PR interval in conducted beats with eventual loss of conduction. Broad, notched QRS with associated ST-T-wave abnormalities leads I, aVL, V5–V6. SV2 + RV6 greater than 45.

Synthesis

Atrial tachycardia with variable conduction. Wenckebach phenomenon. LBBB with associated ST-T-wave changes. Increased precordial voltage suggestive of LVH.

TEST ANSWERS: 17, 50, 51, 74, (78), 104.

Comment: The diagnosis of atrial tachycardia with "block" would have been very difficult in this patient had there not been a period of increased block (decreased conduction), which uncovered the P waves "buried" in the QRS complex during 2:1 AV conduction. One could have easily mistaken this rhythm for sinus with first-degree AV block. There is a gradual prolongation in the PR intervals of the conducted beats until a P wave fails to conduct to the ventricles, an example of the Wenckebach phenomenon. Remember that an AV conduction ratio of 2:1 is a physiologic property of the AV node at atrial rates approaching 200 beats per minute. The superimposed Wenckebach phenomenon produced a higher conduction ratio and is nonphysiologic. First-degree AV block should not be diagnosed in this example because of the presence of higher degrees of block. This combination of conduction abnormalities and rhythm disturbance is often seen in digitalis intoxication.

An additional finding in this example is the markedly increased precordial QRS voltage. Some studies report that LVH may still be diagnosed in patients with a left bundle if the sum of the voltage of the S wave in V2 and the R wave in V6 exceeds 45 mm. In the author's opinion, it is better to consider this as suggestive but not diagnostic of LVH.

REFERENCES: Chung pp 110, 130, 289. Vandenberg. Klein RC. Kafka.

A-12

Clinical History

A 26-year-old woman with palpitations. Chest x-ray and echocardiogram are normal.

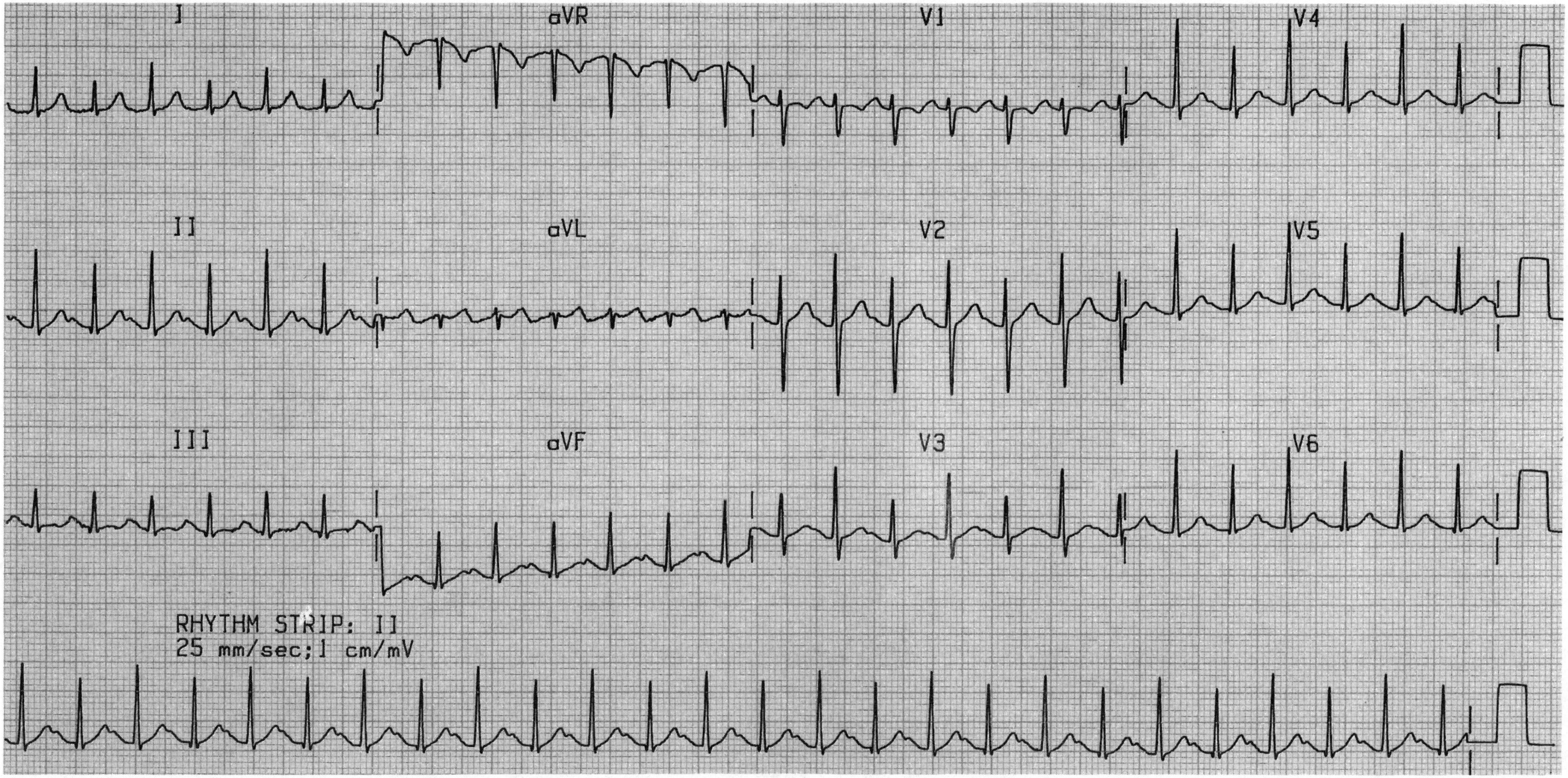

A-12

NARRATIVE INTERPRETATION

Rhythm: **Atrial tachycardia, regular 1:1 conduction, sustained**
Rate: **158**
Intervals: **PR 0.14, QRS 0.06, QT 0.24**
Axis: **+75 degrees**

Abnormalities

Rapid heart rate. Electrical alternans.

Synthesis

Atrial tachycardia, sustained. Electrical alternans.

TEST ANSWERS: 15, 69.

Comment: Note the alternating heights of the QRS complexes, which is characteristic of electrical alternans. This finding is highly suggestive that the arrhythmia uses an atrial-ventricular bypass tract. One review found that such a bypass tract was present in 92 percent of narrow complex tachycardias that exhibited QRS alternans. The presence of electrical alternans is very helpful in distinguishing the rhythm in this tracing as a supraventricular tachycardia, rather than simply a sinus tachycardia. Electrical alternans may also be seen in pericardial tamponade.

REFERENCES: Green. Kalbfleisch. Kremers (1985).

A-13

Clinical History

A 75-year-old asymptomatic woman with a long history of hypertension.

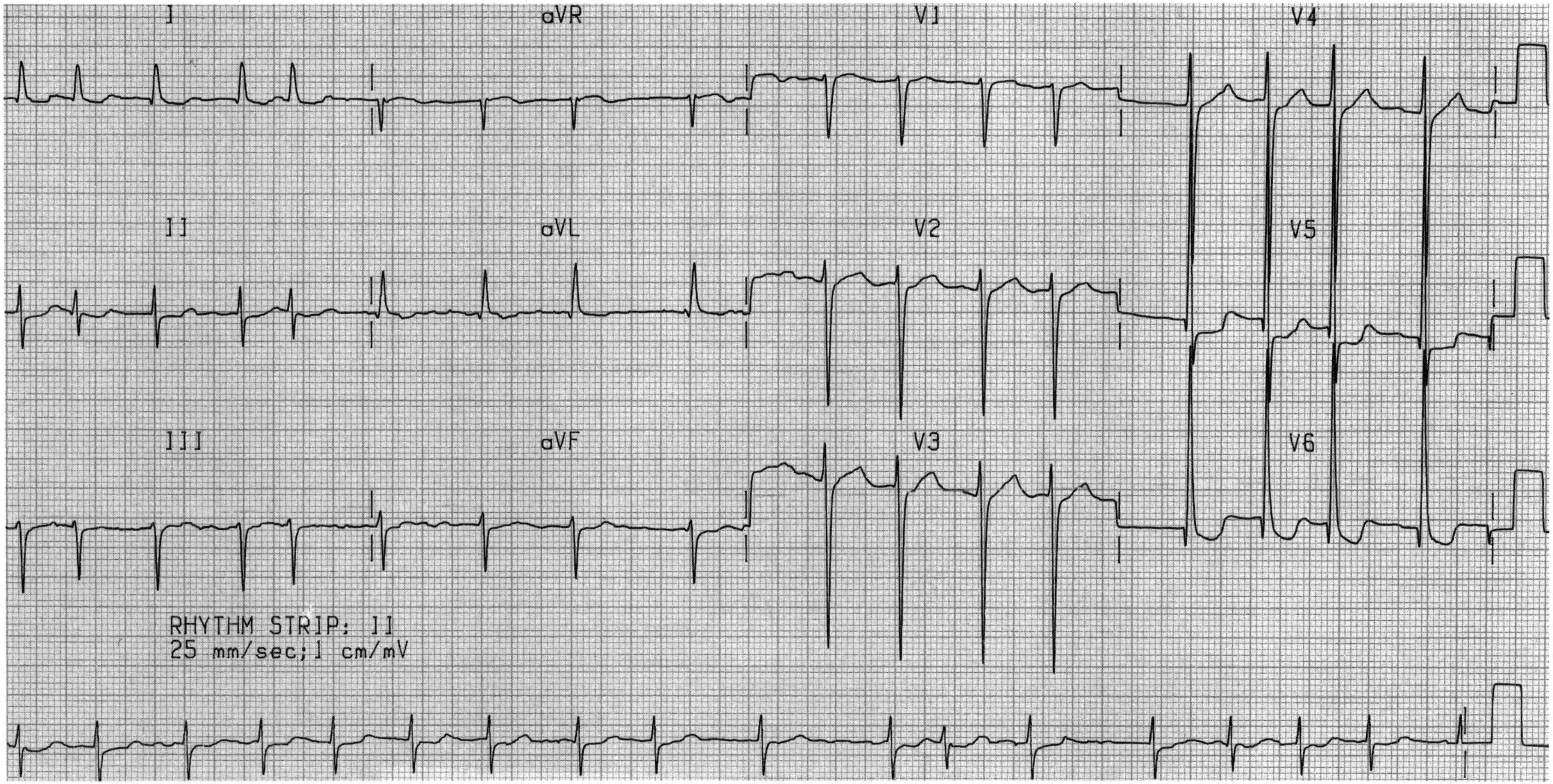

A-13

NARRATIVE INTERPRETATION

Rhythm:	**Atrial fibrillation**
Rate:	**105 (average)**
Intervals:	**PR –, QRS 0.08, QT 0.28**
Axis:	**−30 degrees**

Abnormalities
SV2 + RV5 greater than 35 mm. ST-segment depression leads I, II, aVF, V4–V6. T-wave inversion leads I, aVL, V6.

Synthesis
Atrial fibrillation with controlled ventricular response. LVH by voltage criterion. Associated ST-T-wave abnormalities. Possible ST-T-wave abnormalities suggestive of myocardial ischemia.

TEST ANSWERS: 20, 50, 78, (102), 103.

Comment: Note is made of horizontal ST depression in leads V5 and V6. The classic "strain" ST-segment pattern of LVH is a depressed ST segment with upward concavity associated with T-wave inversion in the left precordial leads. The pattern of the present example is somewhat different and might be seen in a patient with LVH and superimposed ischemia. Serial tracings and clinical history would be invaluable in such a case to make this diagnosis.

A-14

Clinical History

A 16-year-old asymptomatic female high school basketball player.

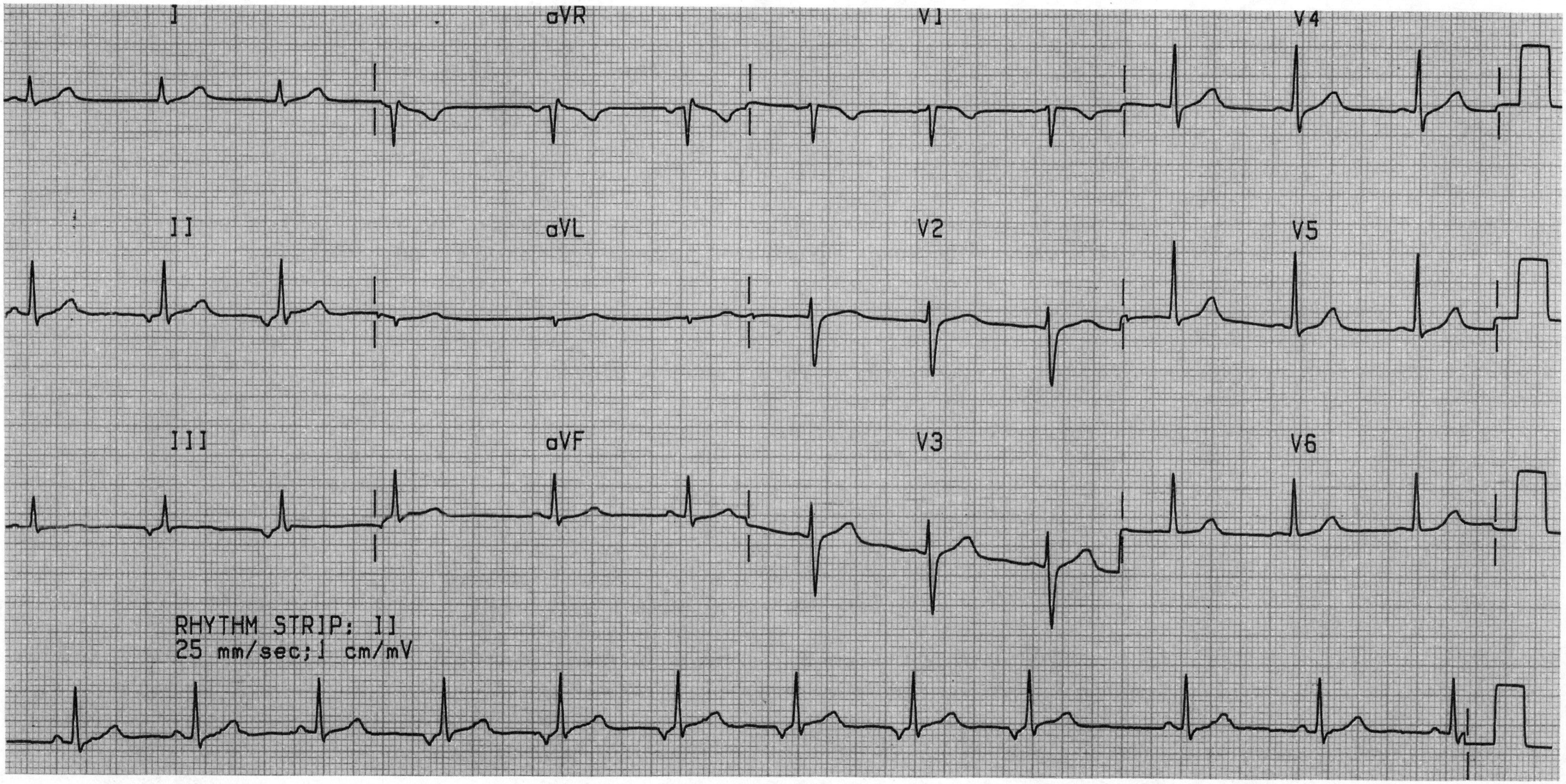

A-14

NARRATIVE INTERPRETATION

Rhythm:	**Sinus with wandering atrial pacemaker to the AV junction**
Rate:	**Sinus rate 74, AV junctional rate 76**
Intervals:	**PR 0.14, QRS 0.08, QT 0.34**
Axis:	**+60 degrees**

Abnormalities

Change in P-wave configuration with development of inverted P waves in lead II with short PR interval.

Synthesis

Sinus rhythm with wandering atrial pacemaker to the AV junction. Otherwise within normal limits.

TEST ANSWERS: 1, 6.

Comment: This is a clinically insignificant rhythm in this young, athletically trained patient. Note that the rate of the ectopic pacemaker is slightly faster than the sinus rate and "usurps" control for a period of time. The first three complexes in leads II and III of the tracing best demonstrate a "wandering" to the AV junction. Note that the second P-wave configuration is intermediate between the normal P wave and the inverted AV junctional morphology. In this athlete, the sinus node is most likely suppressed by vagal influences from physical training, and a subsidiary pacemaker in the AV junction temporarily takes over.

REFERENCE: Zehender.

A-15

Clinical History

A 34-year-old man with Down's syndrome who complains of chest pain.

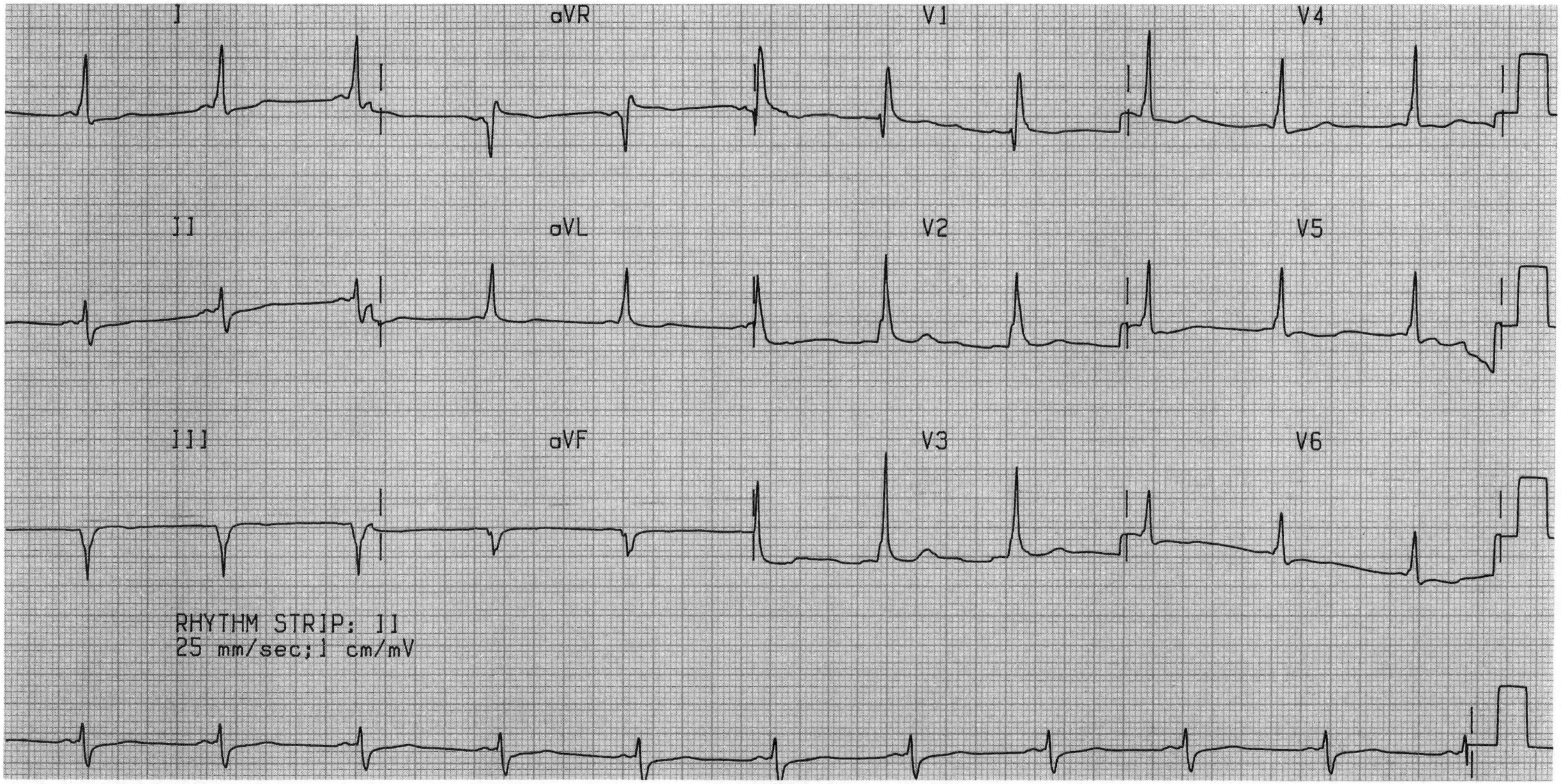

A-15

NARRATIVE INTERPRETATION

Rhythm:	**Sinus**
Rate:	**70**
Intervals:	**PR 0.11, QRS 0.12, QT 0.40**
Axis:	**−45 degrees**

Abnormalities

Short PR interval with delta waves and wide QRS complex and generalized ST-T-wave abnormalities.

Synthesis

Sinus rhythm. Ventricular preexcitation (WPW pattern).

TEST ANSWERS: 1, 49.

Comment: The WPW pattern has been observed in approximately 0.2 percent of otherwise healthy persons. The WPW pattern may be confused with other electrocardiographic diagnoses. Note the pseudoinfarction pattern in leads III and avF, which is suggestive of inferior wall MI. The configuration in lead V1 might also be confused with RBBB. In otherwise healthy persons, the incidence of symptomatic tachyarrhythmias has been estimated to be approximately 12 percent. Studies of hospitalized patients with WPW show an incidence of arrhythmias between 40 and 80 percent. Recent data suggest that preexcitation may disappear over time.

REFERENCES: Barrett. Krahn. Horowitz.

A-16

Clinical History

An 80-year-old man with dyspnea on exertion.

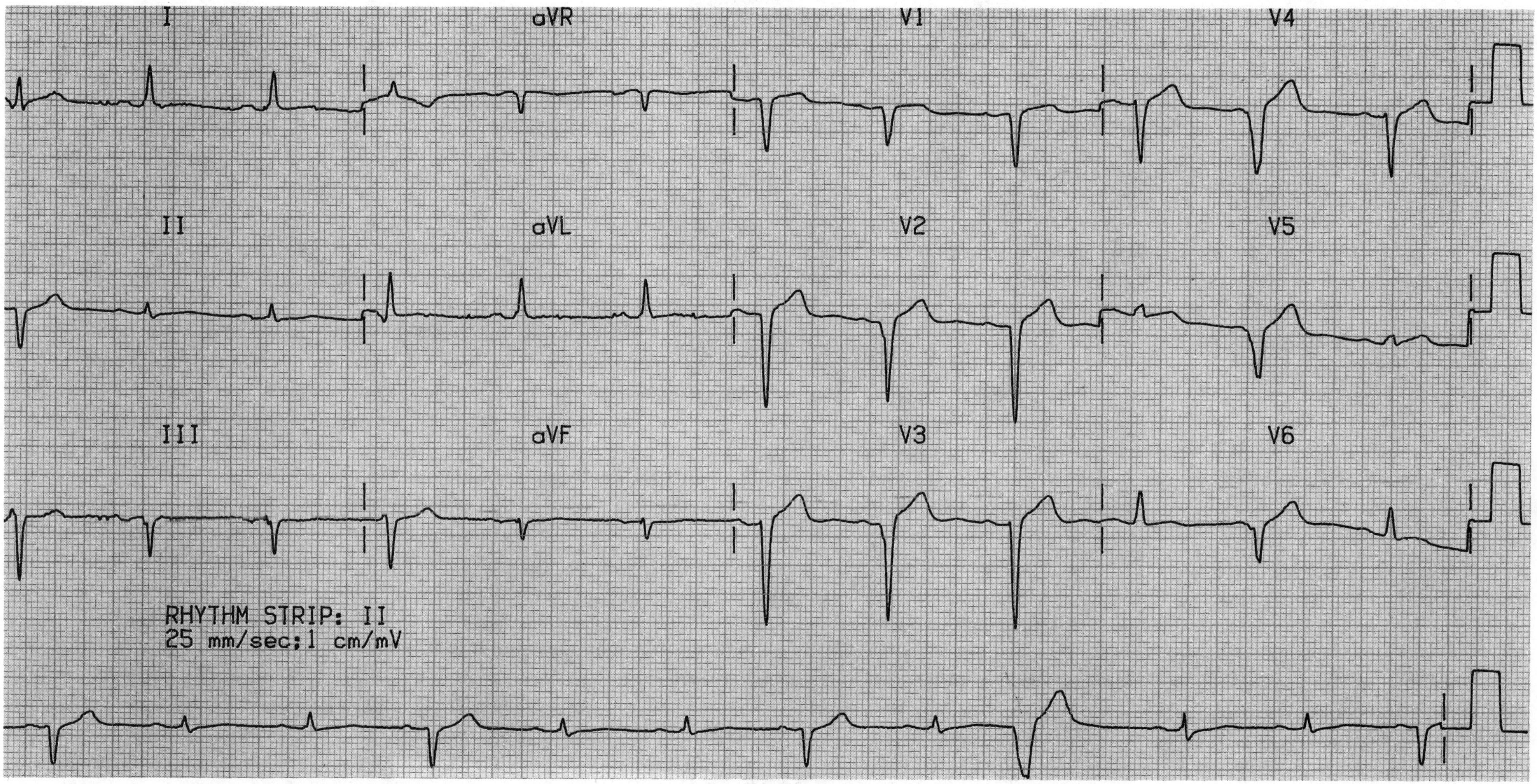

A-16

NARRATIVE INTERPRETATION

Rhythm:	**Sinus**
Rate:	**72**
Intervals:	**PR 0.18, QRS 0.08, QT 0.38**
Axis:	**−15 degrees**

Abnormalities

VPCs. QS waves leads V1–V2. Small R wave lead V3. Fusion beats.

Synthesis

Sinus rhythm. Anterior wall MI of indeterminate age. VPCs uniform. Fusion complexes.

TEST ANSWERS: 1, 26, 56, 82.

Comment: The rhythm strip provides an excellent example of fusion of supraventricular conduction with "late" VPCs. The VPCs are actually uniform, despite having different morphologies because of fusion. The fusion complexes should make one look for a parasystolic focus. The extrasystoles do not, however, exhibit the constant interectopic interval characteristic of parasystole. The fusion complexes may be the result of slight variations in the sinus rate in combination with uniform, fixed coupling of ventricular premature beats.

A-17

Clinical History

A 55-year-old man with a history of a myocardial infarction.

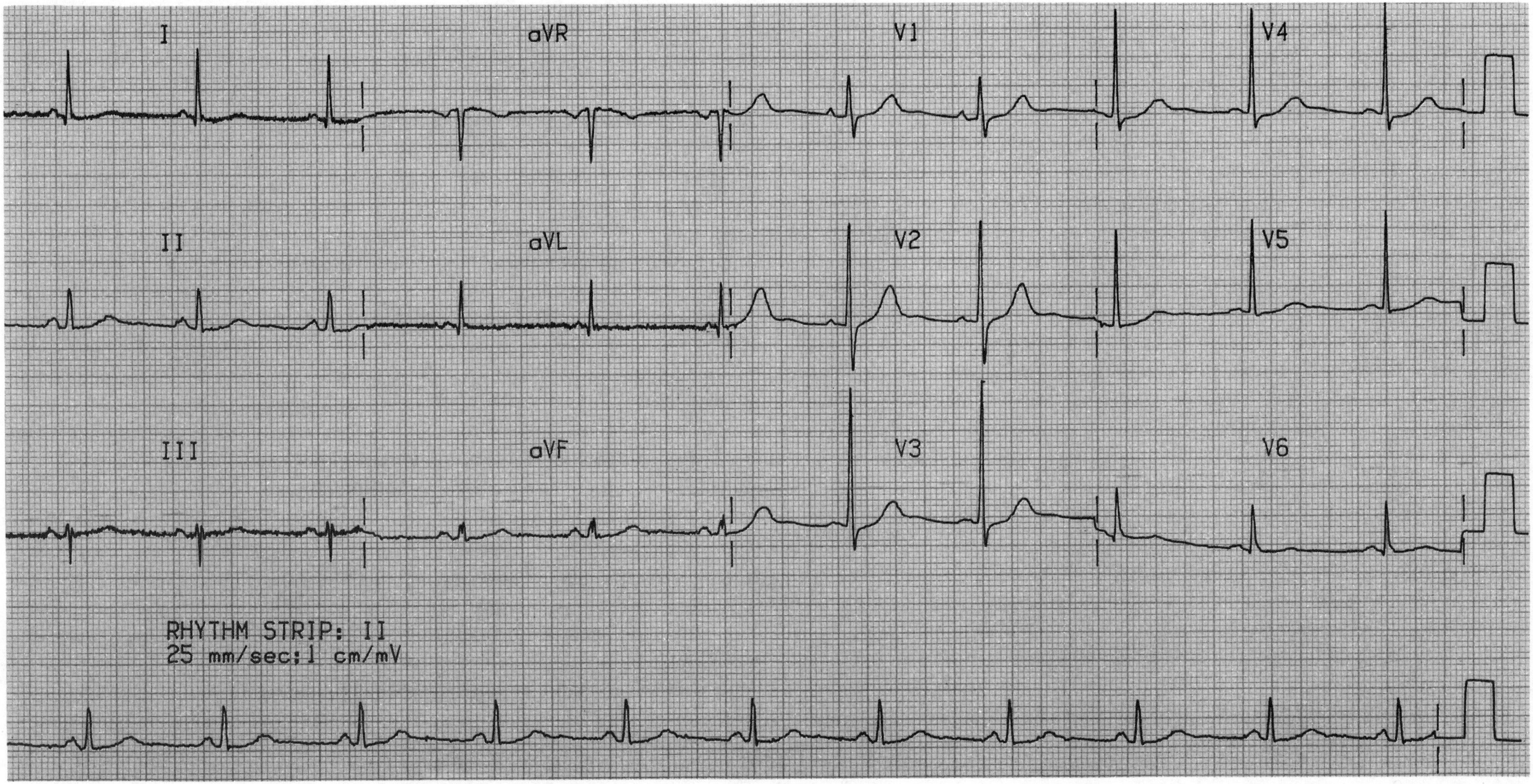

A-17

NARRATIVE INTERPRETATION

Rhythm:	**Sinus**
Rate:	**68**
Intervals:	**PR 0.14, QRS 0.08, QT 0.38**
Axis:	**+15 degrees**

Abnormalities
R greater than S wave leads V1 and V2. Slight ST depression leads I, II, aVF, V2–V5.

Synthesis
Sinus rhythm. Posterior wall MI of indeterminate age. Nonspecific ST abnormalities.

TEST ANSWERS: 1, 94, 106.

Comment: This tracing demonstrates an isolated posterior wall MI. Tall R waves in the right precordial leads may also be seen in persons with RVH. An upright T wave in lead V1 or concomitant evidence of inferior wall MI supports the former diagnosis. This patient had a confirmed posterior wall MI secondary to occlusion of the left circumflex coronary artery.

REFERENCES: Eisenstein. Chaitman. Huey.

A-18

Clinical History

A 64-year-old man who walks into the emergency room complaining of lightheadedness. He has a history of a myocardial infarction.

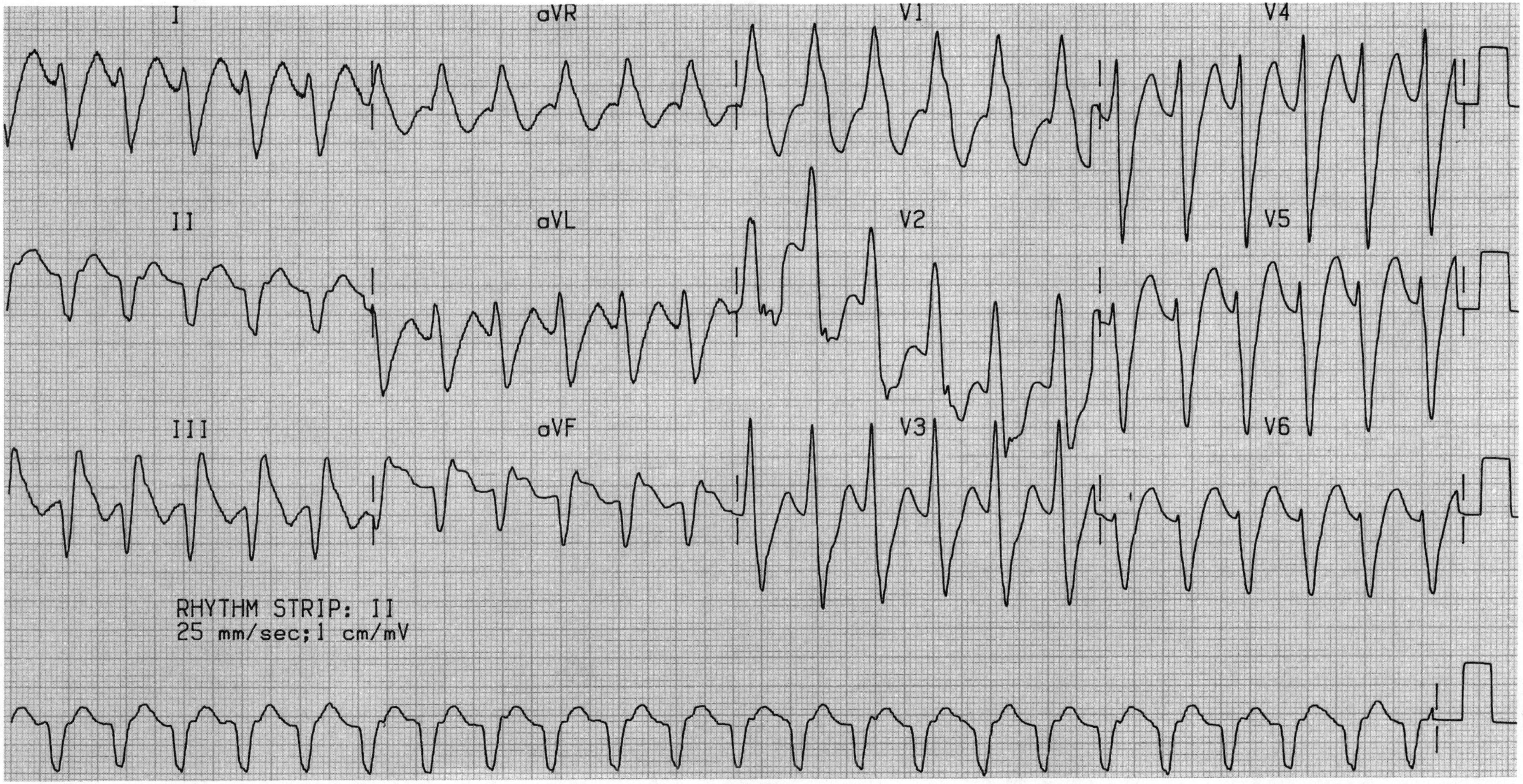

A-18

NARRATIVE INTERPRETATION

Rhythm:	**Wide complex tachycardia suggestive of ventricular tachycardia**
Rate:	**140**
Intervals:	**PR –, QRS 0.16, QT 0.36**
Axis:	**+210 degrees**

Abnormalities
No P waves evident. Wide complex rhythm. Axis rightward of +90 degrees.

Synthesis
Ventricular tachycardia. Right axis deviation.

TEST ANSWERS: 30, 65.

Comment: There has been much written regarding the analysis of wide complex tachycardias. It cannot be overemphasized that these rhythms must be regarded as ventricular in origin until proved otherwise. The fact that the patient was hemodynamically stable should not dissuade one from that electrocardiographic diagnosis. This patient had many indicators that the rhythm was ventricular tachycardia, not supraventricular tachycardia with aberrancy. Characteristics of this rhythm that support a diagnosis of ventricular tachycardia include the markedly prolonged QRS duration and the RS pattern in lead V1.

REFERENCES: Wellens. Akhtar. Brugada. Tchou.

A-19

Clinical History

A 36-year-old man with atypical chest pain and mild dyspnea.

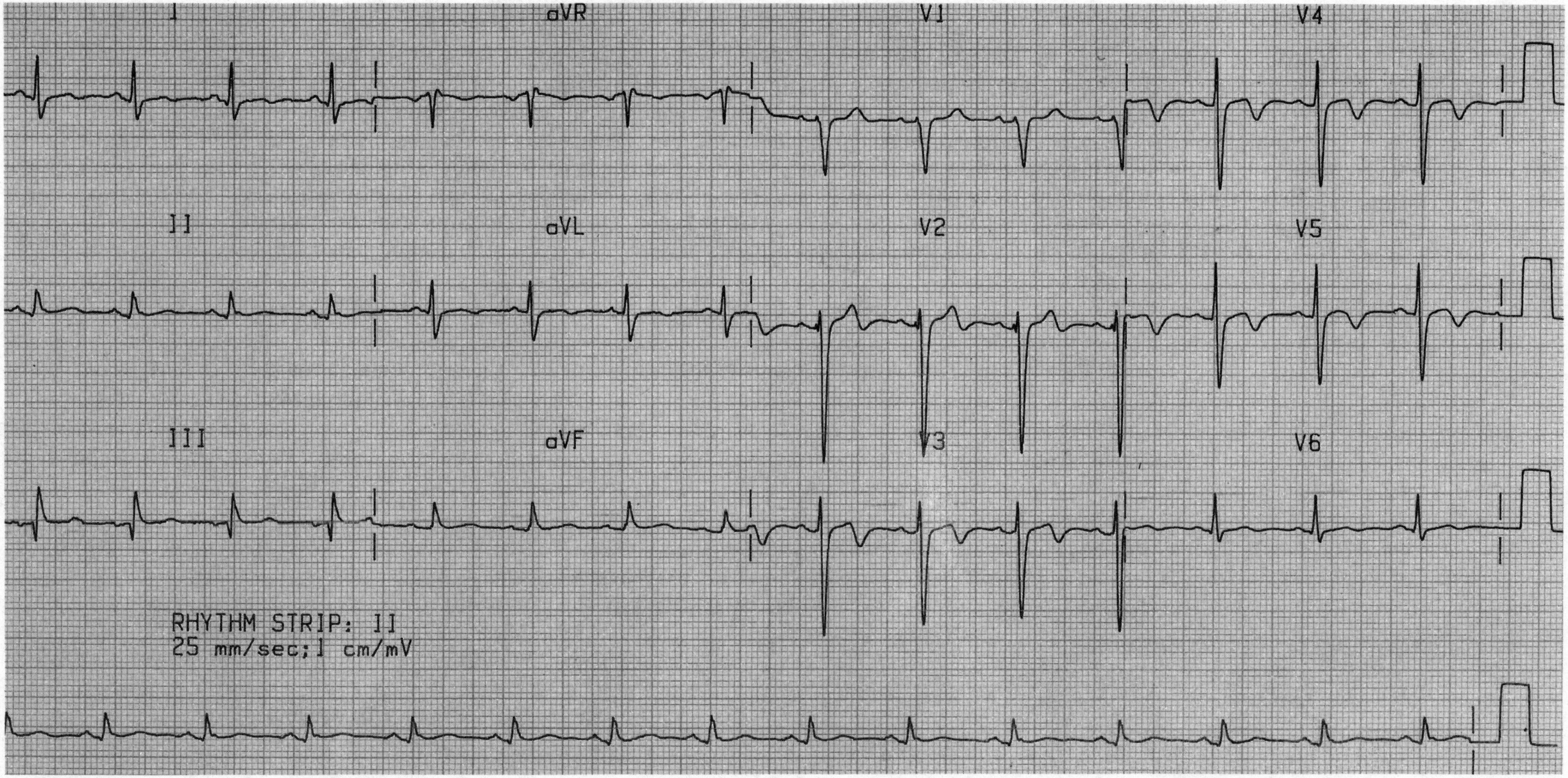

A-19

NARRATIVE INTERPRETATION

Rhythm: Sinus
Rate: 85
Intervals: PR 0.14, QRS 0.08, QT 0.32
Axis: +60 degrees

Abnormalities
ST elevation leads I, aVL, V2–V6. Biphasic T waves leads I, aVL, V2–V3, V6. Inverted T waves leads V4–V5.

Synthesis
Sinus rhythm. ST-T-wave abnormalities suggestive of acute or recent myocardial injury.

TEST ANSWERS: 1, 100.

Comment: Note that these T-wave changes involve the entire precordium, as well as leads I and aVL. They are suggestive of myocardial injury and should not be identified as juvenile T-wave changes, a normal variant. The ST segments in leads I and aVL as well as the entire precordium are slightly elevated and show abnormal downward concavity. Such abnormalities are suggestive of early MI. This patient had further ischemic changes and subsequently developed a non-Q-wave MI. He was found to have a subtotal occlusion of the proximal left anterior descending coronary artery on angiography. The ST abnormalities of pericarditis are occasionally difficult to distinguish from those of myocardial injury. In pericarditis, the ST-segment elevation is usually concave upward and may be associated with PR depression.

A-20

Clinical History

A 69-year-old asymptomatic man with a history of multiple myocardial infarctions, most recently 1 year ago.

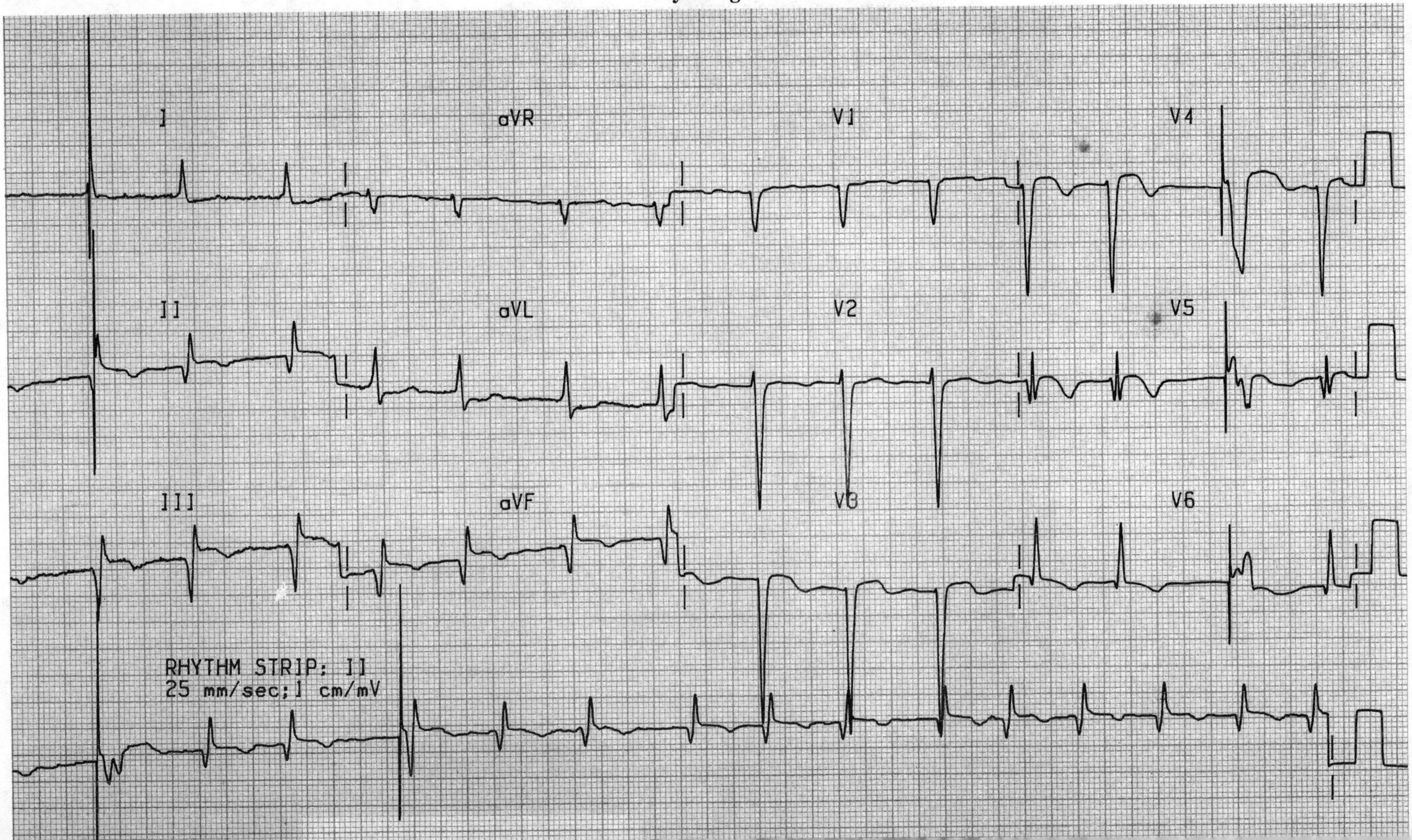

A-20

NARRATIVE INTERPRETATION

Rhythm: **Atrial fibrillation with controlled ventricular response**
Rate: **82 (average)**
Intervals: **PR –, QRS 0.08, QT 0.38**
Axis: **0 degrees**

Abnormalities

Ventricular pacemaker complexes on demand with capture. Pacemaker fusion complex. Q waves II, III, aVF, V5. R waves less than 3 mm leads V1–V4. ST elevation leads II, III, aVF, V3–V6. ST depression leads I, aVL. T-wave inversion leads II, III, aVF, V3–V6.

Synthesis

Atrial fibrillation with controlled ventricular response. Ventricular pacemaker functioning on demand, rate 75 with appropriate capture. Pacemaker fusion complex. Inferior wall MI of indeterminate age. Anteroseptal (extensive anterior) wall MI of indeterminate age. Probable ventricular aneurysm. Clinical correlation or serial tracings required to exclude acute transmural ischemia/infarction.

TEST ANSWERS: 20, 35, 51, 56, 84, (88), 92, 95.

Comment: This tracing points out the importance of serial tracings to confirm the diagnosis of acute injury. Certainly this tracing is compatible with an evolving acute MI. This asymptomatic patient had no new changes on his electrocardiogram, which indicates that the persistent ST elevation beyond 2 weeks of an acute MI was likely due to a ventricular aneurysm. Reverse or poor R-wave progression is generally used as an indicator of anteroseptal MI. The presence of a deep Q wave in lead V5 suggests more extensive necrosis of the anterior wall. Note that the fourth complex on the rhythm strip is a fusion beat that combines depolarization from both atrial conduction and the pacemaker. Note also that the first complex of the 12 lead has a pacemaker spike that occurs just after the initiation of the QRS. In this instance, there is no apparent deformity of the QRS from pacemaker activation; therefore, these complexes have been referred to as "pseudofusion" complexes.

A-21

Clinical History

A 44-year-old asymptomatic man.

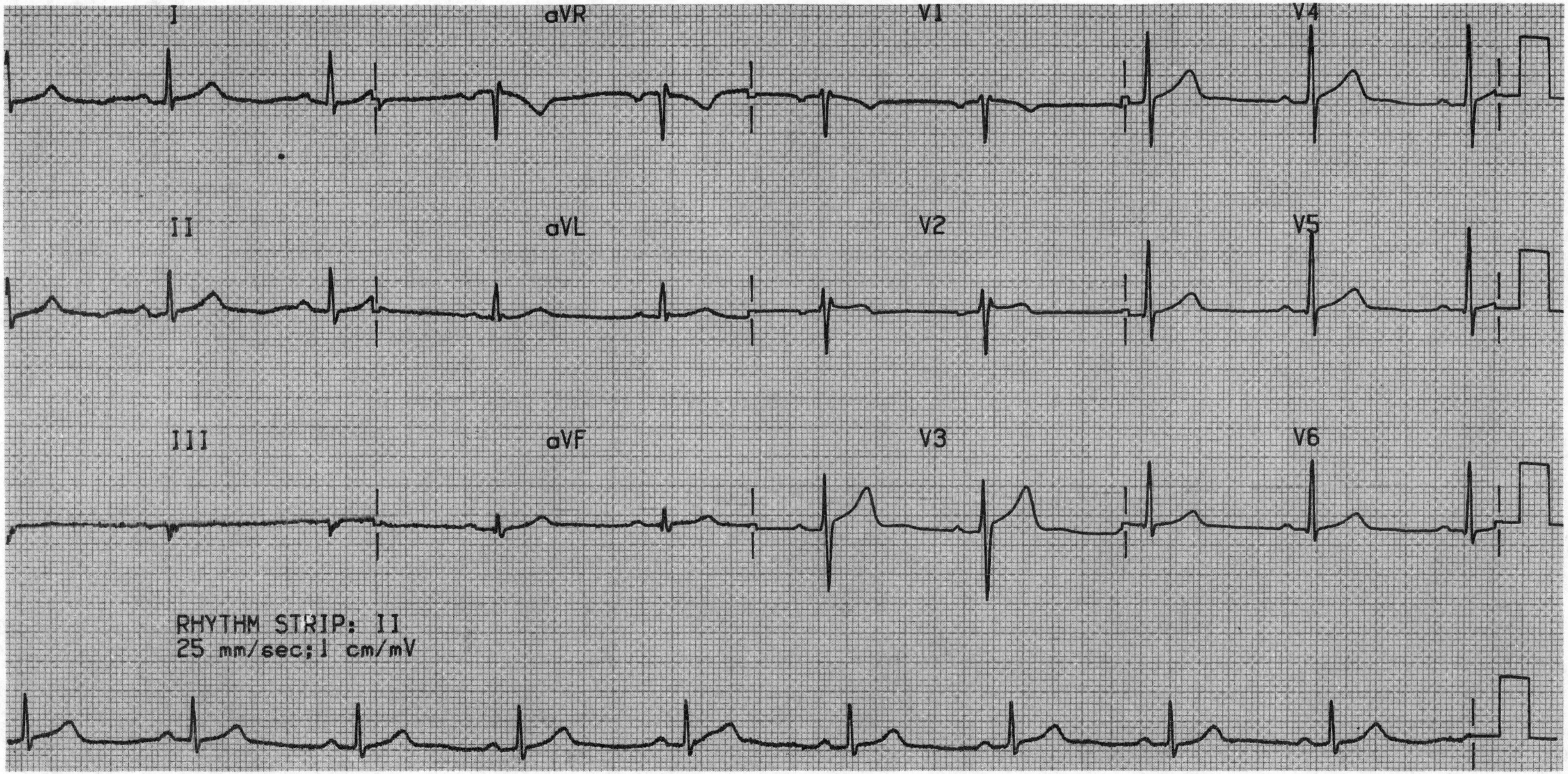

A-21

NARRATIVE INTERPRETATION

Rhythm:	**Sinus bradycardia with first-degree AV block**
Rate:	**53**
Intervals:	**PR 0.21, QRS 0.08, QT 0.40**
Axis:	**+15 degrees**

Abnormalities
Slow heart rate. Prolonged PR interval. RSr′ pattern leads V1–V2.

Synthesis
Sinus bradycardia. First-degree AV block. RSr′ pattern, normal variant.

TEST ANSWERS: 3, 42, 98.

Comment: The RSR′ pattern in lead V1 without any additional evidence of conduction abnormality has been reported in 2.4 percent of normal persons. The secondary R wave has been attributed to activation of the right ventricular outflow tract. Criteria differentiating this pattern as normal have included a primary R wave less than 8 mm, a secondary R wave less than 6 mm, and an R′ amplitude less than the R wave. The normal variant demonstrated in this tracing should not be confused with incomplete RBBB. The diagnosis of incomplete RBBB includes characteristic secondary ST-T-wave abnormalities and is likely to have a more prominent terminal R wave. The borderline first-degree AV block is not obvious in all leads but may be identified in the lead II rhythm strip.

REFERENCES: Chou p 93. Friedman p 164.

A-22

Clinical History

A 68-year-old man with hypertension.

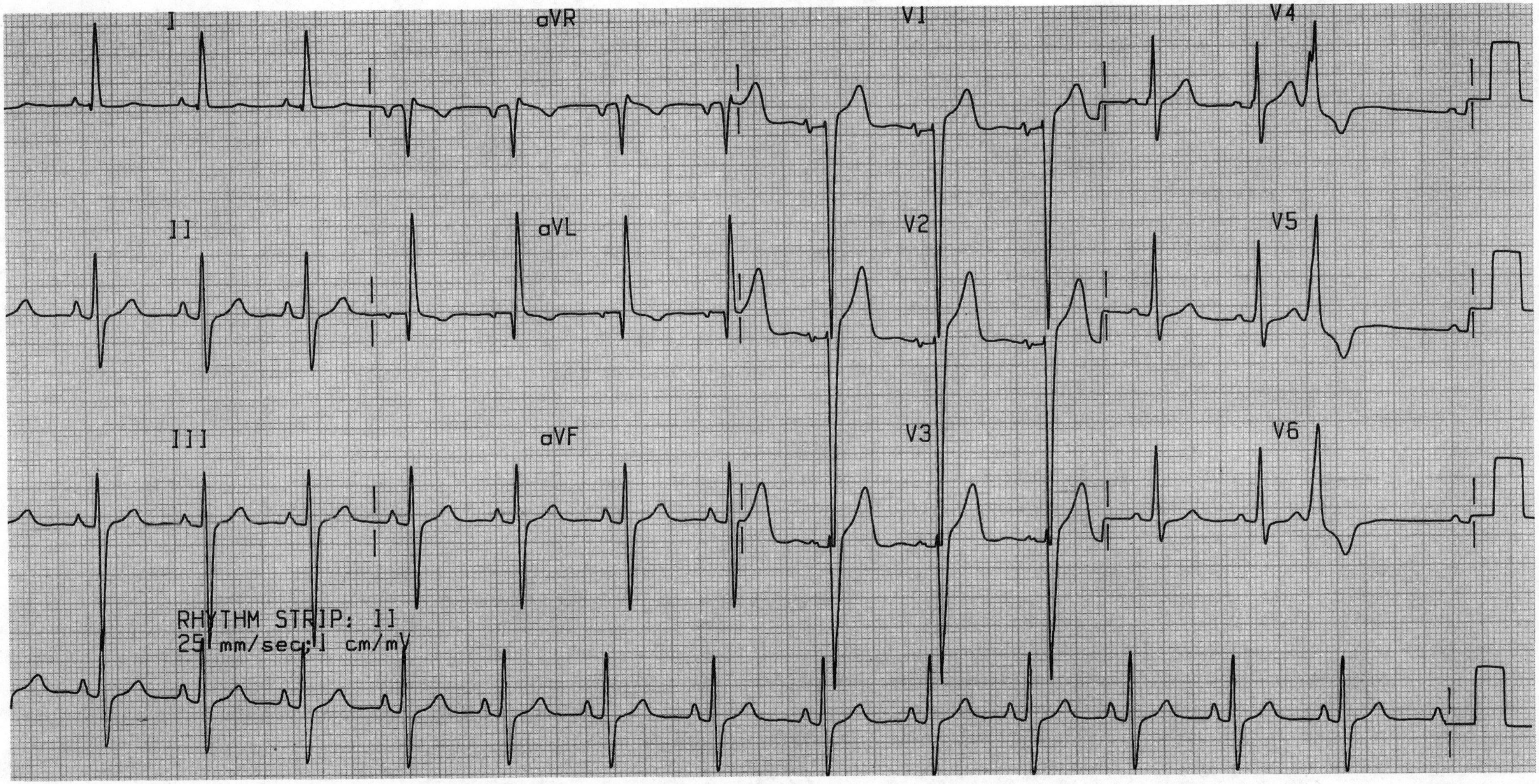

A-22

NARRATIVE INTERPRETATION

Rhythm: **Sinus**
Rate: **80**
Intervals: **PR 0.16, QRS 0.10, QT 0.36**
Axis: **− 30 degrees**

Abnormalities

R wave lead aVL greater than 15 mm. SV2 + RV5 greater than 35 mm. R wave V1–V3 less than 3 mm. T-wave inversion lead aVL. VPC.

Synthesis

Sinus rhythm. VPC. LVH with associated ST-T-wave abnormalities. Poor R-wave progression.

TEST ANSWERS: 1, 26, 66, 78, 103.

Comment: This patient has voltage criteria for LVH. Both the precordial and limb lead voltage easily exceed normal limits. Poor R-wave progression is noted secondary to a leftward shift of the transitional zone from the hypertrophied left ventricle. The axis is at the leftward limit of normal, which also supports a diagnosis of LVH. The T-wave inversion in lead aVL is likely secondary to LVH. Also note that the Q wave in aVL should not be interpreted as indicative of a lateral wall MI.

A-23

Clinical History

A 50-year-old woman with hypertension. A year ago her electrocardiogram was normal.

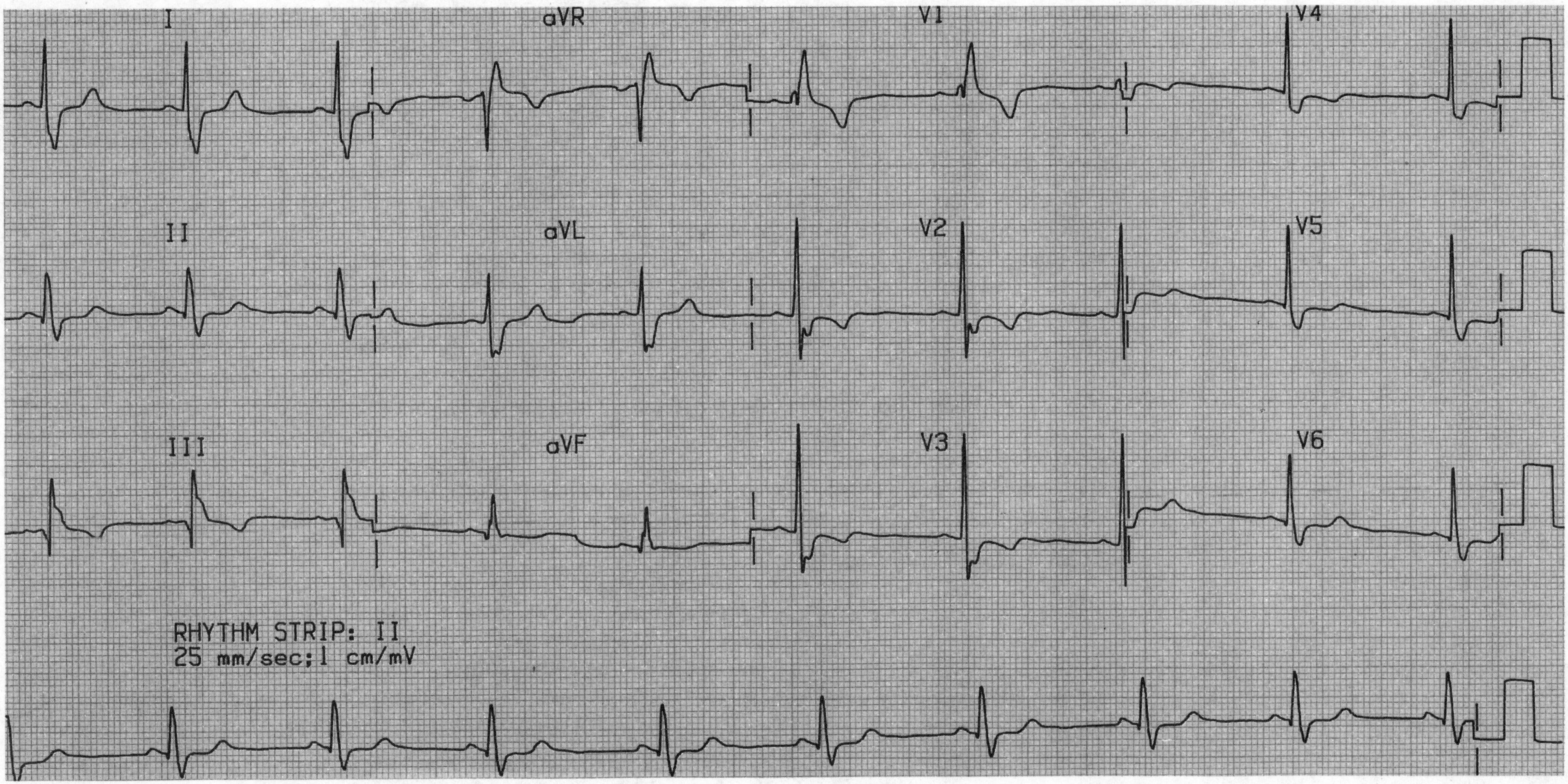

A-23

NARRATIVE INTERPRETATION

Rhythm: **Sinus bradycardia**
Rate: **58**
Intervals: **PR 0.16, QRS 0.12, QT 0.34**
Axis: **+60 degrees**

Abnormalities

Slow heart rate. Broad notched QRS with rsR′ pattern lead V1, and T-wave inversion in leads V1–V3.

Synthesis

Sinus bradycardia. RBBB with associated ST-T-wave abnormalities.

TEST ANSWERS: 3, 70, 104.

Comment: "New" RBBB is most often seen in persons who either have or will develop clinical cardiovascular disease. The Framingham study found the 10-year incidence of cardiovascular mortality to be threefold higher in persons with newly acquired RBBB compared with age-matched controls without RBBB. In contrast, a subset of healthy persons younger than 40 years of age with new RBBB remained free of cardiovascular disease.

REFERENCE: Schneider (1980).

A-24

Clinical History

A 55-year-old man who is 8 days status post coronary artery bypass surgery. He complains of mild palpitations.

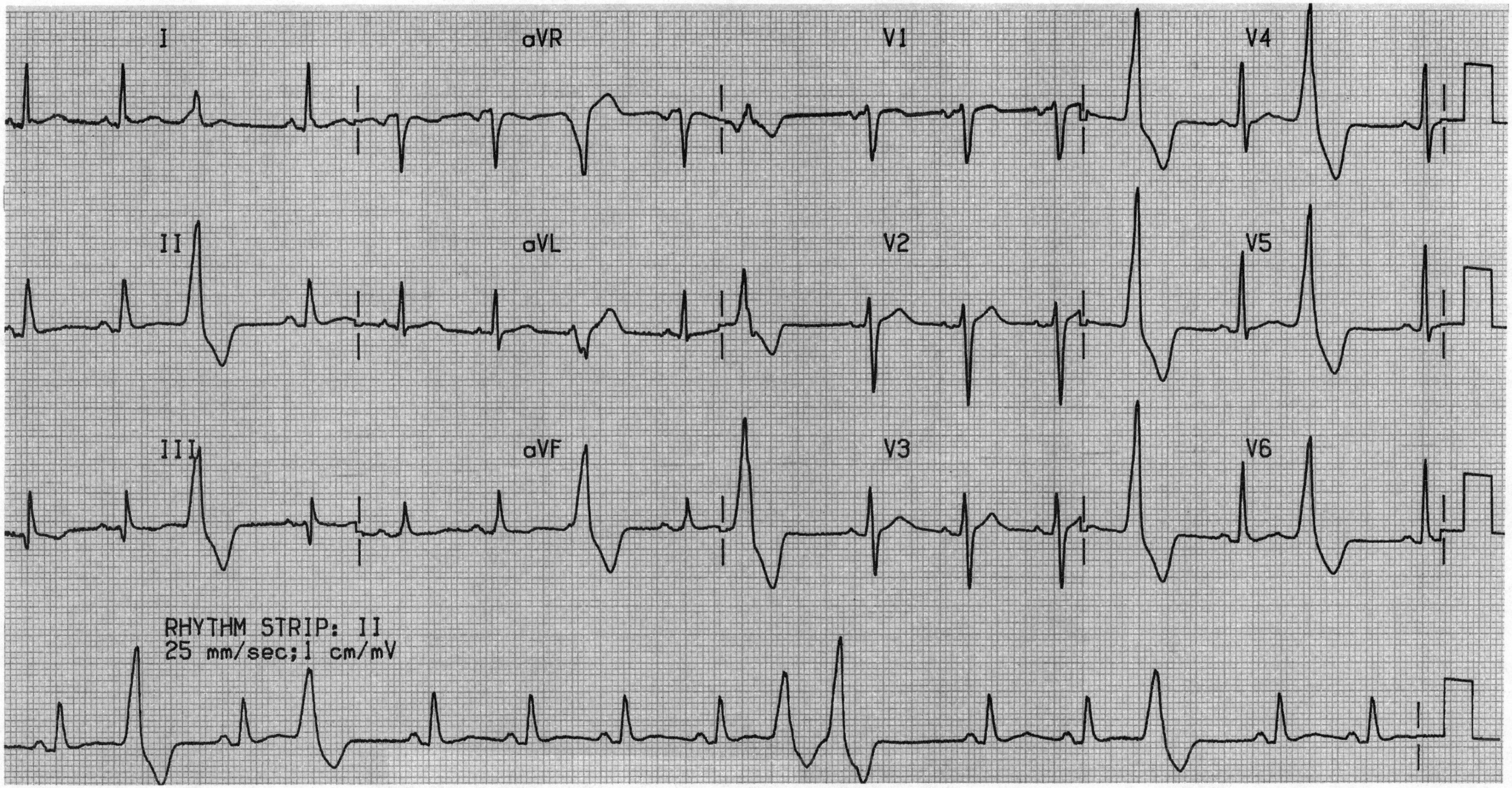

A-24

NARRATIVE INTERPRETATION

Rhythm: **Sinus**
Rate: **88**
Intervals: **PR 0.16, QRS 0.08, QT 0.32**
Axis: **+45 degrees**

Abnormalities
VPCs. Paired VPCs. Slight ST elevation leads I, II, III, aVF, V1–V6.

Synthesis
Sinus rhythm. VPCs, multiform. Paired VPCs on rhythm strip. Nonspecific ST abnormalities.

TEST ANSWERS: 1, 27, 28, 106.

Comment: This patient demonstrates frequent ventricular ectopy and nonspecific ST abnormalities after cardiac surgery. The diffuse ST changes are likely secondary to postoperative pericardial inflammation. A definitive diagnosis of pericarditis cannot be made on this tracing. Interestingly, the presence of complex ventricular ectopy after coronary artery bypass surgery does not carry an adverse prognosis. In one study of 92 postoperative patients, complex ventricular arrhythmias were common (57 percent of patients). These patients were no more likely to develop sudden death, syncope, or other complications than patients without ventricular ectopy.

REFERENCE: Rubin (1985).

A-25

Clinical History

A 79-year-old asymptomatic man with a history of coronary heart disease.

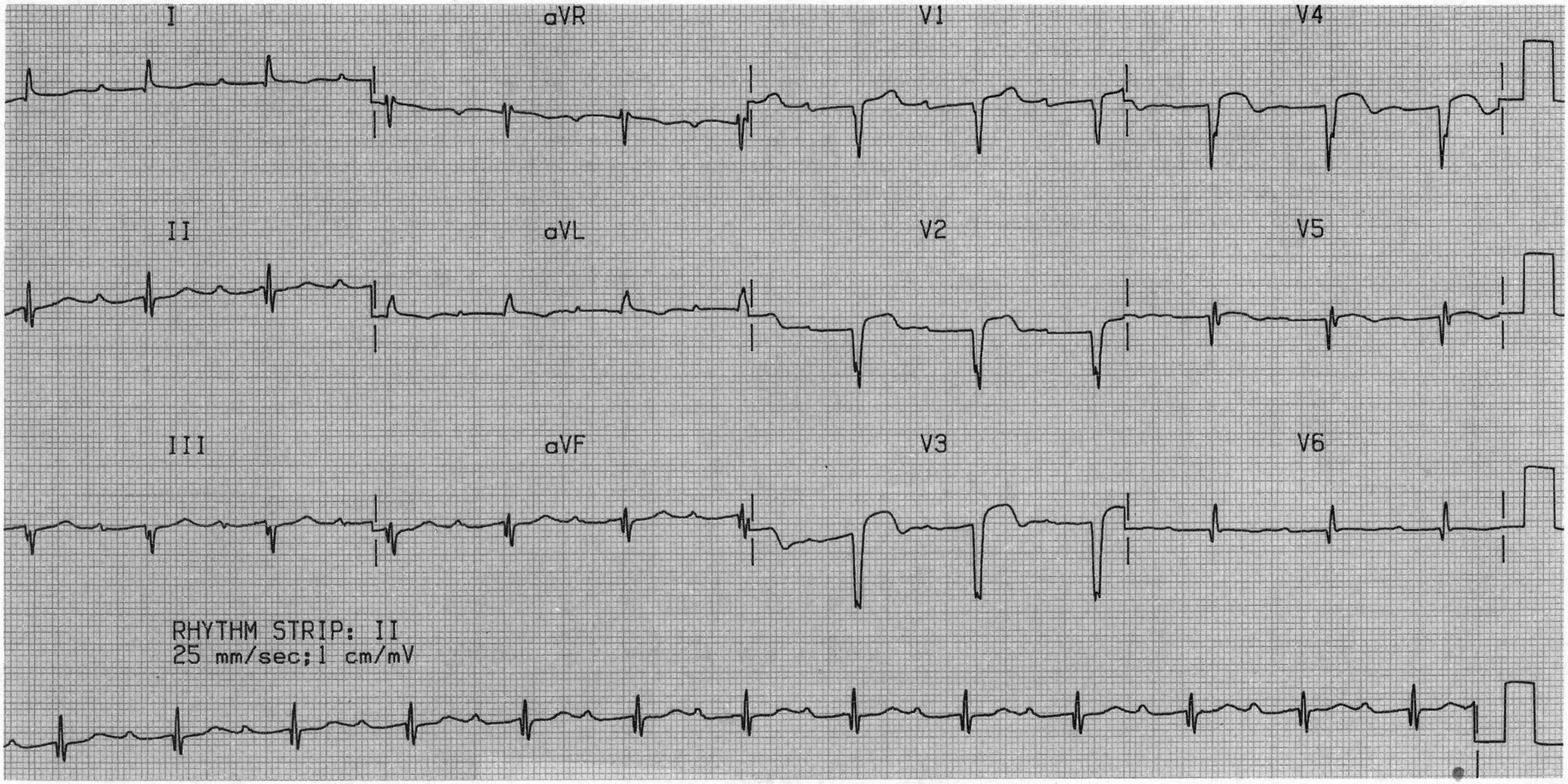

A-25

NARRATIVE INTERPRETATION

Rhythm: **Sinus with first-degree AV block**
Rate: **80**
Intervals: **PR 0.36, QRS 0.08, QT 0.36**
Axis: **−15 degrees**

Abnormalities

Prolonged PR interval. Q waves leads II, III, aVF, V5, V6. QS leads V1–V4. ST elevation leads I, aVL, V1–V6.

Synthesis

Sinus rhythm with first-degree AV block. Inferior wall MI of indeterminate age. Extensive anterior wall MI of indeterminate age. Probable ventricular aneurysm.

TEST ANSWERS: 1, 42, 88, 92, 95.

Comment: A left ventricular aneurysm may develop following acute MI. ST elevation lasting more than 2 weeks following acute MI is likely to persist and is indicative of aneurysm formation. The diagnosis, however, cannot be made definitively by electrocardiography. Ideally, the presence of an aneurysm should be confirmed with imaging techniques. The patient in this example had suffered multiple myocardial infarctions and the persistent ST-segment elevation in the prior anterior and lateral wall infarction zones was indicative of a ventricular aneurysm. This was demonstrated by echocardiography.

A-26

Clinical History

A 34-year-old man with dyspnea and diastolic heart murmur.

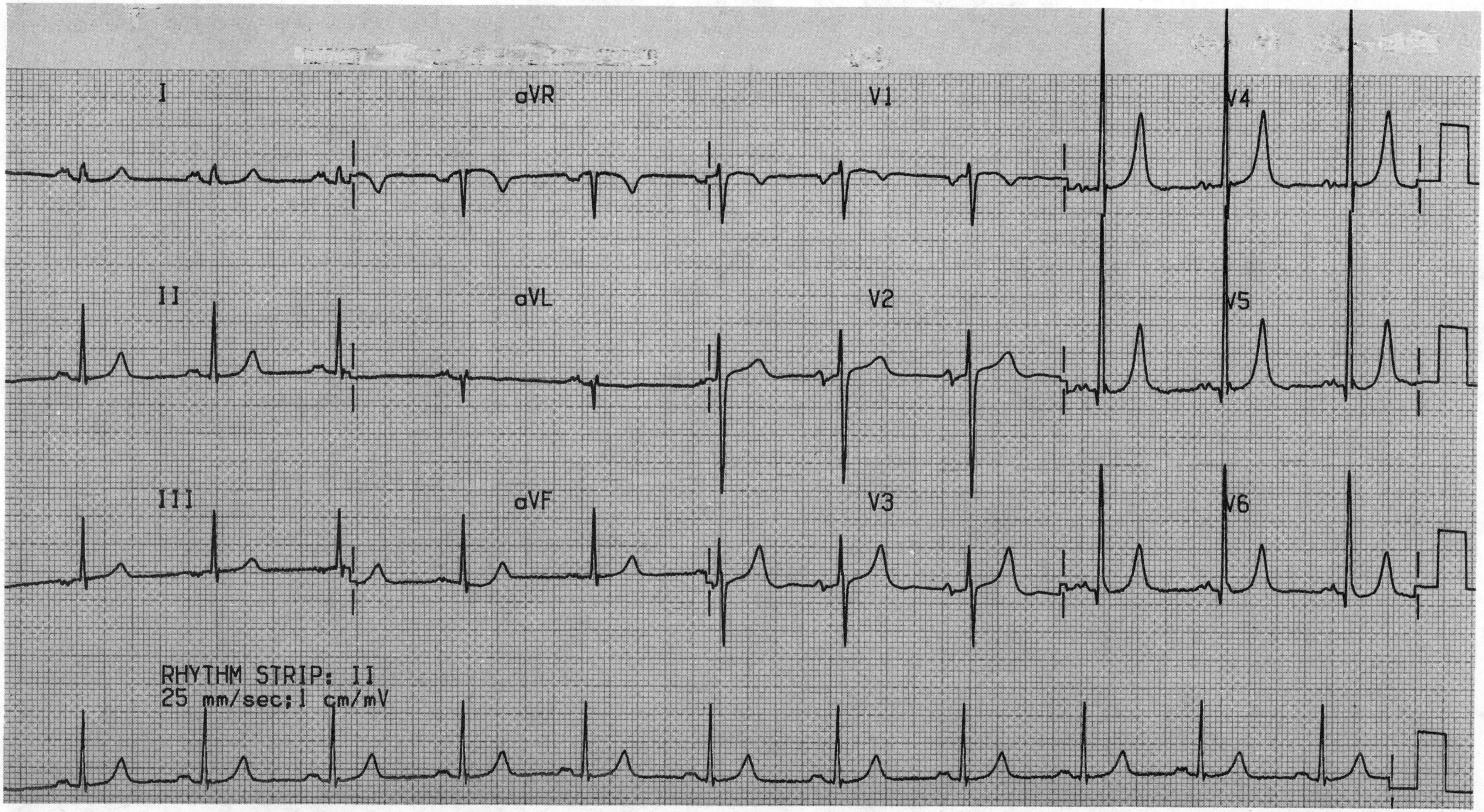

A-26

NARRATIVE INTERPRETATION

Rhythm: **Sinus**
Rate: **65**
Intervals: **PR 0.18, QRS 0.08, QT 0.36**
Axis: **+75 degrees**

Abnormalities

Abnormal P terminal force V1. Broad, notched P wave lead II. SV2 + RV5 equals 50 mm.

Synthesis

Sinus rhythm. Left atrial abnormality. LVH by voltage criteria.

TEST ANSWERS: 1, 60, 78.

Comment: This patient had echocardiographically demonstrated left atrial dilatation. The abnormal P terminal force in lead V1 is easily noted. On careful examination a second criterion for left atrial enlargement is present, namely a broad, notched P wave in lead II with a peak-to-peak interval of the notches of 40 ms. Note that increased voltage for LVH is present in this young man as precordial voltage exceeds age-adjusted limits for LVH. This patient had left ventricular and left atrial enlargement on the basis of aortic insufficiency.

REFERENCES: Alpert (1989). Hazen. Manning. Walker.

A-27

Clinical History

A 90-year-old asymptomatic man. He takes no medications.

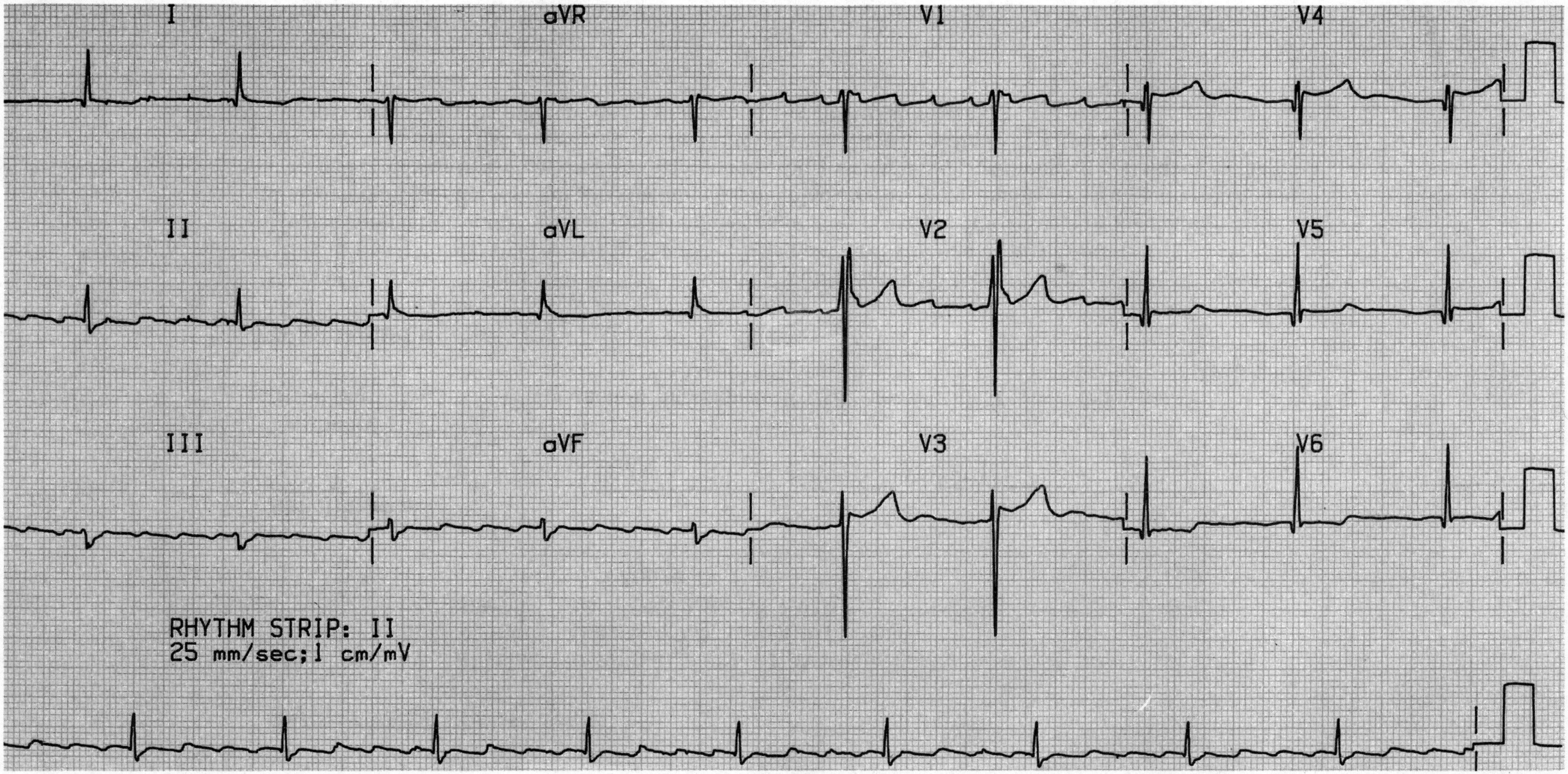

A-27

NARRATIVE INTERPRETATION

Rhythm:	**Atrial flutter with 4:1 AV conduction**
Rate:	**Atrial rate 240, ventricular rate 60**
Intervals:	**PR –, QRS 0.10, QT 0.42**
Axis:	**−15 degrees**

Abnormalities
RSR′ V1–V2. Low T voltage limb leads. Biphasic T waves leads V5–V6.

Synthesis
Atrial flutter with 4:1 AV conduction. Incomplete RBBB. Nonspecific T-wave abnormalities.

TEST ANSWERS: 19, 51, 71, 106.

Comment: Under normal circumstances, patients with atrial flutter will have a physiologic conduction delay at the AV node that results in 2:1 AV conduction. This should not be interpreted as AV "block." Higher conduction ratios usually imply either conduction disease or the effects of medications such as digitalis, beta blockers, or certain calcium channel blockers. It is reasonable to assume that this elderly man had conduction system disease that explains the 4:1 conduction. Although the T waves in the limb leads are at least partially obscured by the flutter waves, there appears to be virtually no T-wave voltage and it is necessary to comment on this feature of the electrocardiogram.

A-28

Clinical History

A 59-year-old man with 45 min of chest discomfort.

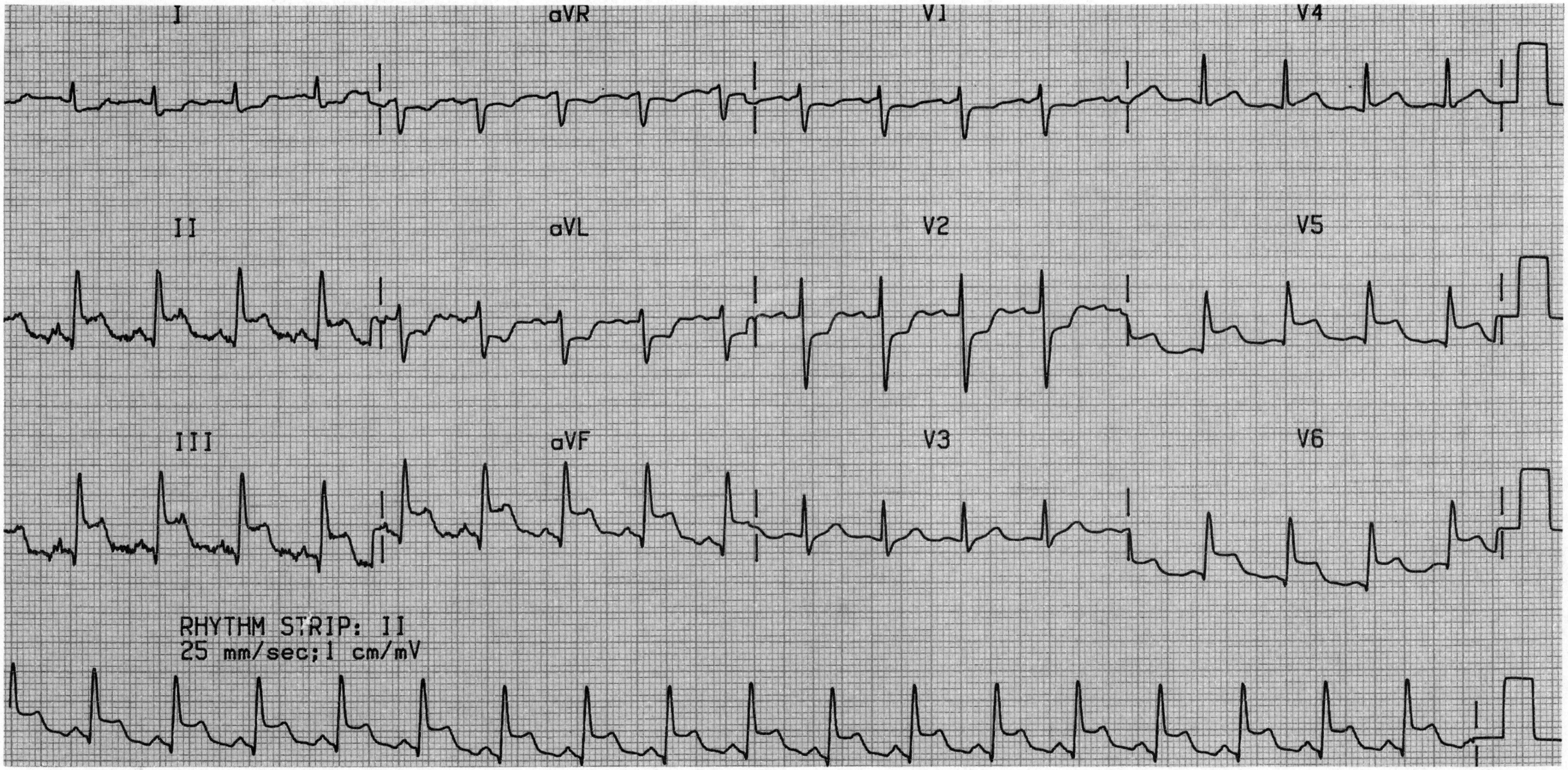

A-28

NARRATIVE INTERPRETATION

Rhythm: **Sinus tachycardia**
Rate: **105**
Intervals: **PR 0.16, QRS 0.08 QT 0.32**
Axis: **+75 degrees**

Abnormalities

Rapid heart rate. ST elevation leads II, III, aVF, V4–V6. ST depression leads I, aVL, V1–V2.

Synthesis

Sinus tachycardia. Inferior lateral wall MI with ST abnormalities of acute myocardial injury. Possible acute posterior wall MI versus anterior myocardial ischemia, or reciprocal changes.

TEST ANSWERS: 4, 91, (93), 100, 101.

Comment: This patient demonstrates acute ST-segment abnormalities consistent with acute MI involving the inferior and inferolateral walls. Early posterior wall infarction is also possible on the basis of ST depression in the anterior precordial leads. This cannot be confirmed with a single electrocardiogram. It has been debated whether the precordial ST depression is a reciprocal electrical phenomenon or a manifestation of anterior ischemia or represents posterior infarction. Often this can be determined only with serial electrocardiographic tracings or with subsequent studies of wall motion. Most studies indicate that patients with inferior wall MI who also demonstrate precordial ST depression have a more extensive area of myocardial damage and an adverse prognosis.

REFERENCES: Schweitzer (1990). Mirvis.

A-29

Clinical History

A 66-year-old woman with palpitations.

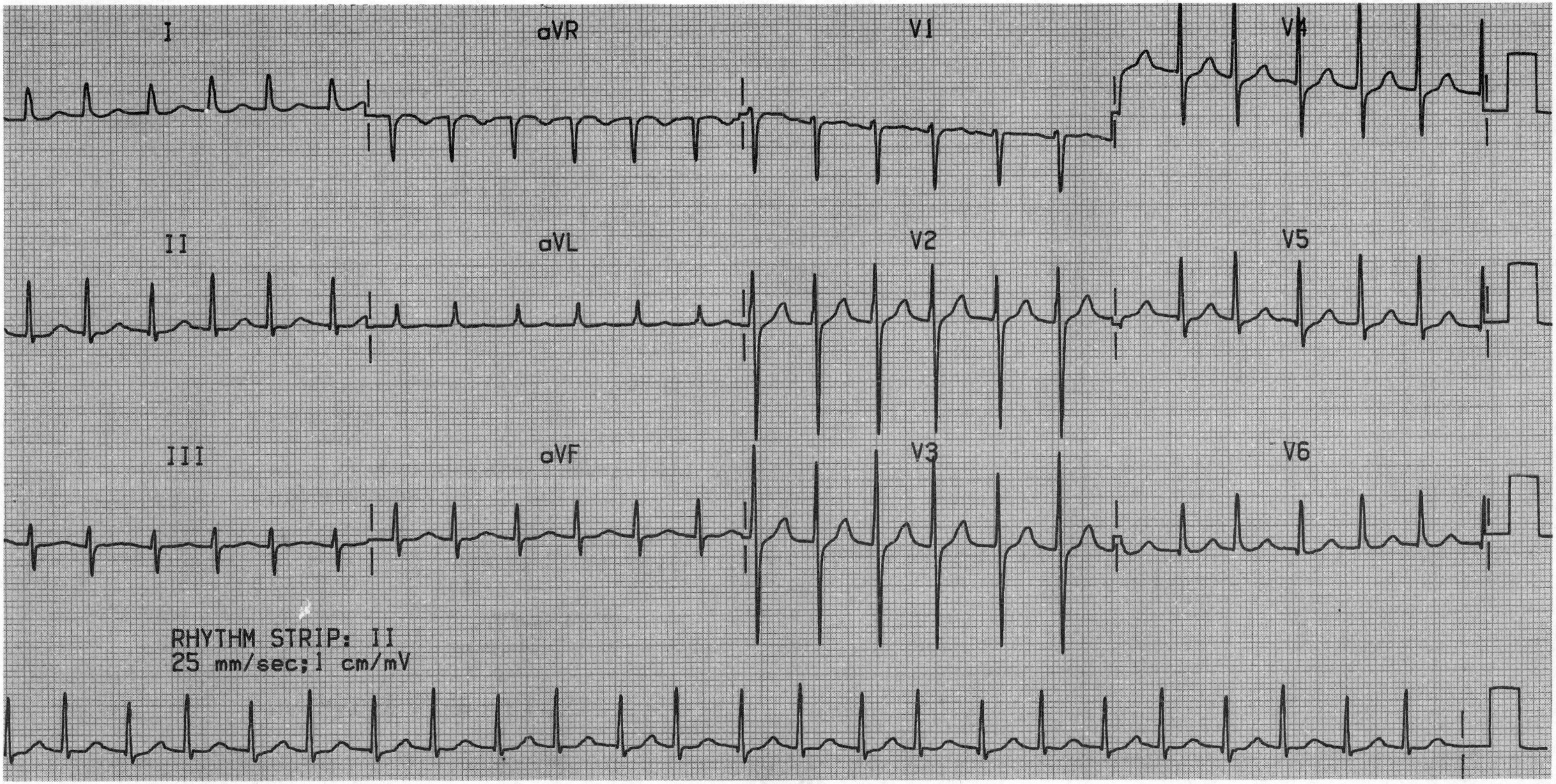

A-29

NARRATIVE INTERPRETATION

Rhythm: **Atrial fibrillation**
Rate: **145 (average)**
Intervals: **PR –, QRS 0.08, QT 0.30**
Axis: **+15 degrees**

Abnormalities

Slight ST depression leads I, II, aVL, aVF, V3–V6.

Synthesis

Atrial fibrillation with a rapid ventricular response. Nonspecific ST abnormalities.

TEST ANSWERS: 20, 50, 106.

Comment: On first glance, the reader might misinterpret this rhythm as supraventricular tachycardia because it appears quite regular. On closer inspection, there is slight variation of the RR intervals and no organized P-wave activity, indicative of atrial fibrillation. The rapid ventricular response is physiologic in the absence of AV blocking agents or intrinsic conduction disease.

A-30

Clinical History

A 66-year-old man admitted for elective cardiac catheterization. He has a loud systolic murmur.

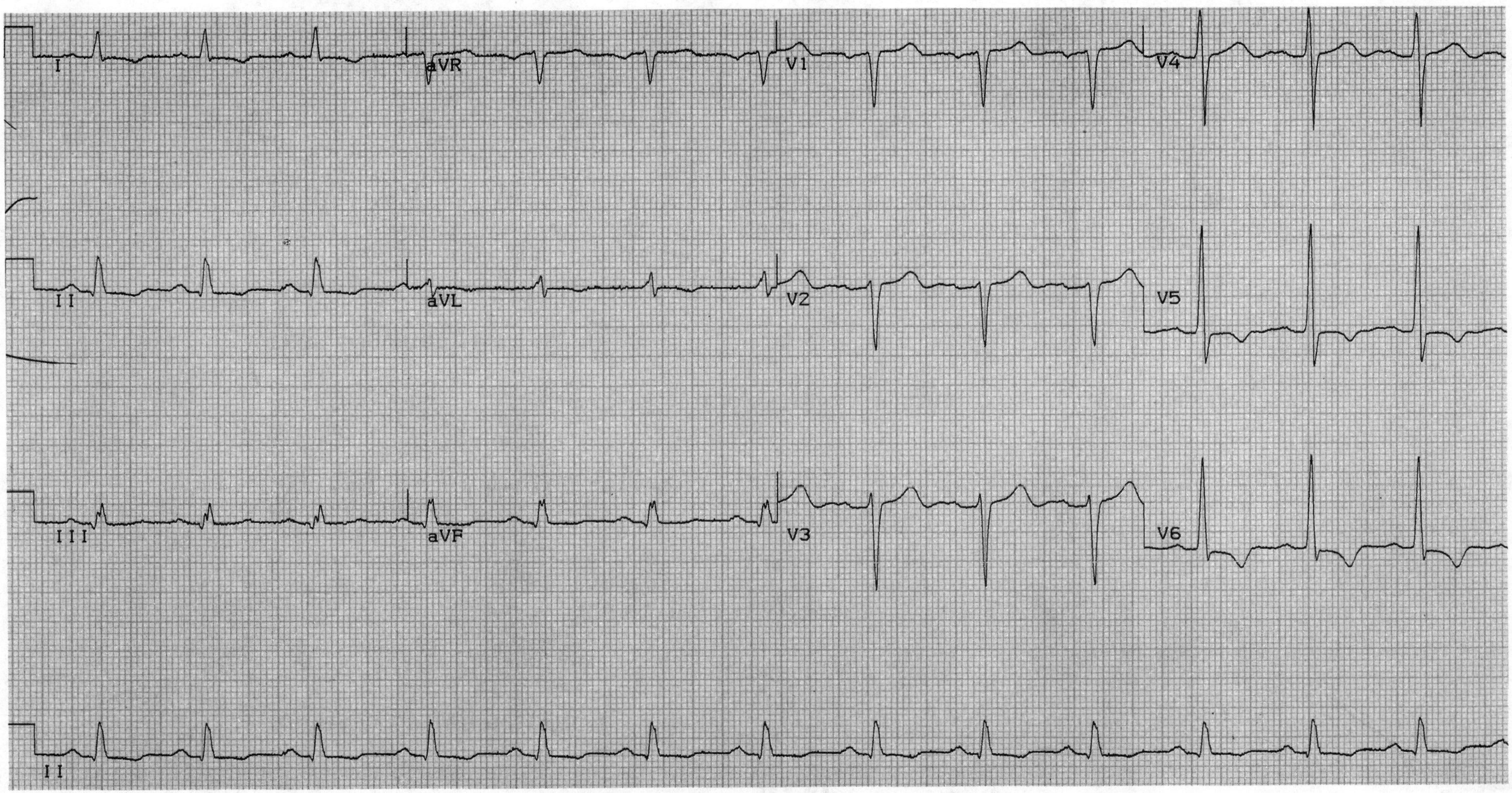

A-30

NARRATIVE INTERPRETATION

Rhythm: **Sinus**
Rate: **80**
Intervals: **PR 0.18, QRS 0.11, QT 0.40**
Axis: **+60 degrees**

Abnormalities

SV2 + RV5 greater than 35. T-wave inversion leads I, II, V5–V6. Prolonged QRS duration.

Synthesis

Sinus rhythm. LVH. Associated ST-T-wave abnormalities and intraventricular conduction delay.

TEST ANSWERS: 1, 76, 78, 103.

Comment: The reader should not become careless and forget to check the standardization of each electrocardiogram. On initial inspection there are no voltage criteria for LVH in this tracing. However, the tracing is recorded at one-half standard. This patient had obvious precordial voltage and associated ST-T-wave criteria for LVH. Clinically, he had marked cardiomegaly due to aortic stenosis and insufficiency.

A-31

Clinical History

A 74-year-old man admitted to the CCU.

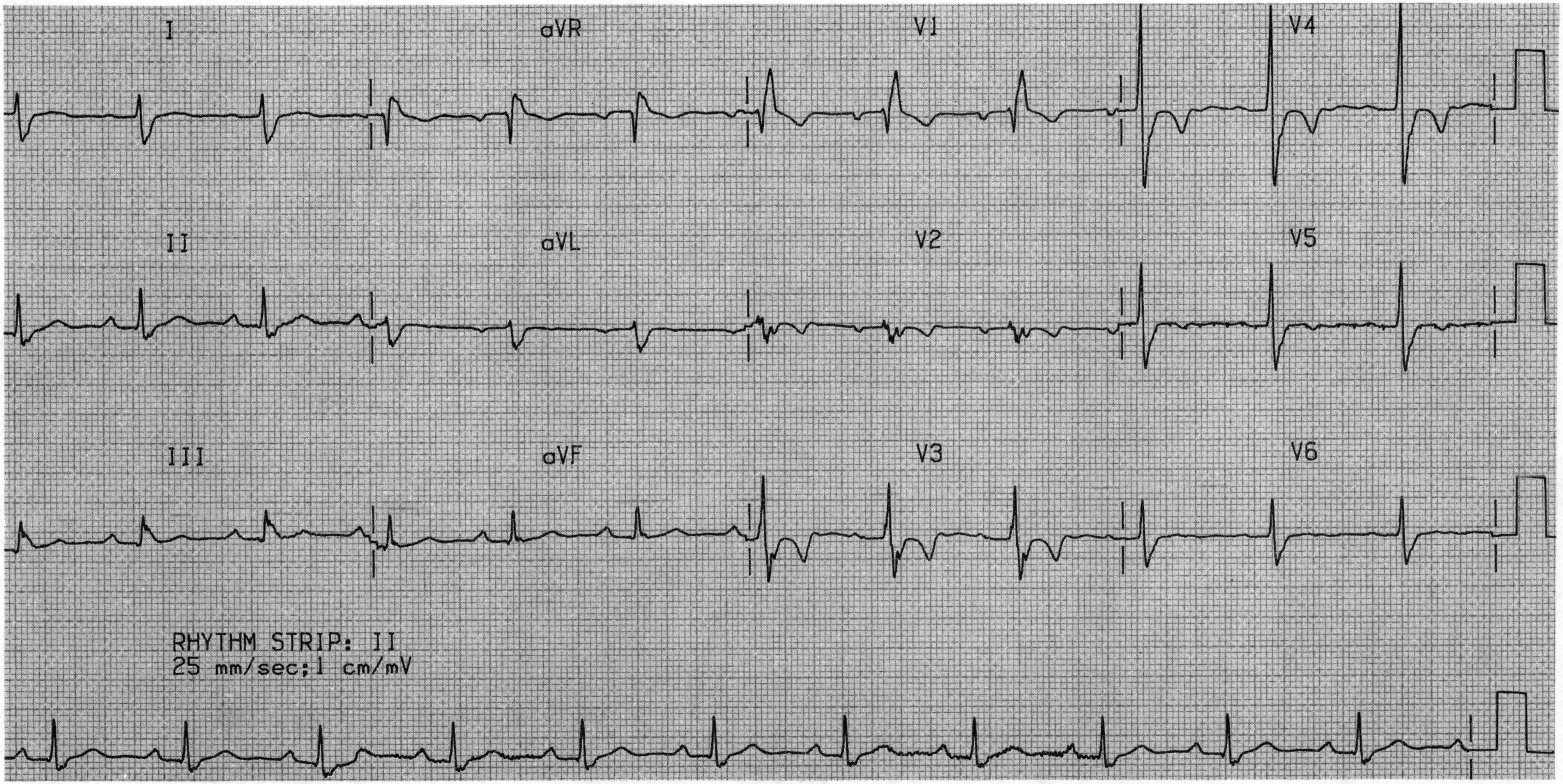

A-31

NARRATIVE INTERPRETATION

Rhythm:	**Sinus**
Rate:	**65**
Intervals:	**PR 0.24, QRS 0.12, QT 0.36**
Axis:	**+105 degrees**

Abnormalities
Axis rightward of +90 degrees. Prolonged PR interval. Broad QRS with rSR′ and T-wave inversion leads V1–V2.

Synthesis
Sinus rhythm. First-degree AV block. RBBB. Associated ST-T-wave abnormalities. Right axis deviation. Left posterior fascicular block.

TEST ANSWERS: 1, 42, 65, 70, 73, 104.

Comment: In patients with RBBB, the QRS axis should be interpreted using the first 0.06 s. In this example, the axis is abnormally rightward and is consistent with left posterior fascicular block (LPFB). Additional diagnostic criteria of LPFB include a small initial R wave in aVL and narrow Q waves in the inferior limb leads. This patient has evidence of trifascicular block based on the presence of RBBB, LPFB, and first-degree AV block. This electrocardiogram should not be "overread" for abnormalities. The secondary ST-T-wave changes in V1–V5 are associated with the RBBB and should not be interpreted as suggestive of MI. True MI became quite evident on additional tracings (see next example).

A-32

Clinical History

A 74-year-old man admitted to the CCU who has developed chest discomfort.

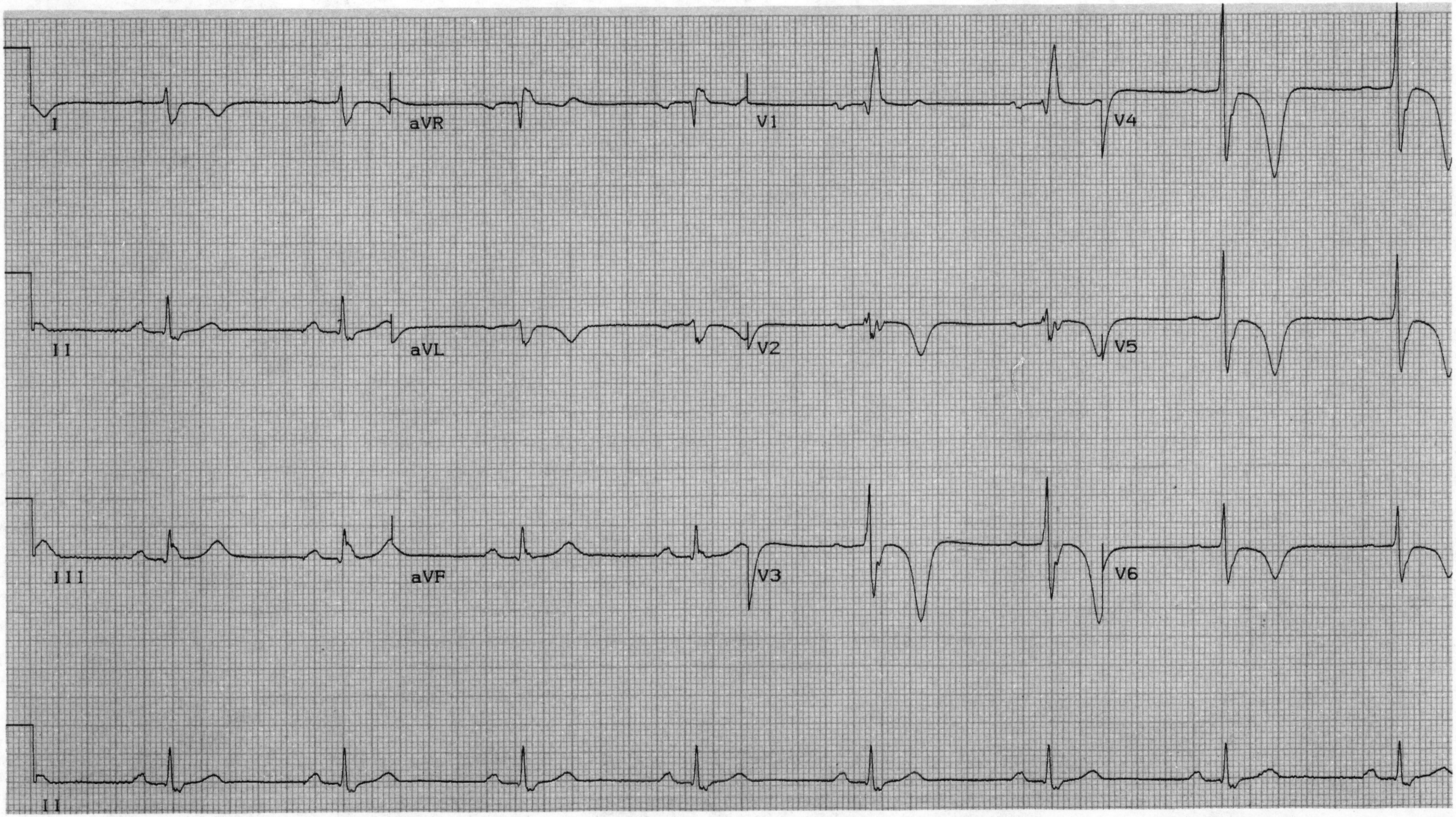

A-32

NARRATIVE INTERPRETATION

Rhythm: **Sinus bradycardia with first-degree AV block**
Rate: **48**
Intervals: **PR 0.24, QRS 0.14, QT 0.52**
Axis: **+105 degrees**

Abnormalities

Slow heart rate. Prolonged PR interval. Axis rightward of +90 degrees. Broad QRS with rSR′ lead V1. Deep T-wave inversion leads I, aVL, V2–V6. T wave upright lead V1. ST segment straight with slight elevation leads I, aVL, V1–V6.

Synthesis

Sinus bradycardia. First-degree AV block. RBBB. Right axis deviation. Left posterior fascicular block. ST-T-wave abnormalities suggesting myocardial injury.

TEST ANSWERS: 3, 42, 65, 70, 73, 100, (102).

Comment: This tracing demonstrates extensive anterior and lateral wall myocardial ischemia or early injury in the presence of a prior RBBB and left posterior fascicular block. The significant findings are the markedly inverted T waves in the lateral leads and across the precordium. Note also the upright T in lead V1, where inversion would be expected in uncomplicated RBBB. The ST-T-wave findings are no longer secondary to the conduction abnormality and reflect coronary insufficiency. The findings are highly suggestive of this diagnosis but are much more diagnostic when compared with the patient's prior tracing in the previous example.

A-33

Clinical History

A 49-year-old asymptomatic woman.

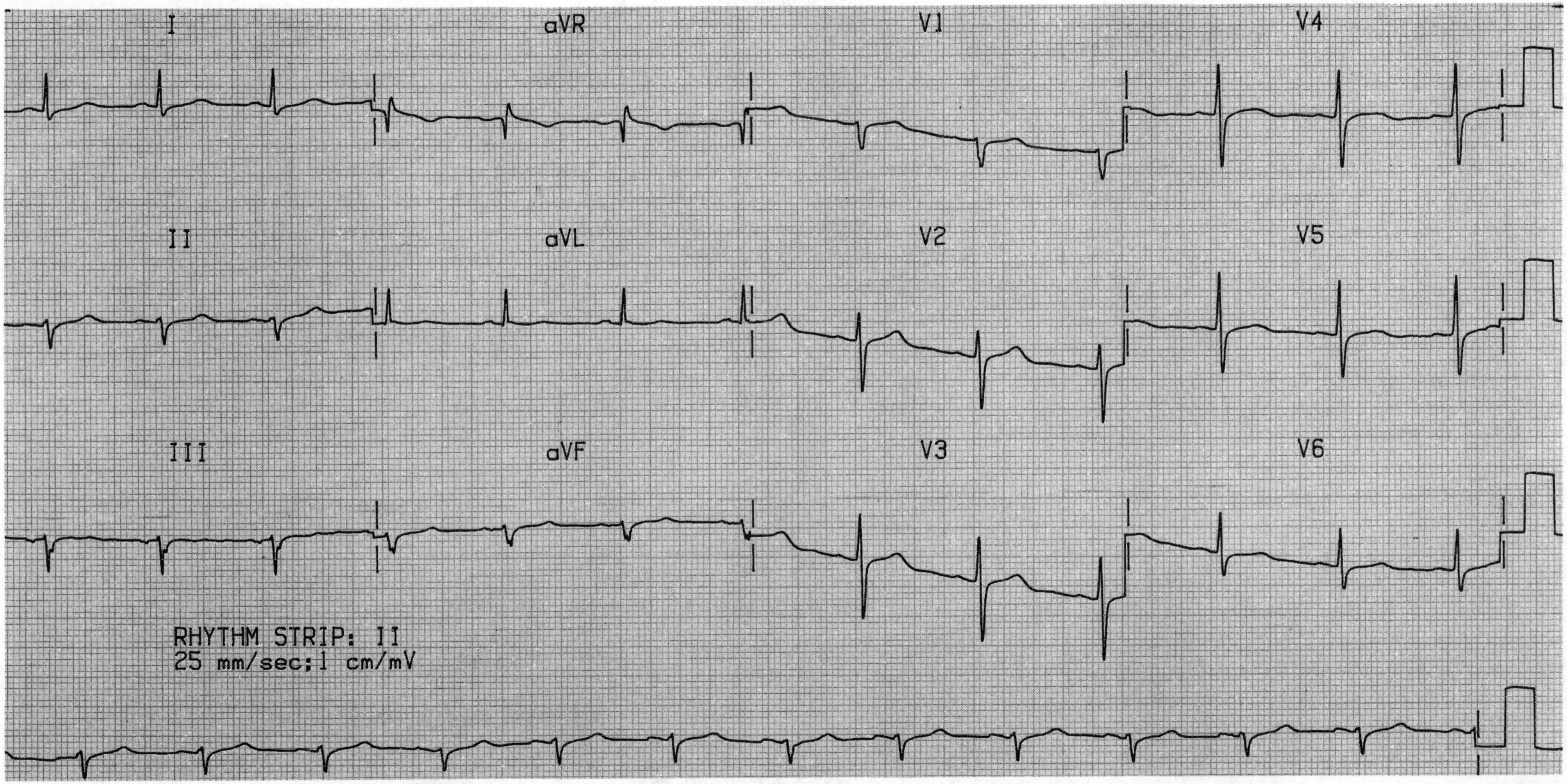

A-33

NARRATIVE INTERPRETATION

Rhythm:	**Sinus**
Rate:	**75**
Intervals:	**PR 0.16, QRS 0.08, QT 0.36**
Axis:	**−45 degrees**

Abnormalities
Axis leftward of −30 degrees.

Synthesis
Sinus rhythm. Left axis deviation. Left anterior fascicular block.

TEST ANSWERS: 1, 64, 72.

Comment: This patient has left anterior fascicular block (LAFB) as her only electrocardiographic abnormality. In population studies the prevalence of LAFB has ranged from 1 to 14 percent. The prognosis of patients with LAFB is no different from that of persons without this abnormality. It is important to realize that not everyone with left axis deviation has LAFB. Other conditions causing left axis deviation include inferior wall MI, chronic pulmonary disease (pseudo left axis deviation), LVH, and a variety of congenital cardiac anomalies.

REFERENCES: Barrett. Perloff (1979). Friedman p 625.

A-34

Clinical History

A 49-year-old woman with severe dyspnea.

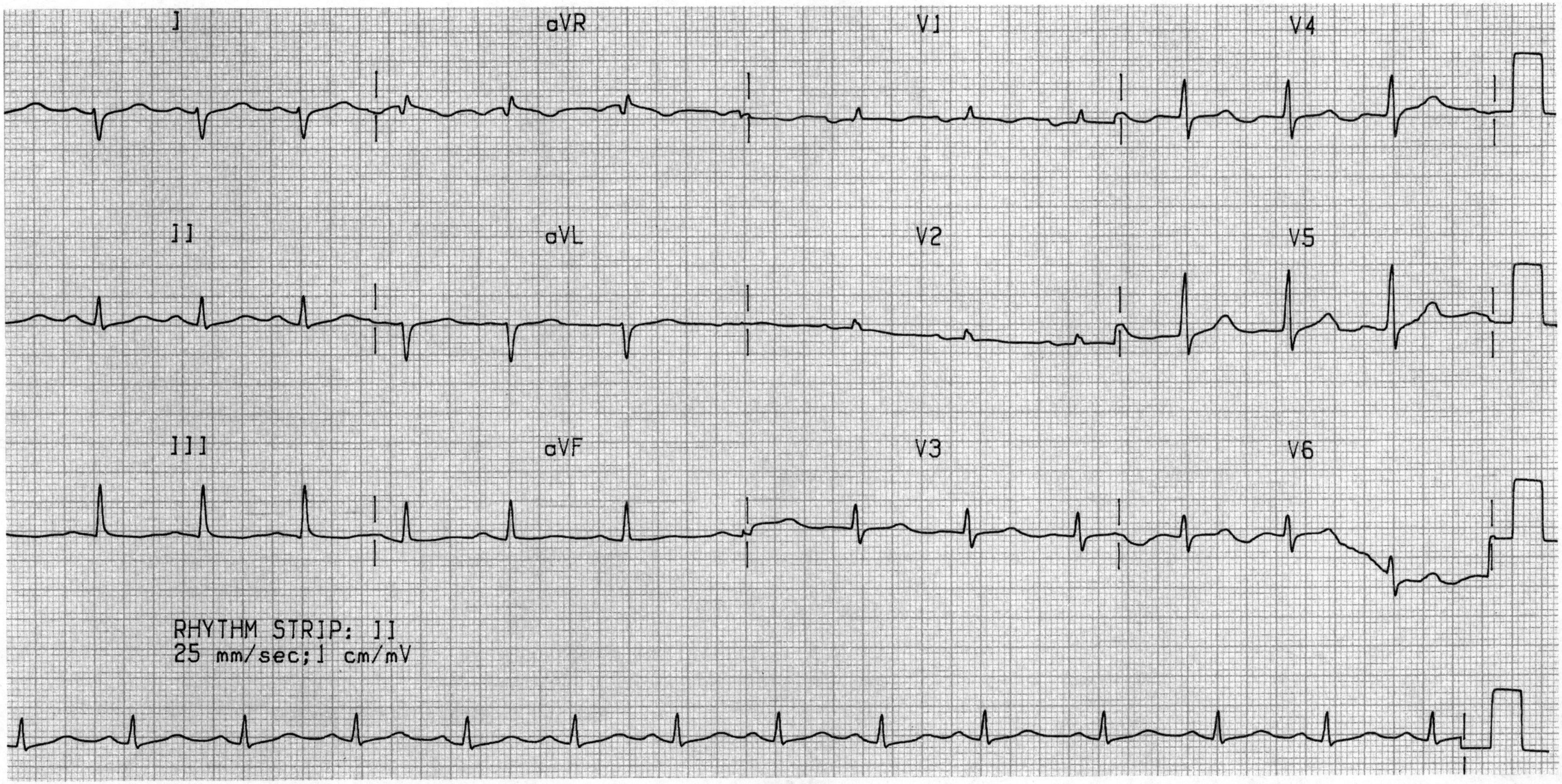

A-34

NARRATIVE INTERPRETATION

Rhythm:	**Sinus with first-degree AV block**
Rate:	**85**
Intervals:	**PR 0.22, QRS 0.08, QT 0.40**
Axis:	**+120 degrees**

Abnormalities
Prolonged PR interval. qR lead V1. Prominent R wave lead V2. Axis rightward of +90 degrees.

Synthesis
Sinus rhythm. First-degree AV block. Right axis deviation. RVH.

TEST ANSWERS: 1, 42, 65, 79.

Comment: This patient had severe primary pulmonary hypertension with RVH. Marked right axis deviation is evident with prominent R forces in the right precordial leads. Other causes of rightward axis besides RVH include left posterior hemiblock and lateral wall MI.

REFERENCES: Chou pp 104–108. Surawicz.

A-35

Clinical History

A 65-year-old man with lightheadedness.

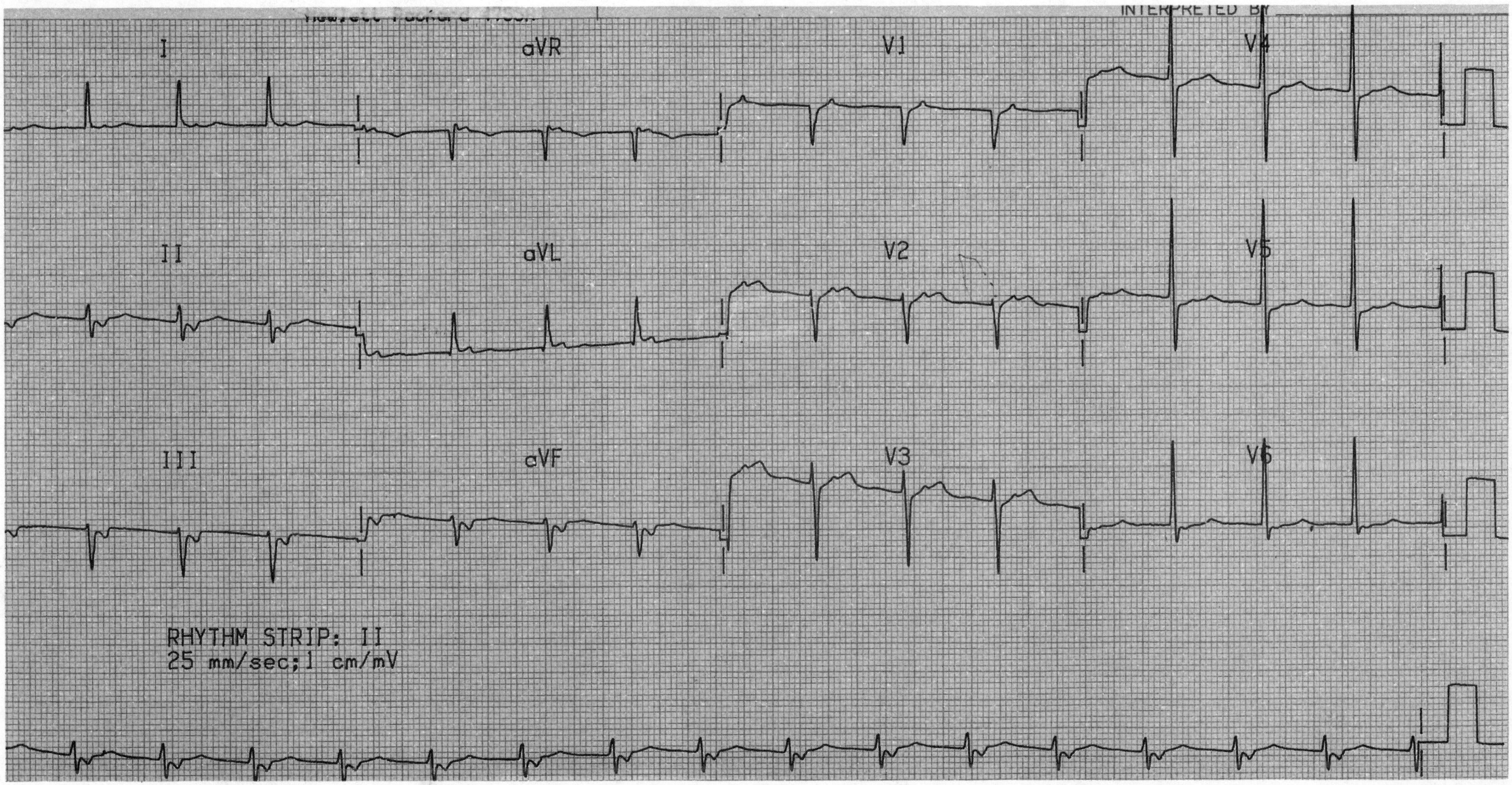

A-35

NARRATIVE INTERPRETATION

Rhythm: **Accelerated AV junctional rhythm**
Rate: **95**
Intervals: **PR –, QRS 0.08, QT 0.34**
Axis: **−45 degrees**

Abnormalities

Inverted P waves leads II, III, aVF. Axis leftward of −30 degrees. Slight ST depression leads V3–V6.

Synthesis

Accelerated AV junctional rhythm. Left axis deviation. Left anterior fascicular block. Nonspecific ST-segment abnormalities.

TEST ANSWERS: 23, 64, 72, 106.

Comment: The inverted P waves that occur after the QRS are indicative of a junctional focus. The rhythm is an "accelerated" junctional rhythm because of the heart rate. Normally the AV junction functions as a subsidiary escape pacemaker at a rate of 35 to 50 beats per minute. The increased rate of this example is the result of increased automaticity at the AV junction. Another term for this rhythm is *nonparoxysmal junctional tachycardia*. Accelerated AV junctional rhythm is usually seen in patients with underlying cardiac disease such as acute MI, myocarditis, or COPD or after cardiac surgery. It is also often a result of digitalis toxicity.

A-36

Clinical History

A 70-year-old man following cardiac surgery.

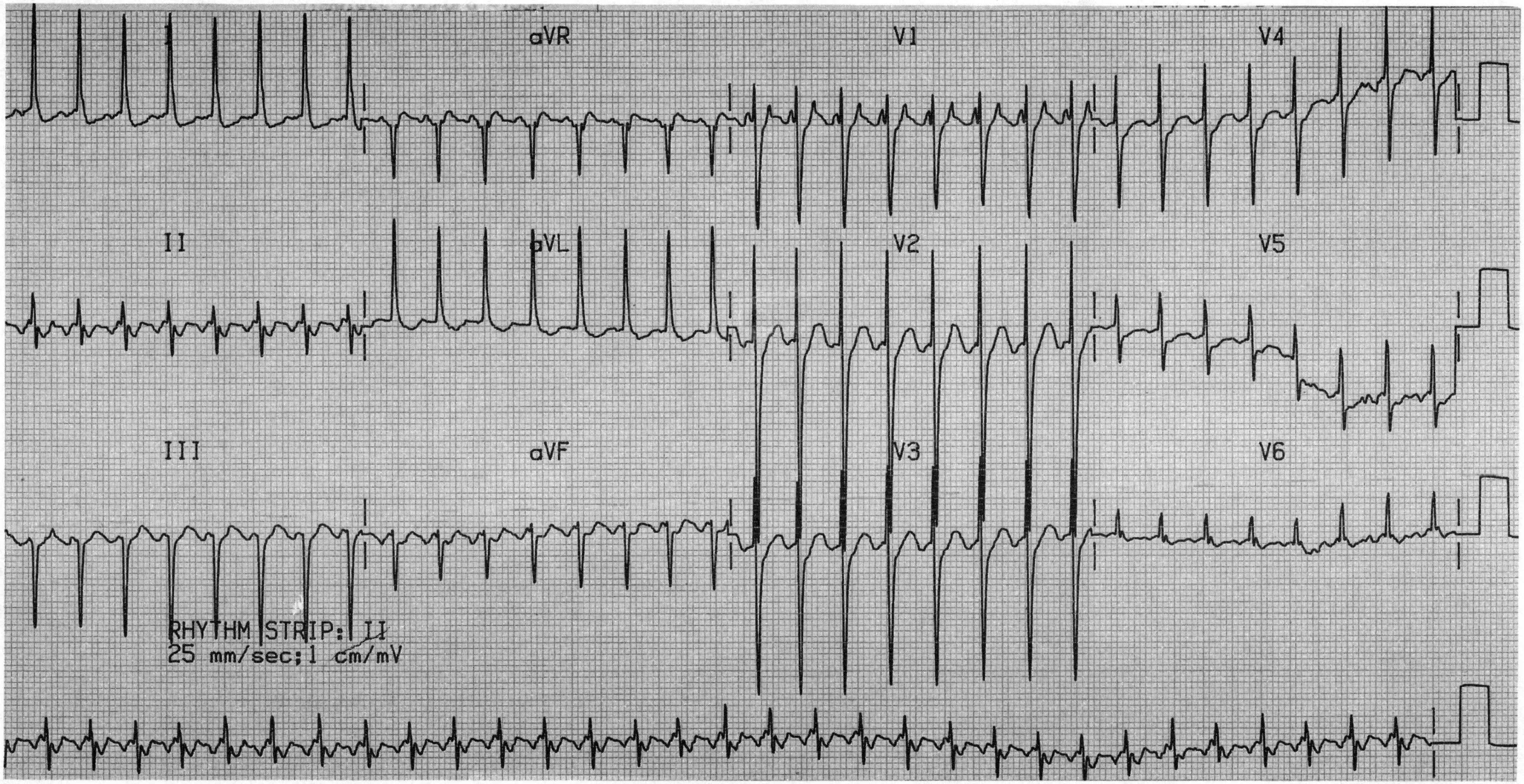

A-36

NARRATIVE INTERPRETATION

Rhythm: **Atrial flutter**
Rate: **Atrial rate 380, ventricular rate 190**
Intervals: **PR –, QRS 0.08, QT –**
Axis: **–30 degrees**

Abnormalities

R wave aVL greater than 11 mm. ST depression leads I, aVL, V2–V6. T wave flat leads I, aVL, V6.

Synthesis

Atrial flutter with 2:1 AV conduction. LVH by voltage criteria. Associated ST-T-wave abnormalities.

TEST ANSWERS: 19, 50, 78, 103.

Comment: This patient has developed atrial flutter following cardiac surgery. The rapid atrial rate is indicative of type II atrial flutter. Type I and type II flutter are characterized by atrial rates of 240 to 340 and 340 to 433 beats per minute, respectively. Type I flutter may be converted to sinus rhythm with electrical cardioversion, antiarrhythmic agents, or rapid atrial pacing. In contrast, type II atrial flutter cannot be affected by pacing. Remember that with atrial rates in this range, 2:1 AV conduction is a physiologic response of the AV node and does not represent AV nodal disease. The electrical axis in the lead II rhythm strip is seen to vary from normal to slightly leftward. This is probably secondary to respiratory variation.

REFERENCE: Horowitz pp 58–63.

A-37

Clinical History

A 66-year-old man in the CCU.

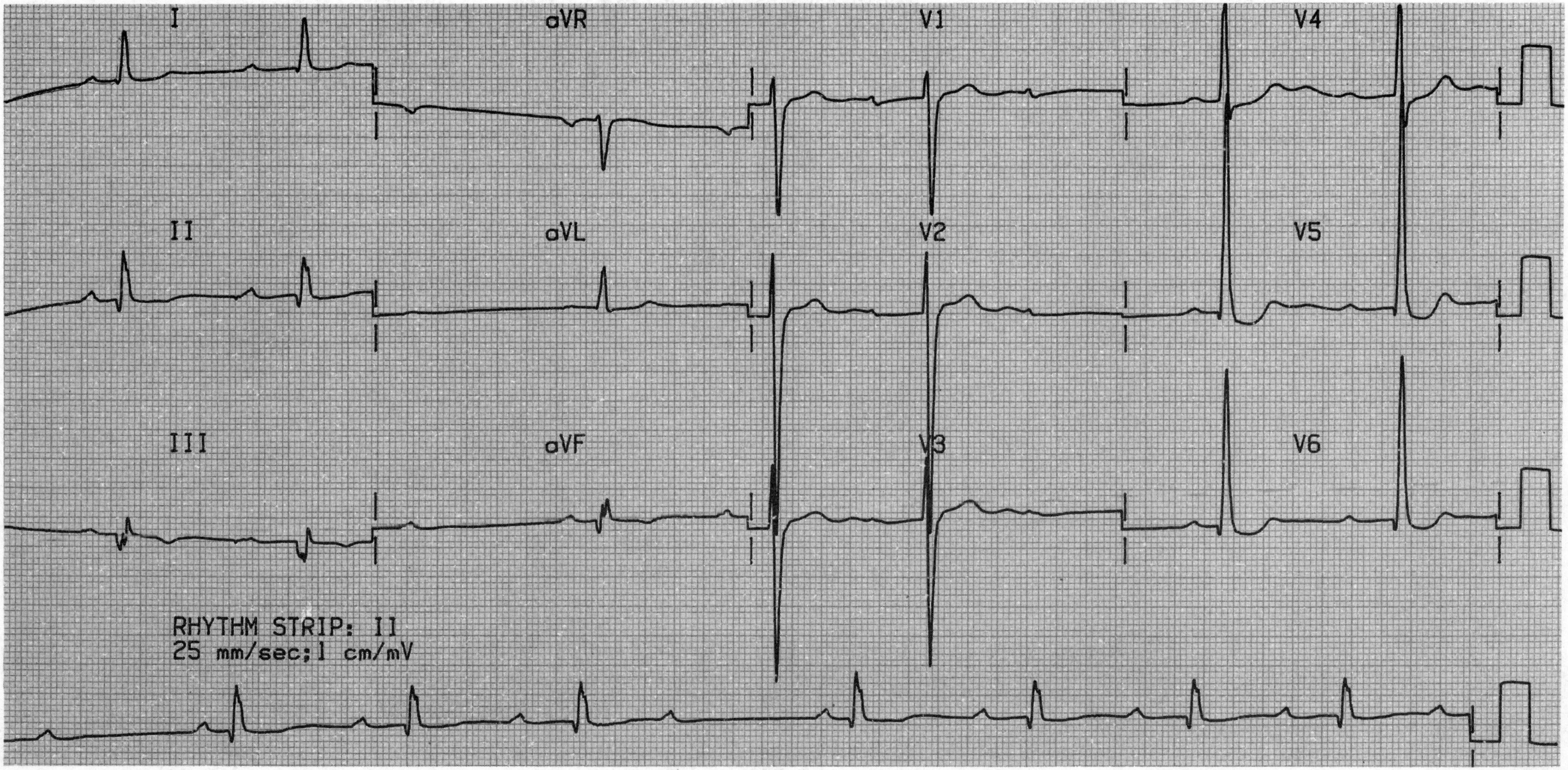

A-37

NARRATIVE INTERPRETATION

Rhythm: **Sinus bradycardia with second-degree AV block, Mobitz type I**
Rate: **55**
Intervals: **PR variable, QRS 0.12, QT 0.44**
Axis: **+30 degrees**

Abnormalities

Slow heart rate. Gradual prolongation of PR interval with eventual failure to conduct P wave. Shortest PR interval is abnormally prolonged. Q waves leads II, III, aVF. Prolonged QRS duration. ST depression leads I, aVL, V4–V6. SV2 + RV5 greater than 35. T-wave inversion leads II, III, aVF.

Synthesis

Sinus bradycardia. Second-degree AV block, Mobitz I (Wenckebach). Inferior wall MI of indeterminate age. LVH. Intraventricular conduction delay (IVCD). ST-T-wave abnormalities associated with LVH or IVCD or both.

TEST ANSWERS: 3, 43, 76, 78, 92, 103, 104.

Comment: This tracing demonstrates a number of electrocardiographic abnormalities. There is progressive prolongation of the PR interval with eventual failure to conduct one P wave to the ventricles; this is diagnostic of Mobitz type I second-degree AV block. The RR interval containing the blocked P wave should also be less than twice the sum of two PP intervals, and the RR intervals become progressively shorter. Note that the PR interval following the blocked P wave is prolonged, although first-degree AV block is generally not diagnosed as part of a sequence involving second-degree AV block. The ST-T-wave abnormalities in this example are probably related both to LVH and the associated IVCD.

A-38

Clinical History

A 45-year-old man with sudden onset of palpitations.

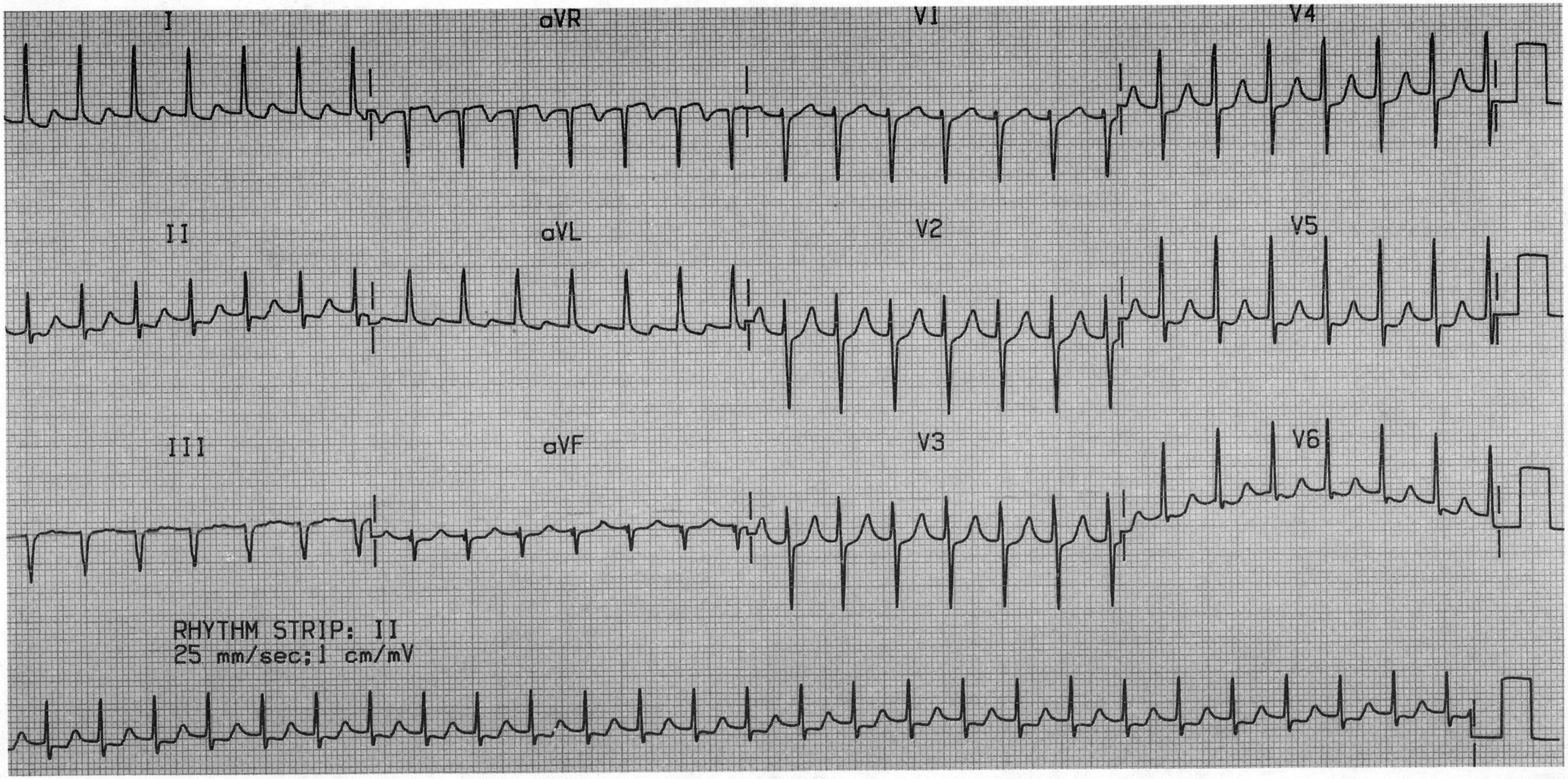

A-38

NARRATIVE INTERPRETATION

Rhythm:	**Supraventricular tachycardia**
Rate:	**160**
Intervals:	**PR –, QRS 0.08, QT 0.28**
Axis:	**−15 degrees**

Abnormalities

Rapid heart rate. ST depression leads I, II, aVL, aVF, V3–V6. Alternating heights of R wave, most prominent in lead V3.

Synthesis

Supraventricular tachycardia. Electrical alternans. Nonspecific ST-segment abnormalities.

TEST ANSWERS: 18, 69, 106.

Comment: This patient has paroxysmal supraventricular tachycardia (PSVT). This is a catchall term for a number of arrhythmias. The characterization of this rhythm as atrial tachycardia is deferred because P waves are not clearly evident. AV nodal reentrant tachycardia is the most common cause of PSVT in adults, where it represents at least 50 percent of patients. This rhythm is characterized by reentry within the AV node and results in a narrow complex arrhythmia of about 140 to 200 beats per minute. Characteristically, the P wave is buried in the QRS complex. Means to treat this arrhythmia include vagal maneuvers such as carotid sinus pressure or asking the patient to perform the Valsalva maneuver. Pharmacologic agents for rapid conversion of this rhythm are highly effective and include intravenous verapamil, adenosine, or short-acting beta blockers. Note also the electrical alternans in lead V3. It has been suggested that this indicates a concealed AV nodal bypass tract is involved in the generation of the arrhythmia.

REFERENCES: Manolis. Keefe. Kalbfleisch.

A-39

Clinical History

A 62-year-old asymptomatic woman seen 2 days after gallbladder surgery.

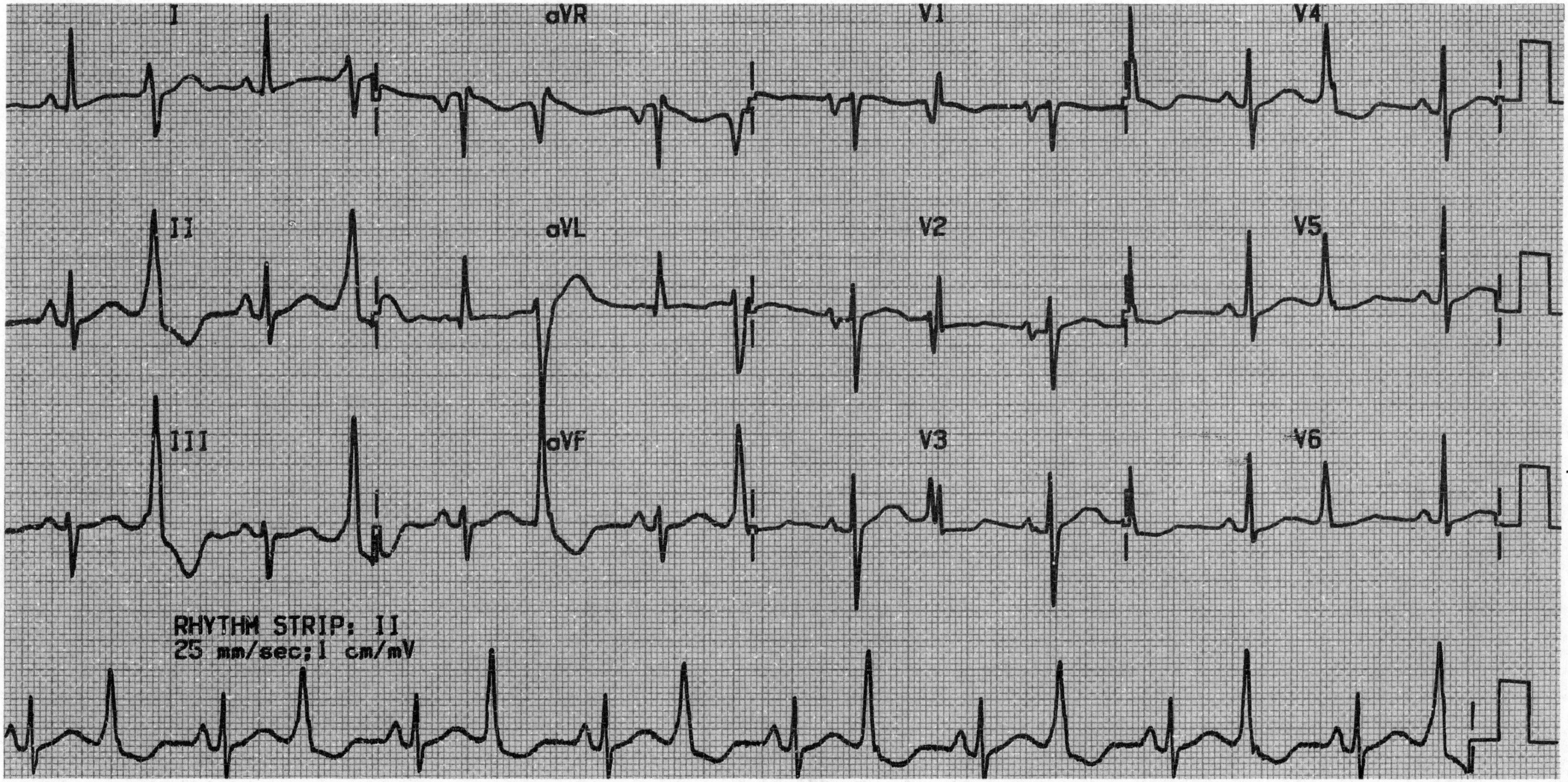

A-39

NARRATIVE INTERPRETATION

Rhythm: **Sinus**
Rate: **92**
Intervals: **PR 0.16, QRS 0.08, QT 0.40**
Axis: **−15 degrees**

Abnormalities

VPCs in bigeminal pattern. Abnormal P terminal force lead V1. T wave flat in lead I, inverted in lead aVL. Slight ST depression lead V6. Lewis index greater than 17 (see below). Prolonged QTc interval.

Synthesis

Sinus rhythm with ventricular bigeminy. Left atrial abnormality. LVH by voltage criteria. Associated ST-T-wave abnormalities. Prolonged QTc.

TEST ANSWERS: 1, 26, 60, 78, 103, 109.

Comment: The rhythm is sinus with ventricular bigeminy. Remember that every other P wave is "buried" within the VPC and the sinus rate is actually twice that of the visualized P waves. Patients with ventricular bigeminy may complain of palpitations or may be asymptomatic. More serious symptoms may arise if the ectopic beats fail to perfuse with the result of a fall in effective cardiac output or blood pressure. LVH may be diagnosed in this example on the basis of a Lewis index of 17 or more (Lewis index: Sum of R minus S wave in lead I and S minus R wave in lead III). This is a highly specific criterion for LVH. The diagnosis is also supported by the presence of left atrial enlargement.

A-40

Clinical History

A 37-year-old man admitted to the coronary care unit with 2 days of chest discomfort. He has a history of treatment for Hodgkin's disease.

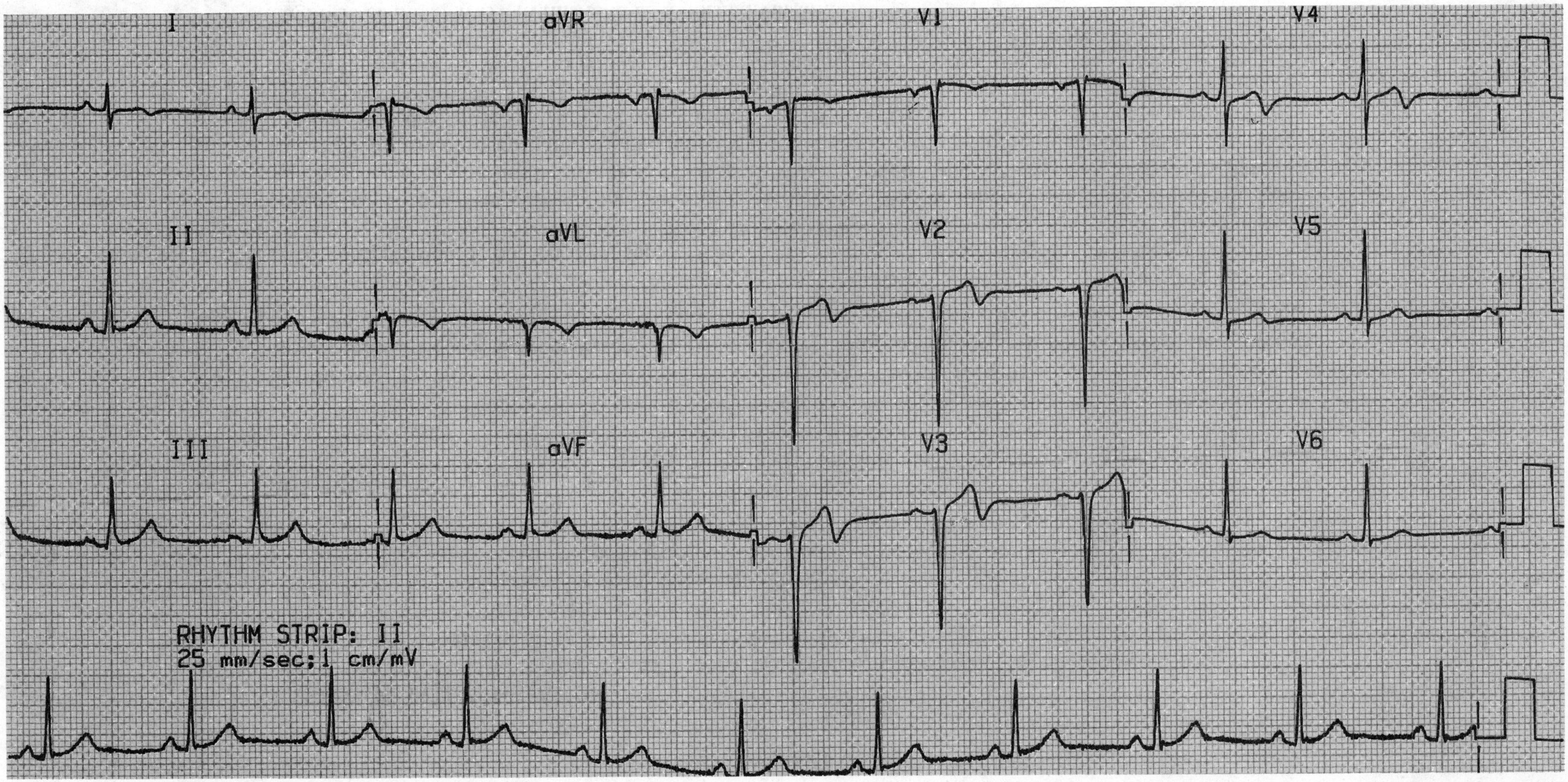

A-40

NARRATIVE INTERPRETATION

Rhythm:	**Sinus**
Rate:	**62**
Intervals:	**PR 0.16, QRS 0.08, QT 0.36**
Axis:	**+90 degrees**

Abnormalities

R wave V1–V3 less than 3 mm. ST elevation leads V2–V4. T-wave inversion leads V2–V5. T wave biphasic lead V5.

Synthesis

Sinus rhythm. Poor R-wave progression. Anteroseptal (anterior) wall MI with ST-T-wave abnormalities suggesting recent myocardial injury.

TEST ANSWERS: 1, 66, 81, (83), 100.

Comment: This patient suffered an acute anteroseptal wall MI. Technically, the poor R-wave progression best localizes the injury to the anteroseptal wall, although the ST-T-wave abnormalities extend a bit further to the anterior wall. He had a history of radiation therapy to the mediastinum for Hodgkin's disease. This has been reported to induce focal coronary obstruction in patients otherwise without coronary atherosclerosis. The Q wave in aVL does not support the diagnosis of lateral wall MI, as there are no supporting Q waves in leads I or V5–V6. Patients with a vertical axis will often demonstrate a QS wave in lead aVL. The negative to biphasic P wave and inverted T wave in aVL also support the diagnosis of the Q wave in this lead as a normal variant.

REFERENCES: Dunsmore. Friedman p 66.

TEST B

B-1

Clinical History

A 73-year-old asymptomatic man with a history of hypertension.

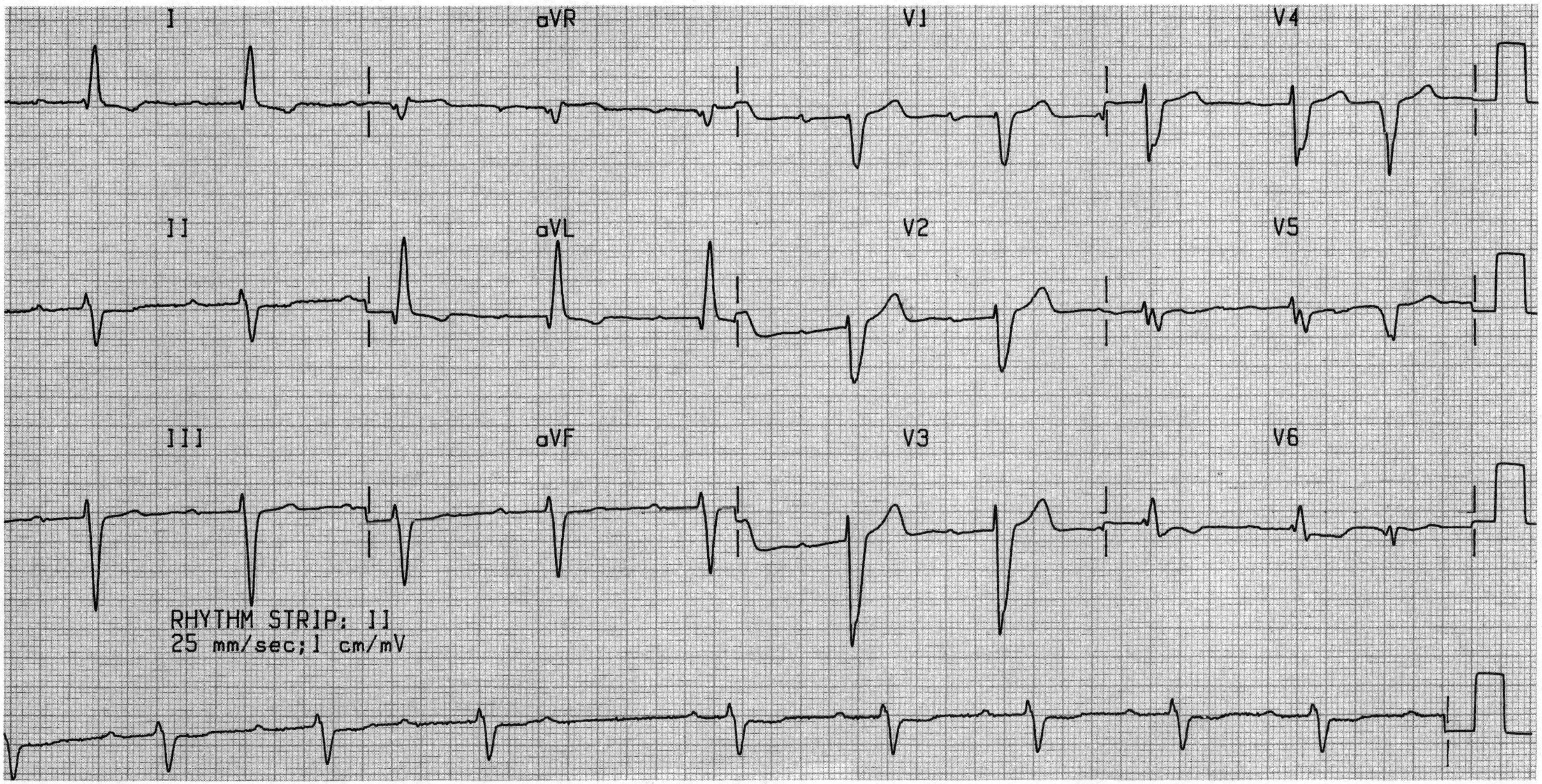

B-1

NARRATIVE INTERPRETATION

Rhythm: **Sinus bradycardia with second-degree AV block, Mobitz type I**
Rate: **58**
Intervals: **PR variable, QRS 0.14, QT 0.40**
Axis: **−45 degrees**

Abnormalities

Slow heart rate. VPC. Incremental prolongation of PR interval with eventual failure to conduct P wave. Broad, notched QRS in leads I, aVL, V6, with T-wave inversion. Axis leftward of −30 degrees.

Synthesis

Sinus bradycardia with second-degree AV block, Mobitz type I. VPC. LBBB with associated ST-T-wave changes. Left axis deviation.

TEST ANSWERS: 3, 26, 43, 64, 74, 104.

Comment: Note that in this example, the shortest PR interval of the Wenckebach sequence is prolonged. However, first-degree AV block should not be diagnosed in the presence of a Wenckebach sequence unless there is a period of stable PR intervals and 1:1 conduction. This patient also demonstrates complete LBBB. A major diagnostic criterion of LBBB is absence of the normal septal activation from left to right. In LBBB the initial forces depolarize the septum from right to left. Accordingly, there cannot be septal Q waves in leftward leads. A Q wave may occasionally be present in aVL in LBBB but should not be present in lead I or V5 and V6. In this example, one might initially consider a Q wave present in lead I, but on closer inspection, a small R wave is evident.

REFERENCE: Willems.

B-2

Clinical History

A 22-year-old military recruit on routine examination.

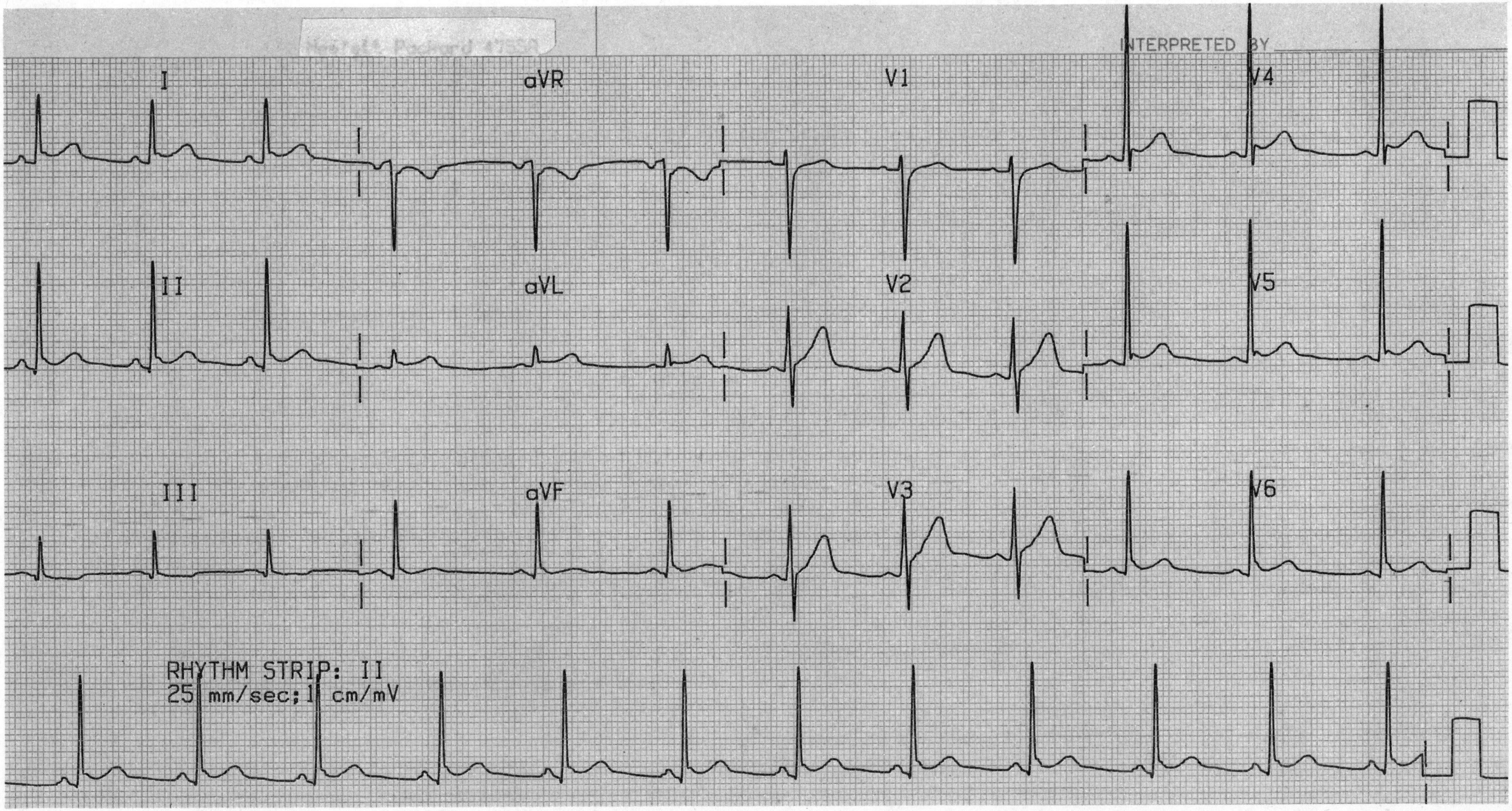

B-2

NARRATIVE INTERPRETATION

Rhythm: **Sinus**
Rate: **72**
Intervals: **PR 0.16, QRS 0.08, QT 0.38**
Axis: **+45 degrees**

Abnormalities

High J point with concave upward ST elevation leads I, II, aVL, aVF, V2–V6.

Synthesis

Sinus rhythm. Normal variant; isolated J-point elevation.

TEST ANSWERS: 1, 96.

Comment: This tracing represents the normal variant of early repolarization seen in some healthy persons. A large study of nearly 50,000 healthy Air Force personnel found that benign ST elevation of the type shown in this electrocardiogram was present in approximately 2 percent. The usual ST segment is isoelectric with the T-P segment and is not elevated above this line by more than 1 to 2 mm. ST-segment elevation greater than this may represent early repolarization, as seen in this example, or acute pericarditis. Interestingly, this patient later developed acute pericarditis with even more marked ST-segment abnormalities (see next tracing).

REFERENCE: Parisi.

B-3

Clinical History

A 23-year-old man with pleuritic chest pain.

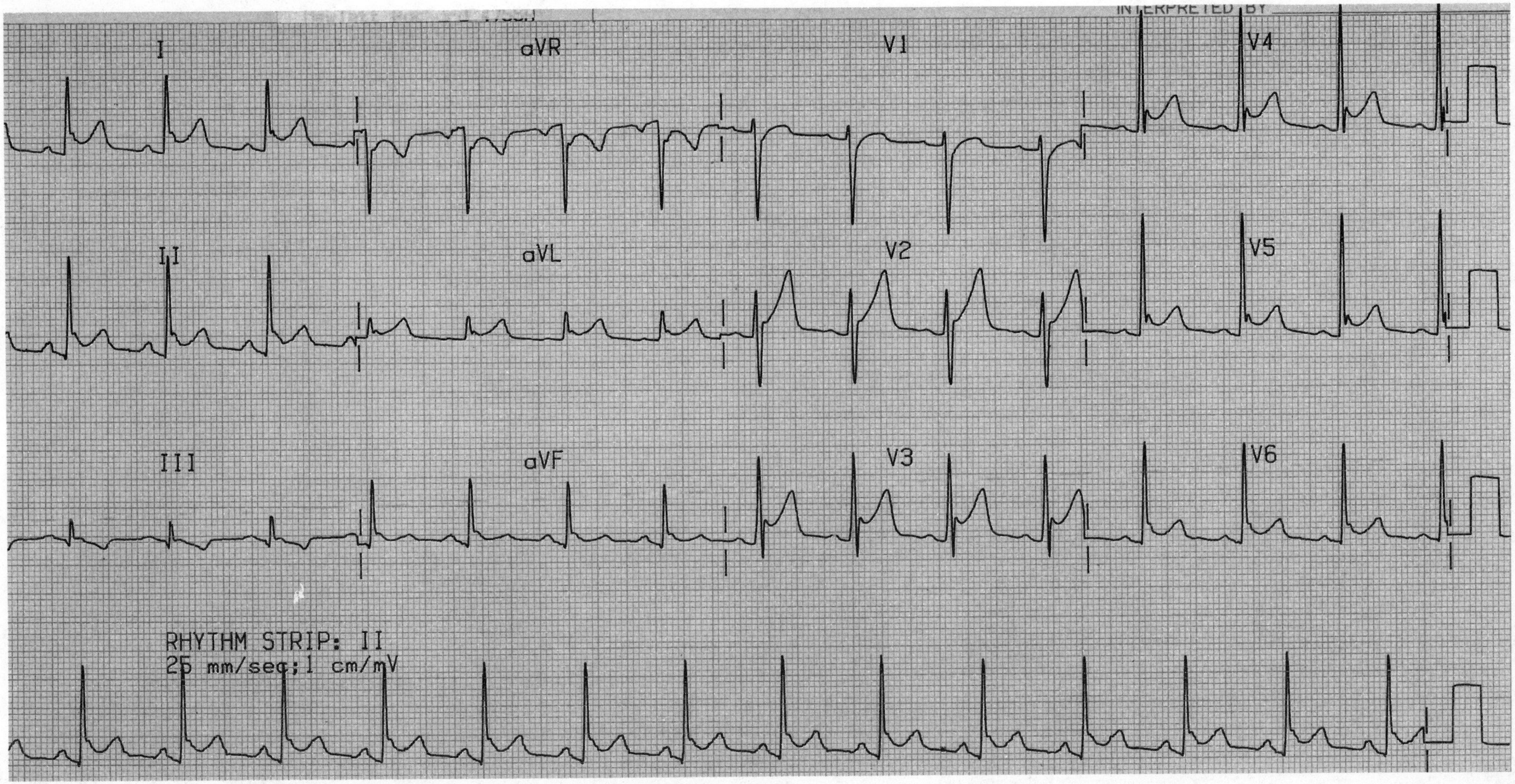

B-3

NARRATIVE INTERPRETATION

Rhythm: **Sinus**
Rate: **85**
Intervals: **PR 0.18, QRS 0.08, QT 0.28**
Axis: **+45 degrees**

Abnormalities

PR depression (most pronounced in) leads II, aVF. J-point elevation throughout. Diffuse ST elevation.

Synthesis

Sinus rhythm. PR depression, J-point elevation, and ST elevation consistent with early, acute pericarditis.

TEST ANSWERS: 1, 63, 105.

Comment: This is an interesting tracing in that this patient had resting ST abnormalities characteristic of early repolarization and subsequently developed acute pericarditis (see previous tracing). It is often difficult to differentiate these two entities. PR depression, if evident, may help to suggest pericarditis; however, this is not a universal finding. It has been suggested that if the ratio of the amplitudes of the ST segment and T wave (ST/T ratio) measured in lead V6 is greater than 0.25, acute pericarditis is present. The diffuse ST elevation, which involves every lead in this example except aVR, distinguishes this from acute myocardial injury, which is usually localized to a specific region of the myocardium.

REFERENCES: Gintzon. Spodick (1976). Wanner.

B-4

Clinical History

A 78-year-old woman with cardiomegaly and bilateral pleural effusions.

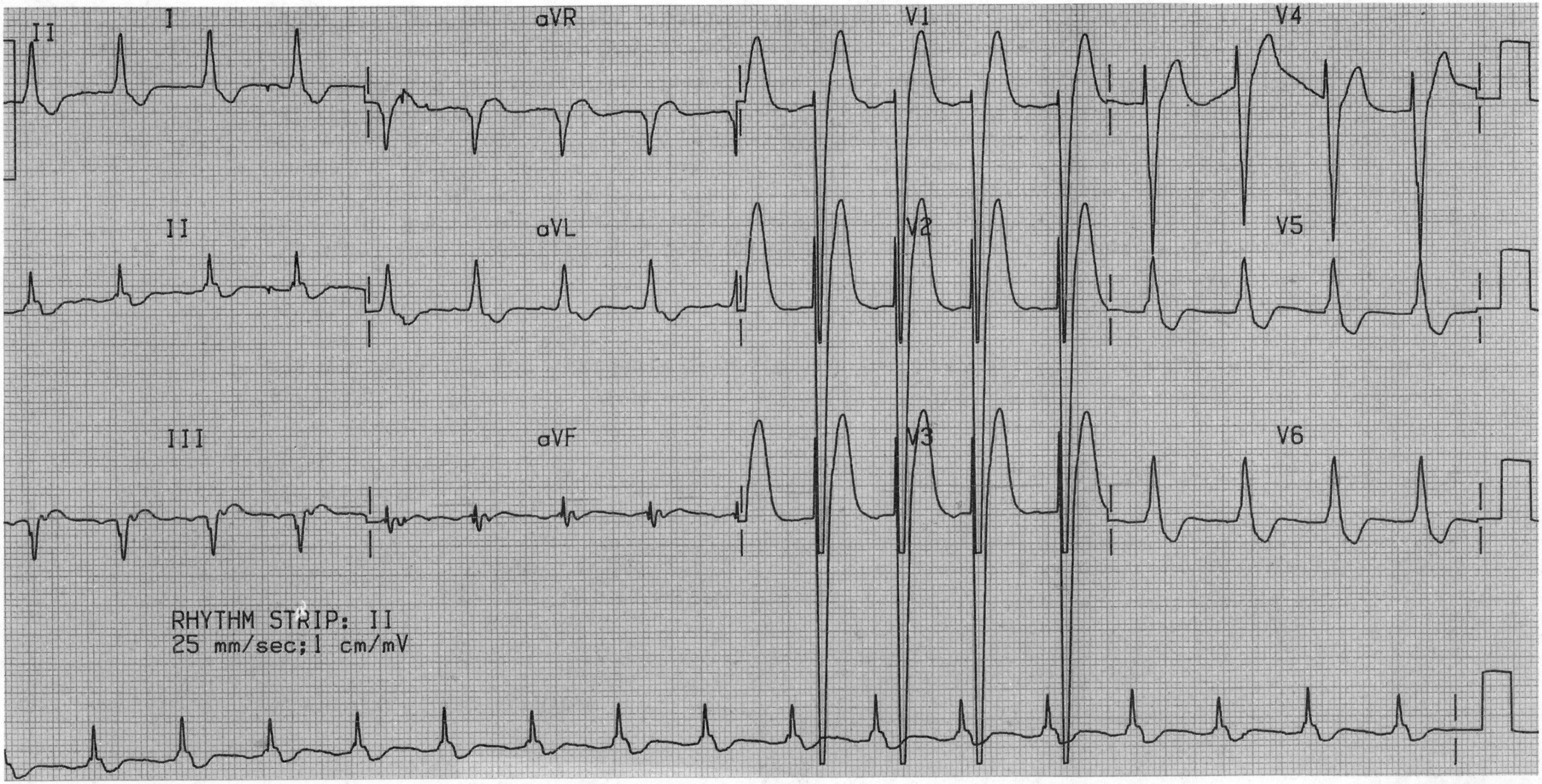

B-4

NARRATIVE INTERPRETATION

Rhythm: **Sinus**
Rate: **99**
Intervals: **PR 0.16, QRS 0.12, QT 0.28**
Axis: **0 degrees**

Abnormalities

Broad, slurred QRS leads I, aVL, V5–V6, with ST depression and T-wave inversion. SV2 + RV5 equals 50 mm.

Synthesis

Sinus rhythm. LBBB with associated ST-T-wave changes. Possible LVH.

TEST ANSWERS: 1, 74, (78), 104.

Comment: The diagnosis of LVH in the presence of LBBB is controversial. LVH and LBBB commonly coexist. Standard electrocardiographic criteria for LVH cannot be used in the presence of LBBB because of voltage changes caused by the conduction abnormality itself. A number of modifications of criteria for LVH in the presence of LBBB have been proposed. One report found that the criterion of SV2 + RV5 greater than 45 mm had a specificity of 100 percent and a sensitivity of 86 percent in patients with LBBB and echocardiographic evidence of LVH. Despite this, the diagnosis of LVH in the presence of LBBB must be made with caution. Therefore, the author has added "possible" LVH in this example.

REFERENCES: Klein RC. Kafka. Vandenberg. Flowers.

B-5

Clinical History

A 78-year-old woman who presents to the emergency department with mild lightheadedness and dyspnea. Her physician reports she has a history of a cardiomyopathy and an abnormal electrocardiogram.

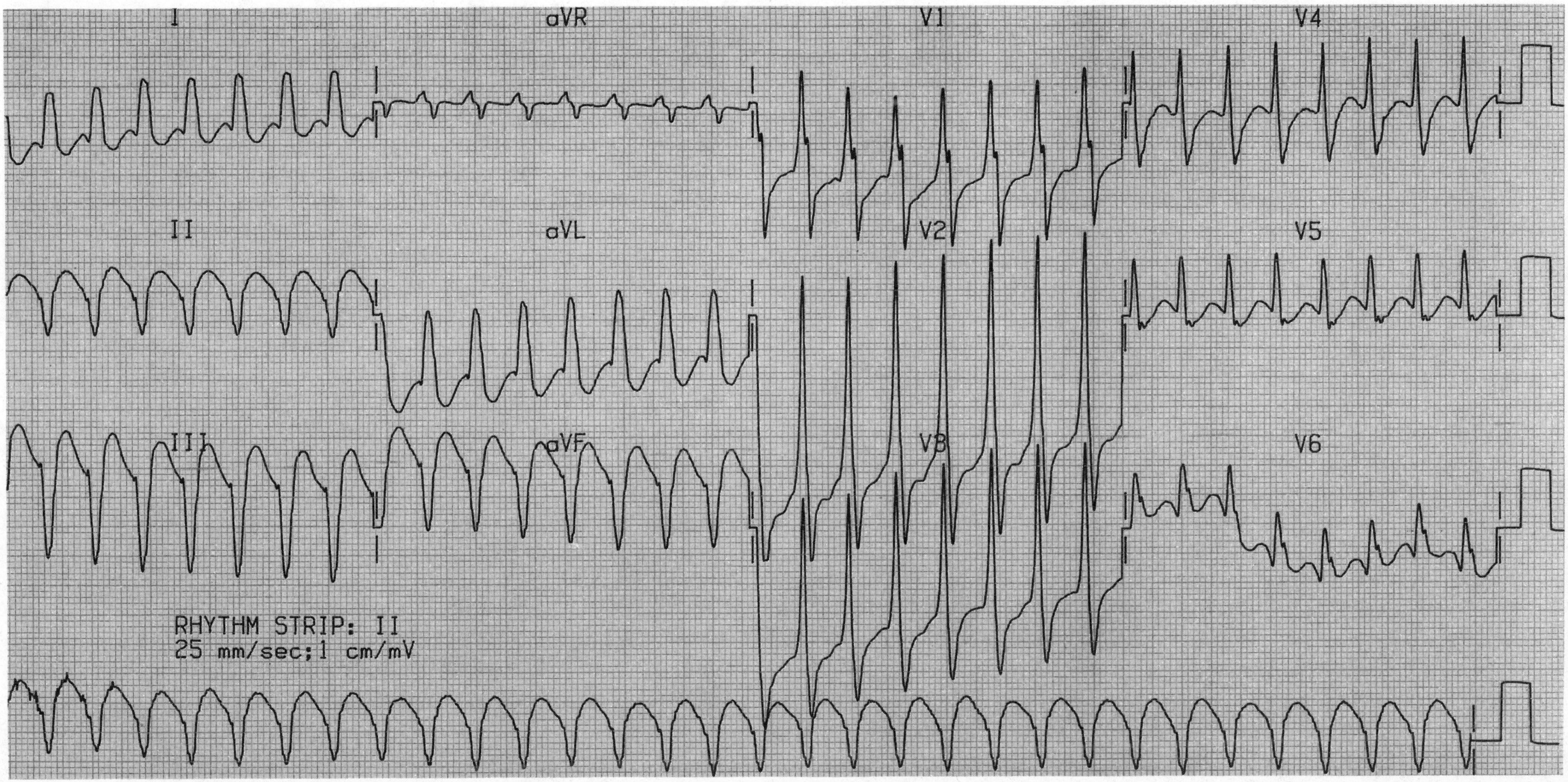

B-5

NARRATIVE INTERPRETATION

Rhythm:	**Wide complex tachycardia consistent with ventricular tachycardia**
Rate:	**185**
Intervals:	**PR –, QRS 0.12, QT –**
Axis:	**−60 degrees**

Abnormalities
Rapid heart rate with wide QRS complex. Axis leftward of −30 degrees.

Synthesis
Ventricular tachycardia. Left axis deviation.

TEST ANSWERS: 30, 64.

Comment: The fact that this patient was not in extremis at presentation should not dissuade the clinician from the true diagnosis of ventricular tachycardia. There are a number of clues that point to the origin of this rhythm as ventricular rather than supraventricular with aberrancy. The configuration of the QRS complex both in V1 and V6 is suggestive of ventricular tachycardia, as is the leftward axis. Despite the attending physician's recollection of an abnormal baseline electrocardiogram, the underlying diagnosis of a cardiomyopathy should always lead the clinician to consider ventricular tachycardia first. It is generally wise to treat an arrhythmia of this type as ventricular tachycardia until proved otherwise. This patient's baseline electrocardiogram may be seen in the previous example.

REFERENCES: Wellens. Brugada. Tchou. Akhtar.

B-6

Clinical History

A 56-year-old woman with a history of rheumatic fever.

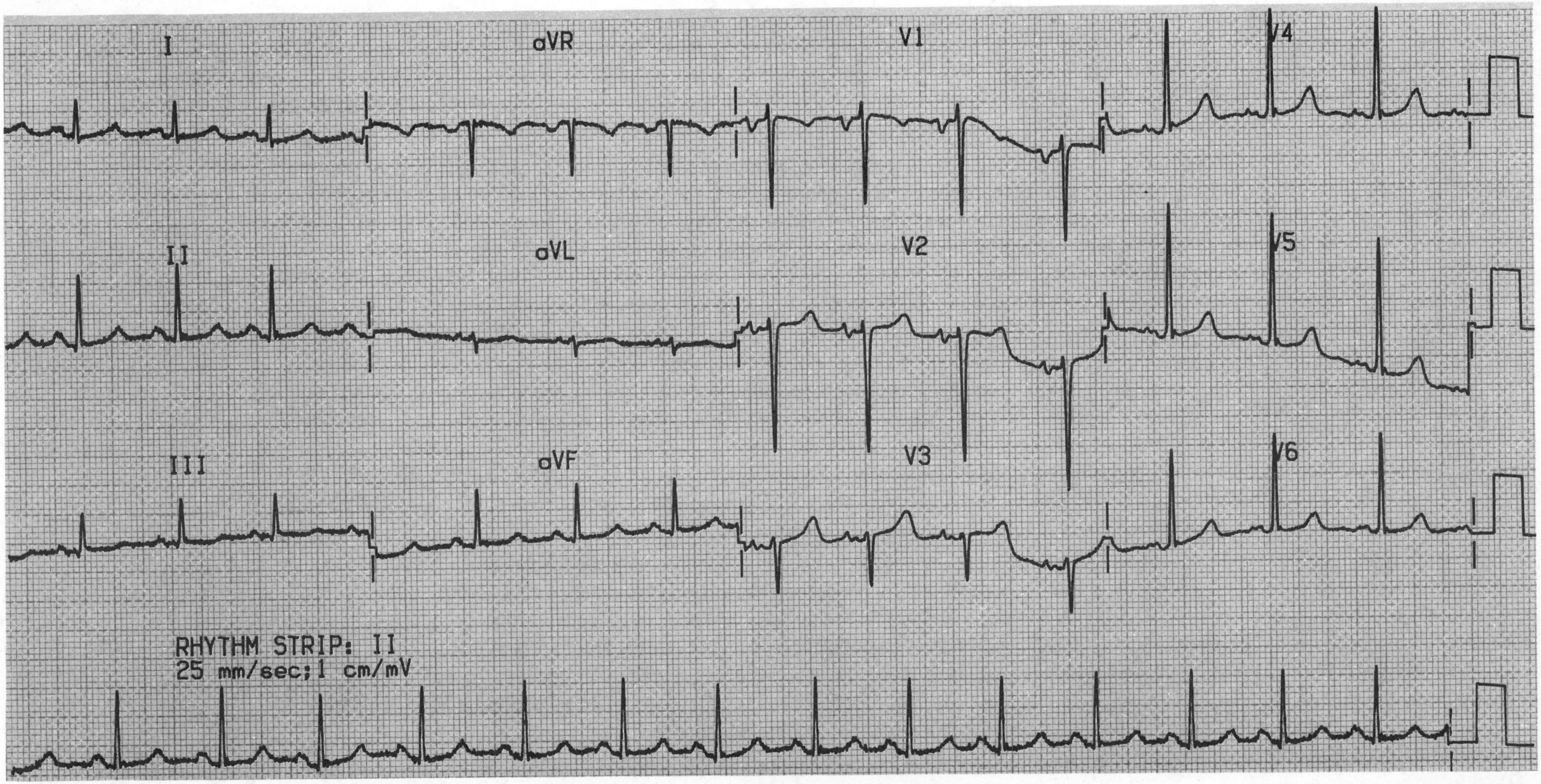

B-6

NARRATIVE INTERPRETATION

Rhythm: **Sinus**
Rate: **88**
Intervals: **PR 0.16, QRS 0.08, QT 0.38**
Axis: **+60 degrees**

Abnormalities

Abnormal P terminal force V1. R wave V1–V3 less than 3 mm. SV2 + RV5 greater than 35 mm.

Synthesis

Sinus rhythm. Left atrial abnormality. Poor R-wave progression. LVH by voltage criteria.

TEST ANSWERS: 1, 60, 66, 78.

Comment: This patient had mitral stenosis with left atrial enlargement confirmed by echocardiography. A deep and wide P terminal force in lead V1 is easily appreciated. A notched P wave is also seen in left atrial abnormality; however, in this example, the peak-to-peak duration of the two notches in lead II is not greater than 40 ms. LVH is not expected from mitral stenosis and was a reflection of this patient's concomitant hypertension. Poor R-wave progression was also likely to be secondary to LVH.

REFERENCE: Hazen.

B-7

Clinical History

A 73-year-old man 2 days following aortic valve surgery. He has been receiving digoxin.

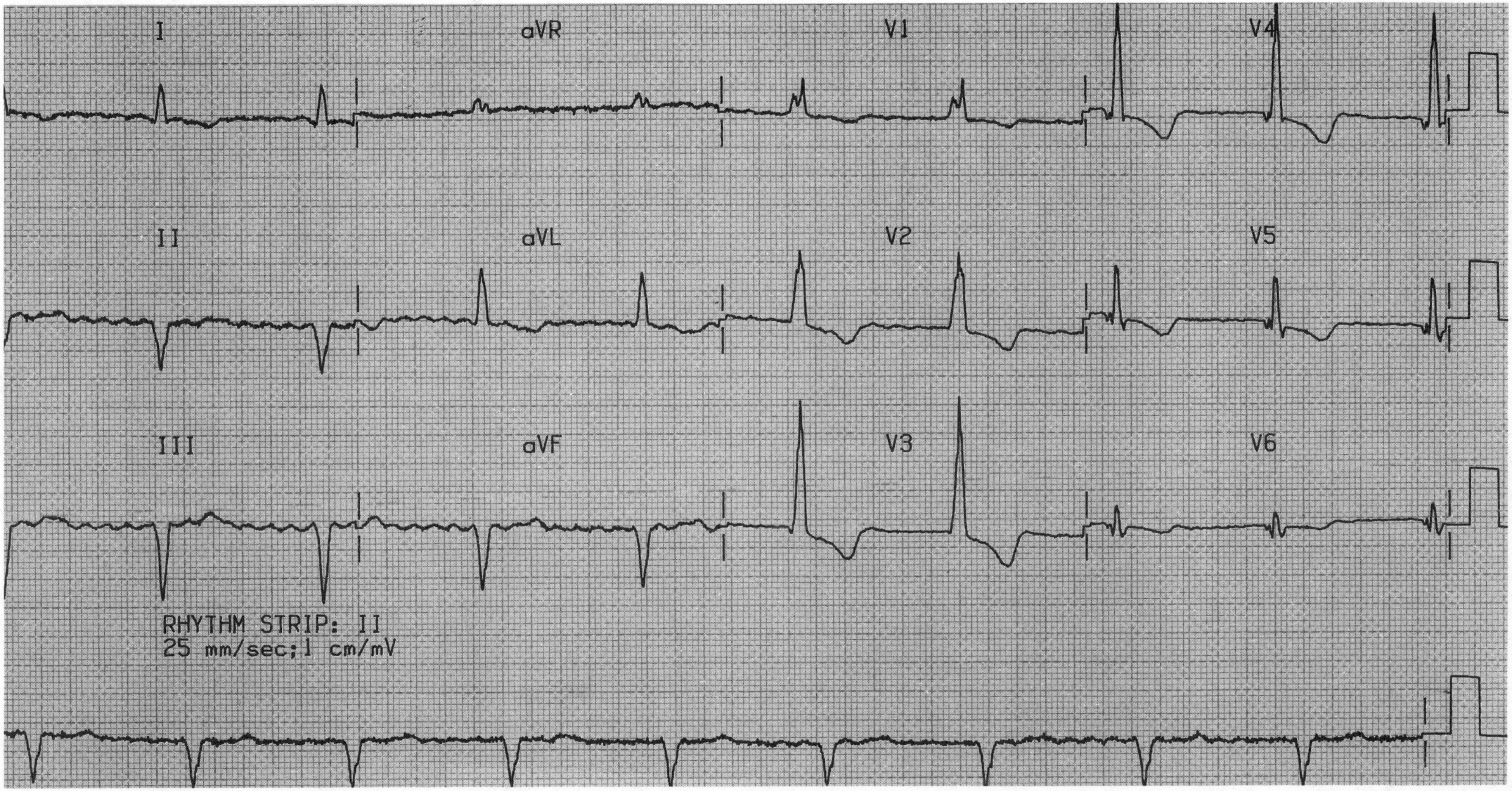

B-7

NARRATIVE INTERPRETATION

Rhythm:	**Atrial fibrillation with complete AV block; AV junctional rhythm**
Rate:	**54**
Intervals:	**PR –, QRS 0.12, QT 0.44**
Axis:	**−75 degrees**

Abnormalities
Broad, notched QRS with RsR′ pattern lead V1 and T-wave inversion leads V1–V3. T-wave inversion leads I, aVL, V4–V6. Axis leftward of −30 degrees.

Synthesis
Atrial fibrillation with complete AV block. AV junctional escape rhythm. RBBB with secondary ST-T-wave abnormalities. Left axis deviation. LAFB. Nonspecific T-wave abnormalities.

TEST ANSWERS: 20, 22, 47, 64, 70, 72, 104, 106.

Comment: The underlying rhythm is atrial fibrillation; however, the irregular conduction to the ventricles is absent because of digitalis toxicity, which has produced complete AV block. A subsidiary pacemaker in the AV junction has responded with an escape rhythm. The rate in the 50s indicates this is an escape rhythm rather than an accelerated AV junctional rhythm. One cannot be certain without prior tracings that the rhythm was not of ventricular origin; however, the rate would most likely be slower in that situation. This patient had a previous RBBB and extreme left axis deviation. There are small R waves in leads II, III, and aVF; therefore, inferior wall MI is not likely, although on occasion LAFB can mask a previous Q wave by inducing an initial inferior vector. One may also note the broad initial R wave in lead V1, which has been suggested to represent posterior wall MI. This must be considered a tenuous ECG diagnosis and is not considered reliable by the author. This patient had no coronary heart disease on catheterization. Therefore, the rS complexes in the inferior leads and the broad R wave in lead V1 were due to the LAFB and RBBB, respectively. A minor additional finding is the nonspecific T-wave inversions in the lateral leads; RBBB does not usually produce these changes.

REFERENCES: Benchimol. Kastor (1967).

B-8

Clinical History

A 33-year-old asymptomatic man.

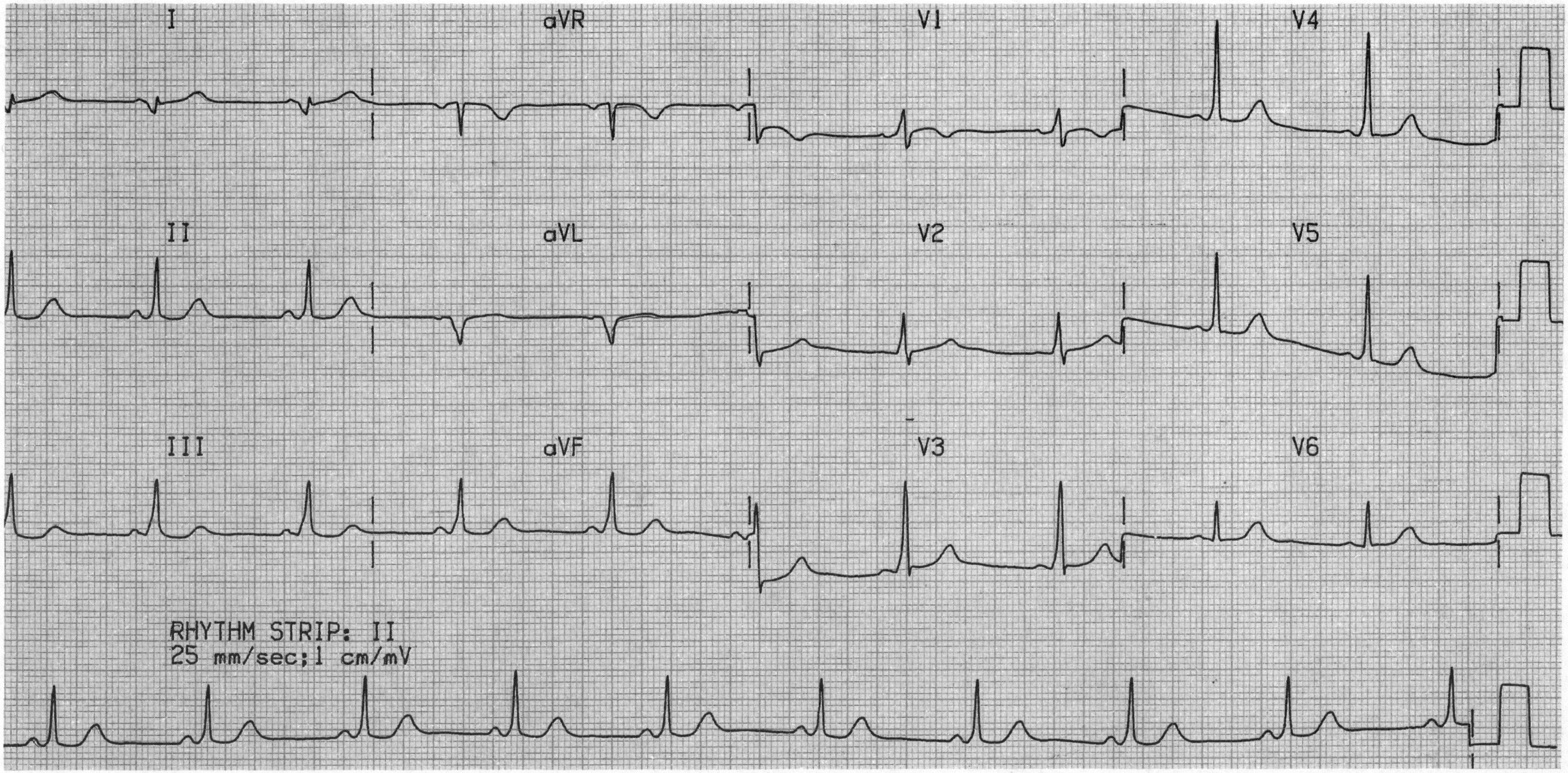

B-8

NARRATIVE INTERPRETATION

Rhythm: **Sinus bradycardia**
Rate: **57**
Intervals: **PR 0.11, QRS 0.10, QT 0.44**
Axis: **+110 degrees**

Abnormalities

Slow heart rate. Short PR interval. Delta waves negative in leads I, aVL, and positive in leads II, III, aVF, V1–V6. Prolonged QRS with generalized ST-T-wave abnormalities.

Synthesis

Sinus bradycardia. Ventricular preexcitation pattern (WPW).

TEST ANSWERS: 3, 49.

Comment: On first glance, the reader might mistakenly interpret this tracing as a lateral and posterior wall MI. On closer examination, the slurred delta wave becomes evident, particularly in lead III. The delta wave is negative in leads I and aVL and positive in the anterior precordial leads, which creates a pseudoinfarction pattern. This pattern is helpful in localizing the bypass tract to a left lateral location.

REFERENCES: Reddy. Goldberger (I and II). Horowitz.

B-9

Clinical History

A 17-year-old male seen in the emergency department following a football injury.

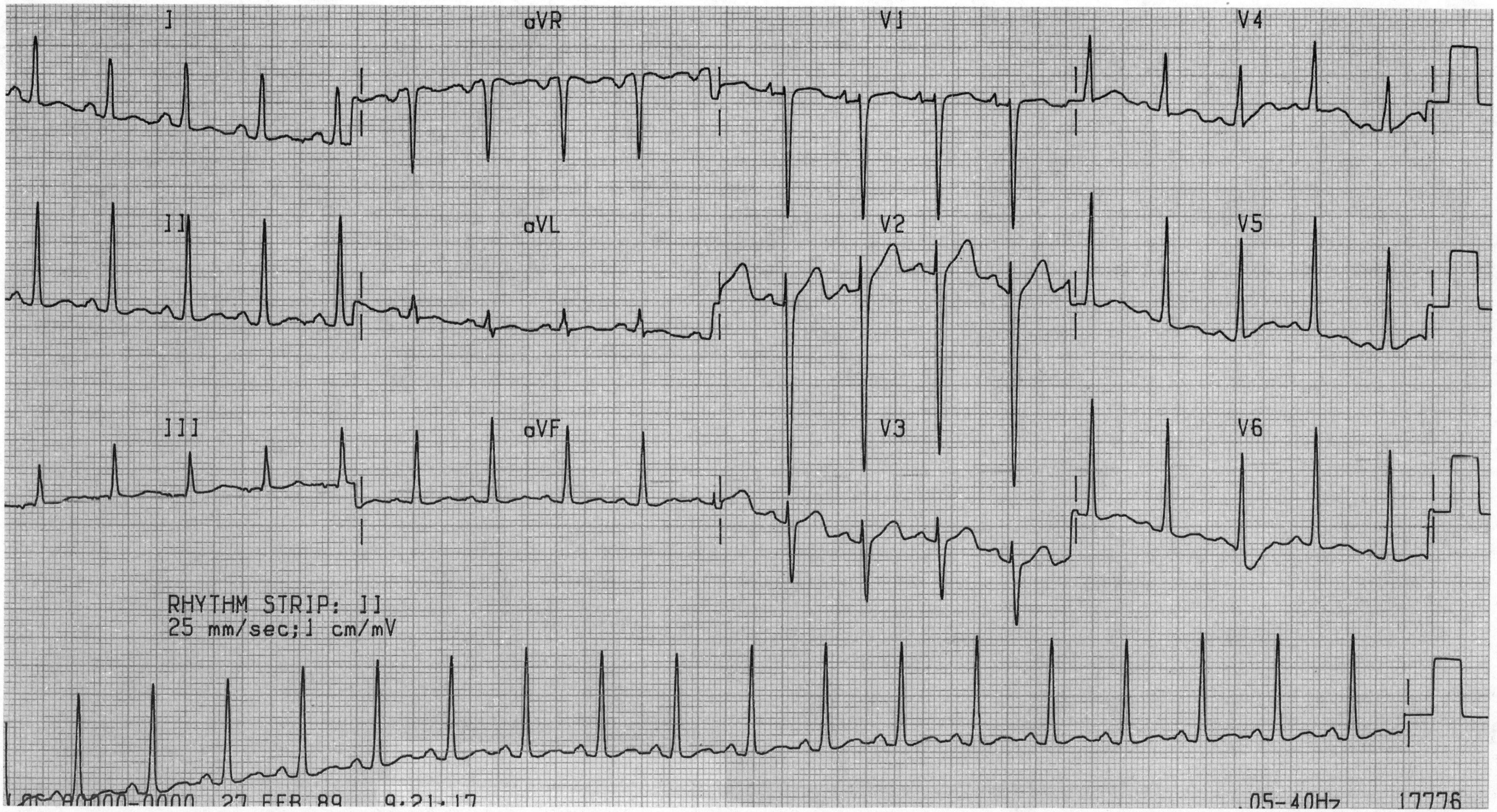

B-9

NARRATIVE INTERPRETATION

Rhythm: **Sinus tachycardia**
Rate: **110**
Intervals: **PR 0.16, QRS 0.08, QT 0.32**
Axis: **+45 degrees**

Abnormalities
Rapid heart rate.

Synthesis
Sinus tachycardia. Otherwise normal electrocardiogram.

TEST ANSWER: 4.

Comment: It is important for the reader to remember that standard voltage criteria for LVH do not apply to persons 30 years of age or younger. One large series that compared voltage criteria for LVH according to age found that the upper limit of normal for SV1 + RV5 (or V6) was 53 mm in patients 16 to 25 years of age compared with 37 mm in patients 31 to 50 years of age.

REFERENCES: Manning. Walker.

B-10

Clinical History

A 54-year-old man admitted for elective cholecystectomy.

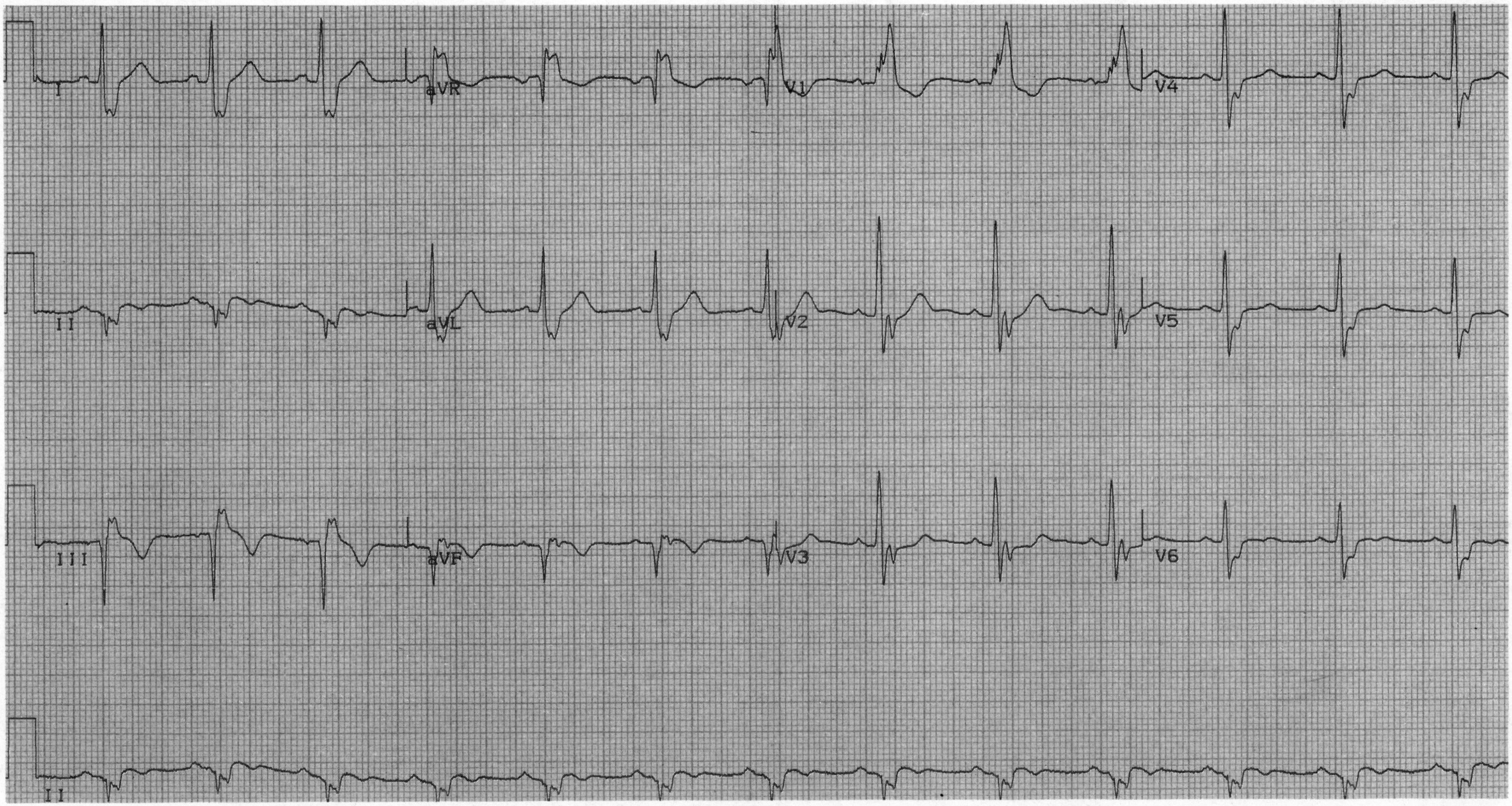

B-10

NARRATIVE INTERPRETATION

Rhythm: **Sinus**
Rate: **78**
Intervals: **PR 0.16, QRS 0.16, QT 0.40**
Axis: **−60 degrees**

Abnormalities

Axis leftward of −30 degrees. Q waves leads II, III, aVF. Broad QRS with rsR′ and T-wave inversion lead V1. T-wave inversion leads II, III, aVF.

Synthesis

Sinus rhythm. Inferior wall MI of indeterminate age. Left axis deviation. RBBB with associated ST-T-wave abnormalities.

TEST ANSWERS: 1, 64, 70, 92, 104, (106).

Comment: This is an interesting tracing because it illustrates the combined presence of inferior wall MI, left axis deviation, and RBBB. In RBBB the first portion of the QRS complex (first 0.06 s) may be interpreted normally. Accordingly, the deep inferior Q waves are diagnostic of this patient's prior inferior wall MI. The left axis deviation is a result of the inferior wall MI and is not secondary to a left anterior fascicular block (LAFB). Note that there are R waves present in leads III and aVF, which indicates that there are inferiorly directed forces. In LAFB these forces should remain in a superior direction and would demonstrate an S wave in these leads. The T-wave inversions in the inferior limb leads are likely secondary to the prior infarction but may be classified as nonspecific.

REFERENCES: Fisher. Milliken. Warner (*Am Heart J*). Friedman p 287.

B-11

Clinical History

A 56-year-old man in the emergency department with "unexplained" tachycardia.

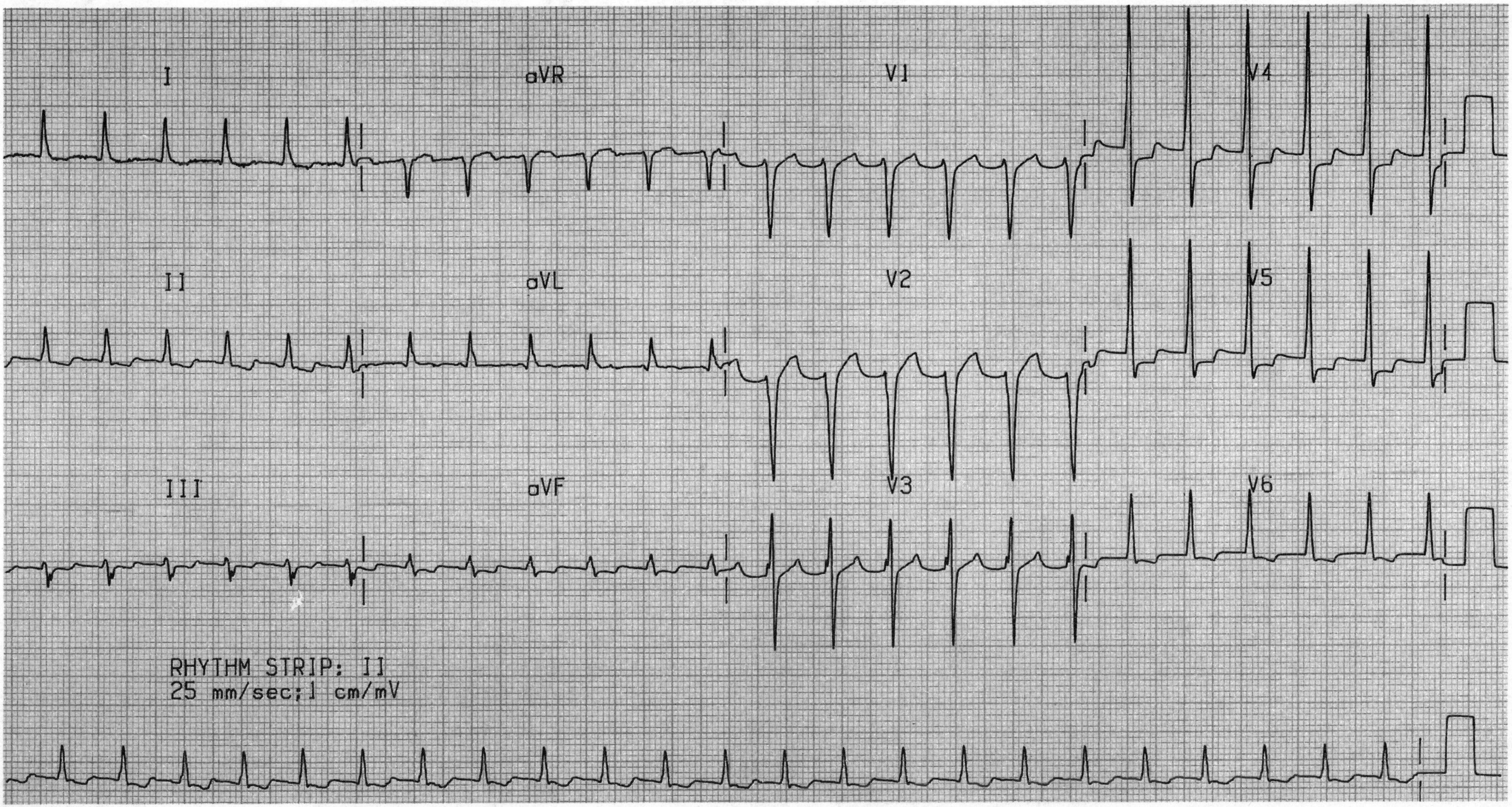

B-11

NARRATIVE INTERPRETATION

Rhythm:	**Supraventricular tachyarrhythmia, probably atrial flutter with 2:1 AV conduction**
Rate:	**Ventricular rate 140, atrial rate 280 (probable)**
Intervals:	**PR –, QRS 0.08, QT 0.26**
Axis:	**+15 degrees**

Abnormalities

Rapid heart rate. ST depression leads I, II, III, aVF, V4–V6. T-wave inversion leads II, III, aVF, V4–V6. SV2 + RV5 greater than 35 mm.

Synthesis

Supraventricular tachyarrhythmia, probably atrial flutter with 2:1 AV conduction. LVH by voltage criteria. Associated ST-T-wave abnormalities.

TEST ANSWERS: (18), 19, (50), 78, 103.

Comment: The differentiation of sinus tachycardia, supraventricular tachycardia, and atrial flutter with 2:1 AV conduction can often be quite difficult on a single electrocardiogram. The reader should suspect atrial flutter whenever the heart rate is around 150 and only a single abnormal P wave is evident. The second P wave of atrial flutter may be "buried" in the QRS complex. In this example, no unequivocal P wave is apparent, although it is suspected to be superimposed on the T wave of the preceding complex. In this situation, the clinician can often determine the rhythm by attempting vagal maneuvers such as carotid sinus pressure. Patients with sinus tachycardia will generally show only slight slowing of the heart rate. Patients with supraventricular tachycardia may convert to regular sinus rhythm, whereas those with atrial flutter may only increase the degree of AV block (see following electrocardiogram).

B-12

Clinical History

A 56-year-old man in the emergency department with "unexplained" tachycardia. He has been administered adenosine.

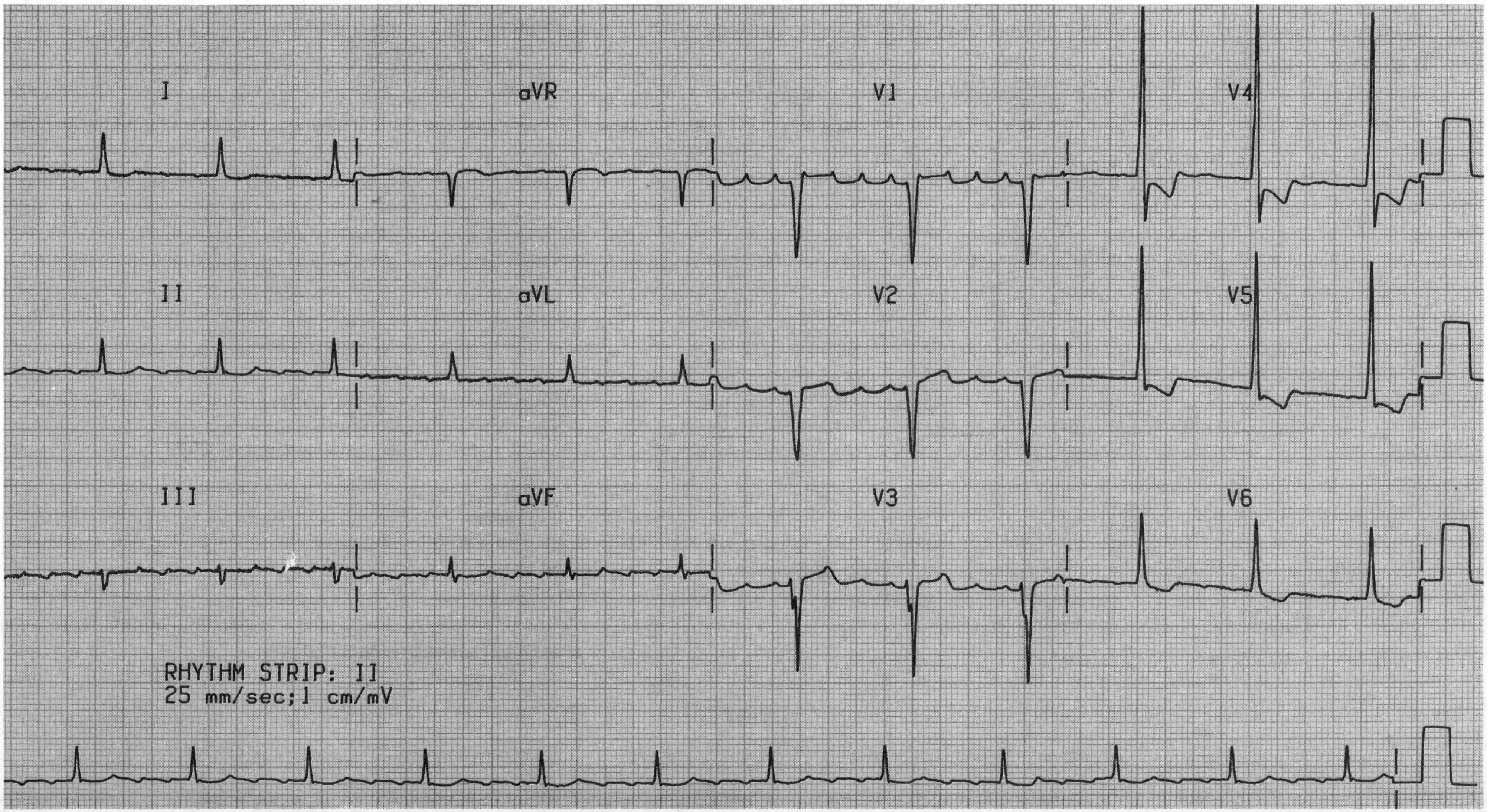

B-12

NARRATIVE INTERPRETATION

Rhythm: **Atrial flutter with 4:1 AV conduction**
Rate: **Atrial rate 296, ventricular rate 74**
Intervals: **PR –, QRS 0.08, QT 0.34**
Axis: **+15 degrees**

Abnormalities

ST depression leads I, II, aVF, V4–V6. T-wave inversion leads V4–V6. R wave less than 3 mm leads V1–V3. SV2 + RV5 greater than 35 mm.

Synthesis

Atrial flutter with 4:1 AV conduction. LVH. Associated ST-T-wave abnormalities. Poor R-wave progression.

TEST ANSWERS: 19, 51, 66, 78, 103.

Comment: The patient in the previous tracing has been administered adenosine, which has produced increased AV block and "uncovered" the atrial flutter waves. The physiologic 2:1 AV conduction of the previous tracing has changed to nonphysiologic 4:1 AV conduction as a result of the medication. Adenosine has multiple cardiac effects in addition to its depressive effect on AV conduction. These include slowing of the SA node, decreasing atrial contractility, and causing coronary vasodilation. Other intravenous medications that can be used in the acute care setting to assist with rhythm determination include verapamil, diltiazem, edrophonium, or short-acting beta blockers such as esmolol.

REFERENCE: Belardinelli.

B-13

Clinical History

A 60-year-old heavy smoker.

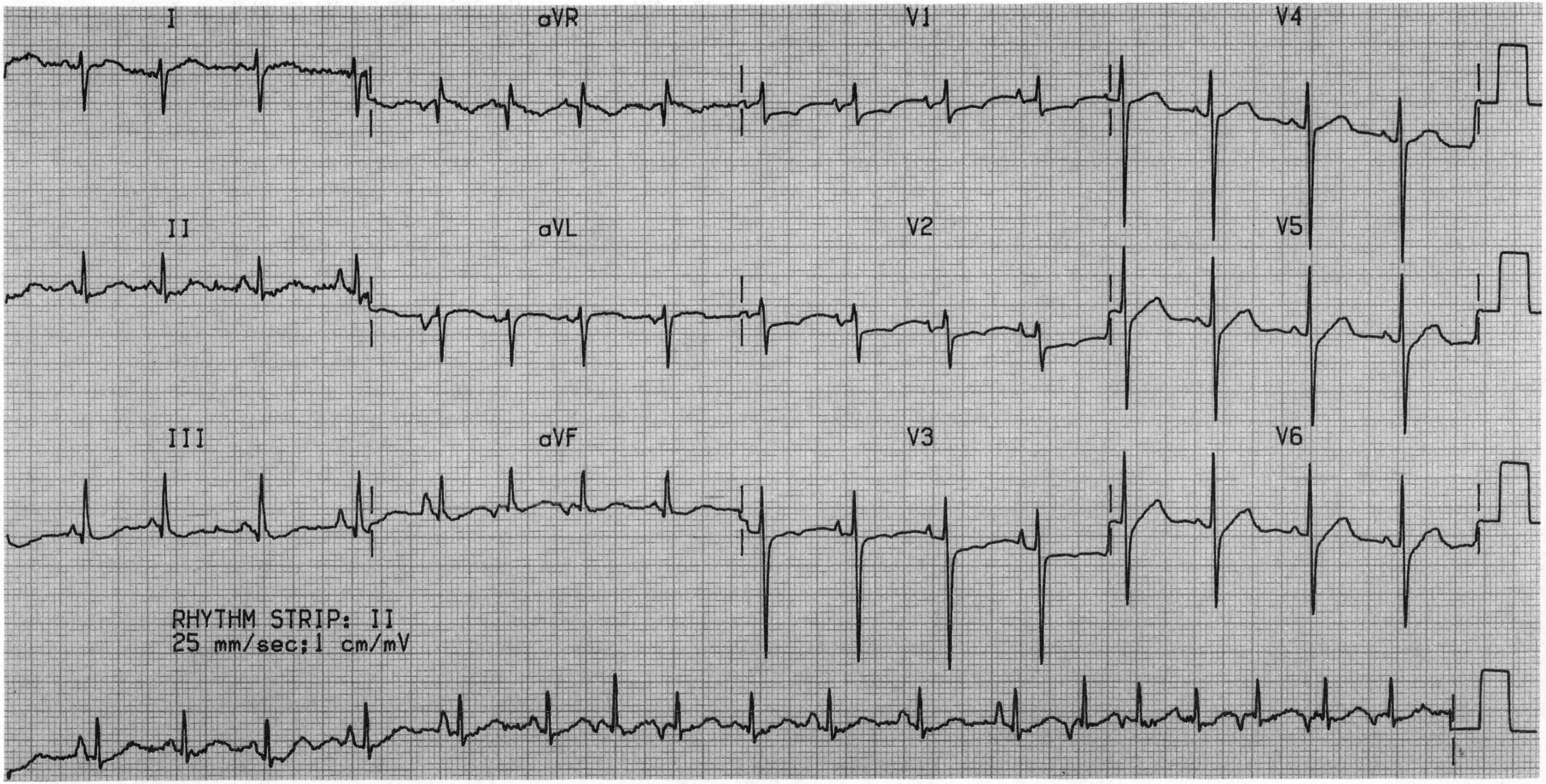

B-13

NARRATIVE INTERPRETATION

Rhythm:	**Multifocal atrial rhythm (MAR), multifocal atrial tachycardia (MAT)**
Rate:	**95 (MAR), 140 (MAT)**
Intervals:	**PR –, QRS 0.08, QT 0.36**
Axis:	**+120 degrees**

Abnormalities

Frequent, multifocal APCs. Period of MAT on rhythm strip. Axis rightward of +90 degrees. ST depression leads II, III, aVF, V1–V3. Tall R wave V1. Deep S waves leads V5–V6.

Synthesis

Multifocal atrial rhythm with period of multifocal atrial tachycardia. Right axis deviation. RVH. Associated nonspecific ST abnormalities.

TEST ANSWERS: 13, 14, 65, 79, 103, (106).

Comment: This tracing demonstrates both the rhythm disturbances and QRS morphology of severe COPD with cor pulmonale. Right axis deviation, tall R waves in the right precordial leads, and deep S waves in the left precordial leads are all a result of RVH. The ST-T abnormalities in the right precordial leads are most likely also related to RVH. Both multifocal atrial rhythm and multifocal atrial tachycardia are rhythm disturbances seen in association with COPD. By definition, multifocal atrial rhythm describes a rhythm of less than 100 beats per minute where there is no dominant atrial mechanism. This distinguishes it from sinus rhythm with frequent APCs where there is a clear sinus focus. Multifocal atrial tachycardia is identified when there are multiple atrial foci at a rate faster than 100 beats per minute. Both are seen in this example.

REFERENCES: Chou p 325. Kastor (1990).

B-14

Clinical History

A 75-year-old man with sepsis.

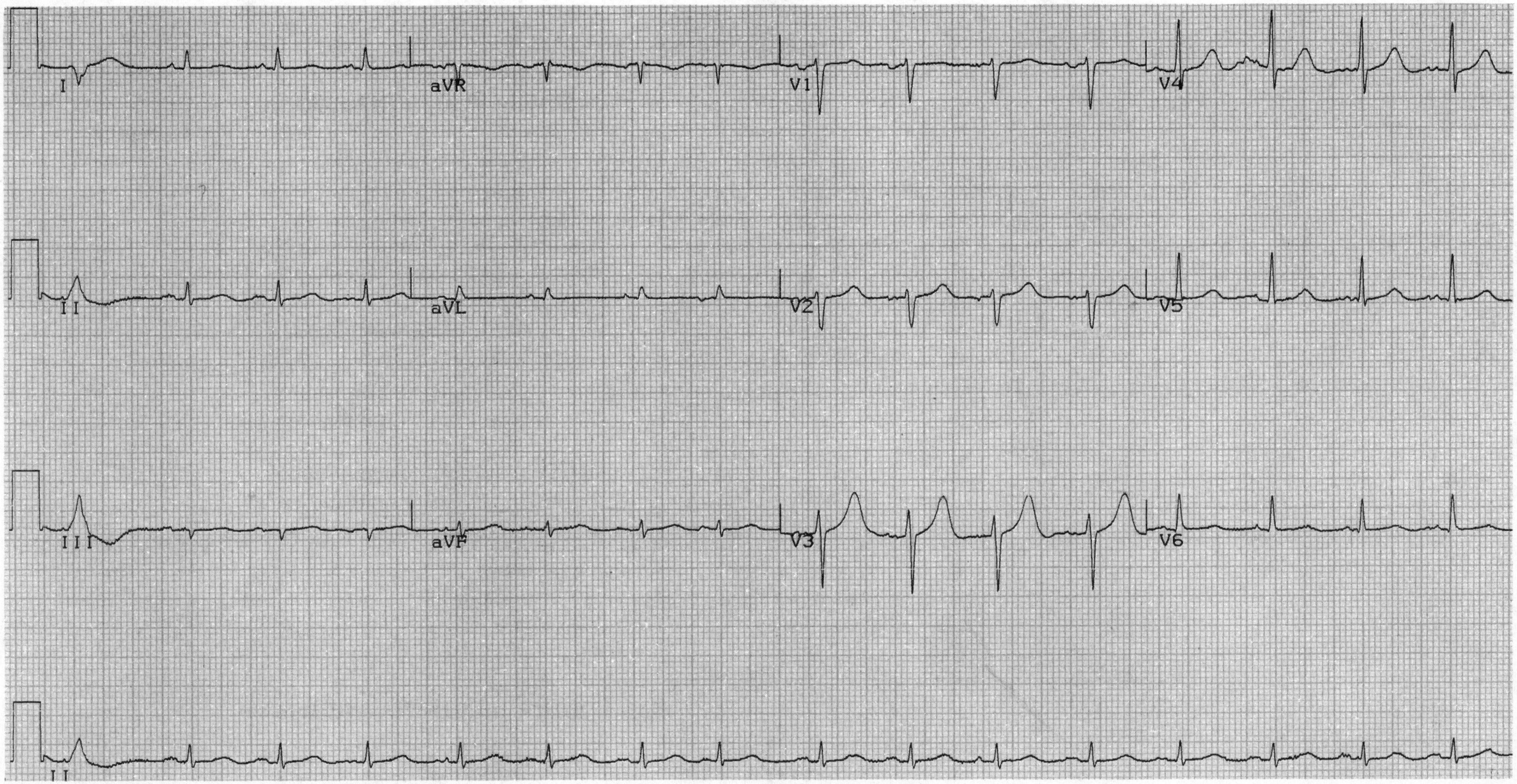

B-14

NARRATIVE INTERPRETATION

Rhythm: Sinus
Rate: 95
Intervals: PR 0.16, QRS 0.08, QT 0.36
Axis: 0 degrees

Abnormalities
Limb lead voltage less than 6 mm. VPC. APC.

Synthesis
Sinus rhythm. VPC. APC. Low-voltage limb leads.

TEST ANSWERS: 1, 10, 26, 67.

Comment: The limb-lead voltage is low in this patient. Causes of low voltage include COPD, pericardial effusion, multiple MIs with loss of viable myocardium, myxedema, amyloidosis, and marked obesity. The first complex of the tracing is most likely a VPC, although technically it cannot be confirmed as such without visualization of the prior complex. On careful inspection APCs are also evident. Note that the eighth complex is premature and shows an altered P-wave configuration.

REFERENCE: Marriott p 21.

B-15

Clinical History

An asymptomatic 18-year-old man.

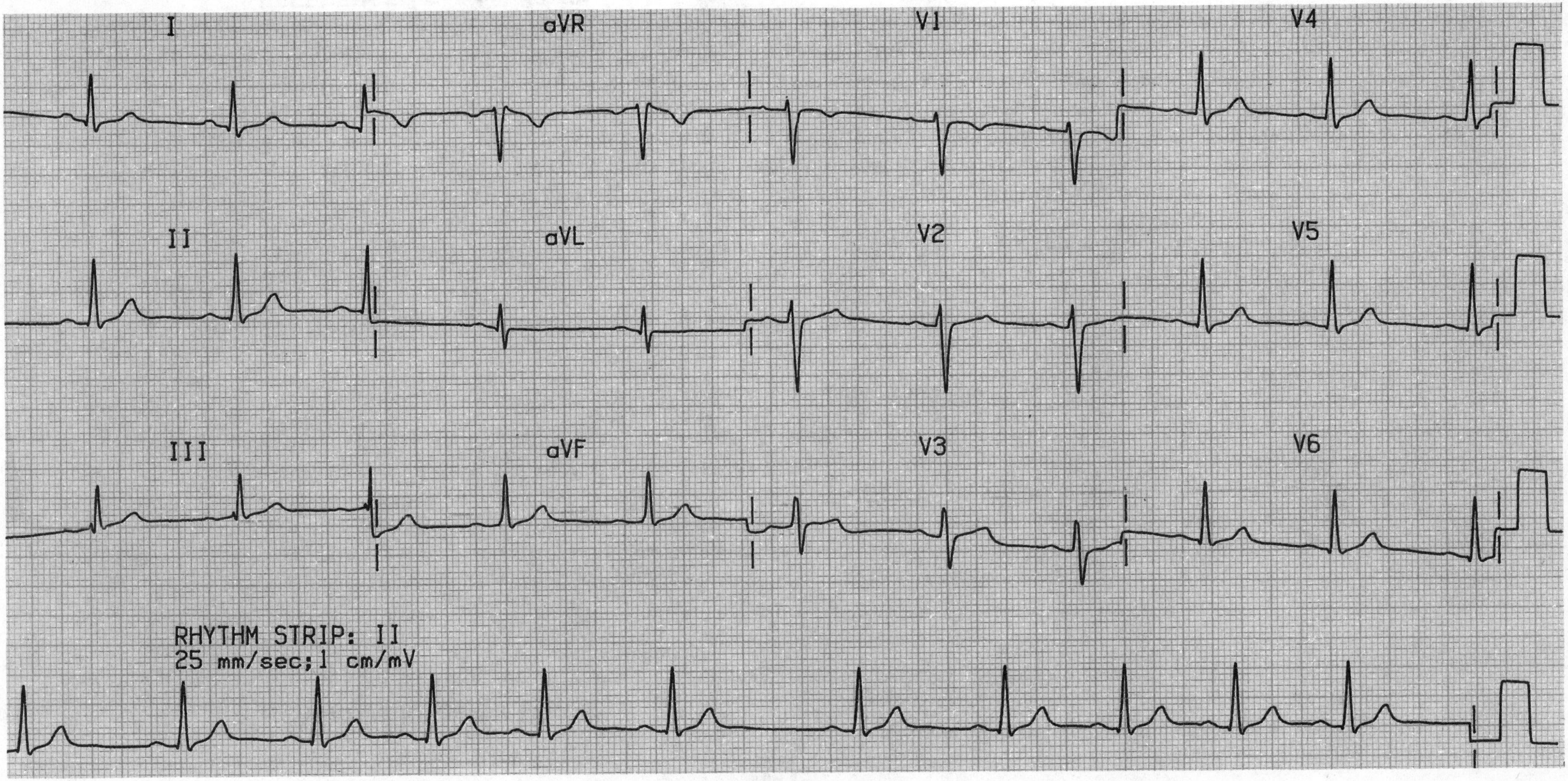

B-15

NARRATIVE INTERPRETATION

Rhythm:	**Sinus, with sinus arrhythmia**
Rate:	**65**
Intervals:	**PR 0.16, QRS 0.08, QT 0.38**
Axis:	**+60 degrees**

Abnormalities
Variation in PP interval of more than 0.16 s.

Synthesis
Sinus rhythm with sinus arrhythmia; otherwise normal electrocardiogram.

TEST ANSWERS: 1, 2.

Comment: Sinus arrhythmia is defined when the basic rhythm is sinus, but the P-to-P interval varies by 16 ms or more. It is usually seen when the intrinsic sinus rate is slow. A gradual lengthening and shortening of the P-to-P intervals differentiates this rhythm from sinoatrial block. Sinus arrhythmia may be divided into respiratory and nonrespiratory forms. Respiratory sinus arrhythmia is a result of alterations in vagal tone induced by the respiratory cycle. Inspiration speeds the heart rate and expiration slows it. Respiratory sinus arrhythmia is most common in younger persons and does not reflect cardiac pathology. Nonrespiratory sinus arrhythmia is unrelated to the respiratory cycle and may result from drugs such as opiates and digitalis. Elderly persons with slow intrinsic heart rates may also show marked nonrespiratory sinus arrhythmia.

REFERENCE: Chung pp 67–69.

B-16

Clinical History

A 59-year-old man in the CCU.

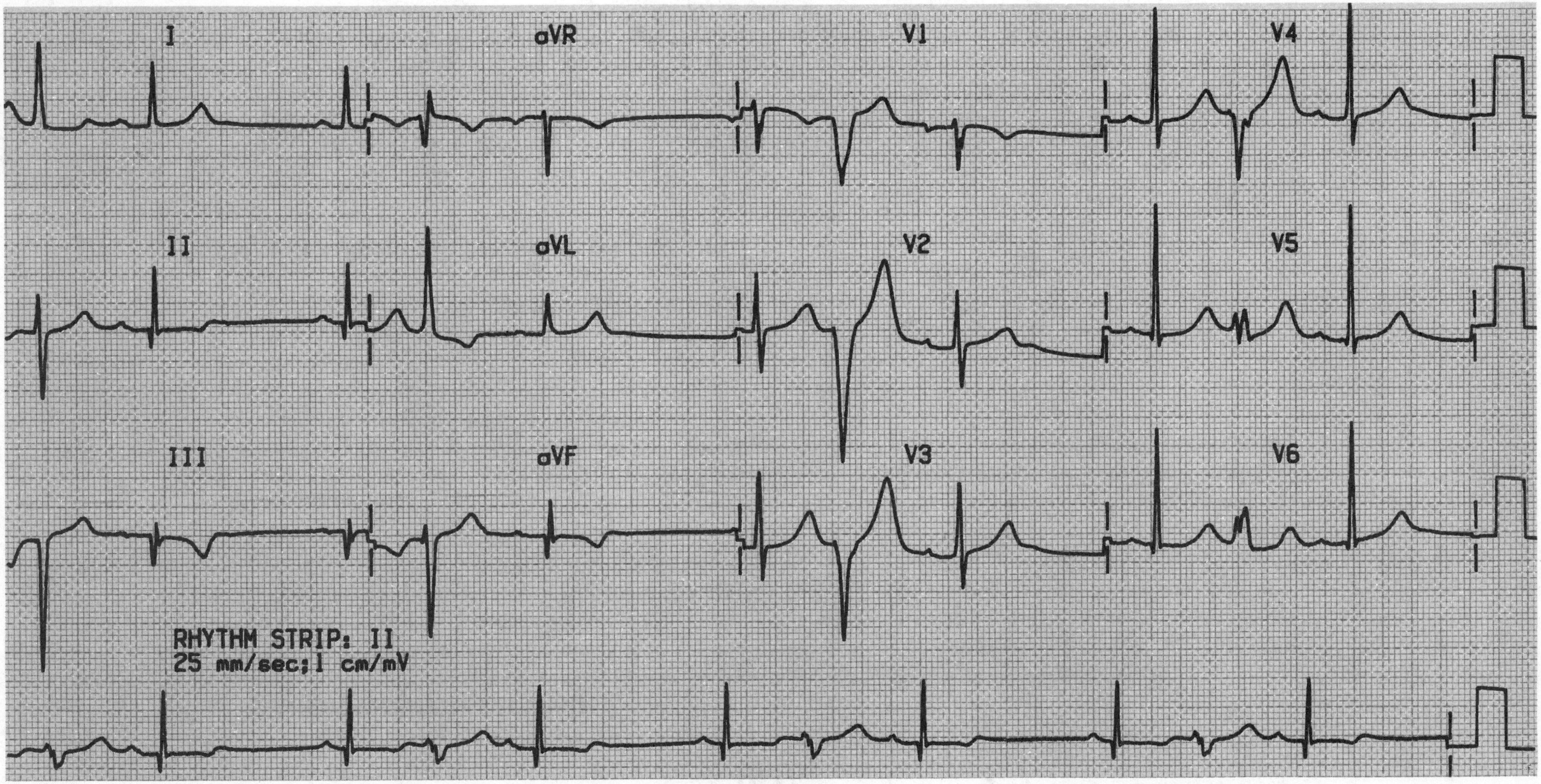

B-16

NARRATIVE INTERPRETATION

Rhythm: **Sinus**
Rate: **46**
Intervals: **PR 0.16, QRS 0.08, QT 0.32**
Axis: **+30 degrees**

Abnormalities

Slow heart rate. Q waves leads II, III, aVF. ST-segment elevation (coved) leads III, aVF. T wave biphasic lead II. T wave inverted leads III, aVF. R wave greater than S wave lead V2. VPCs interpolated with postextrasystolic PR prolongation.

Synthesis

Sinus bradycardia with frequent, uniform, interpolated VPCs. Inferior wall MI with ST-T-wave abnormalities suggesting recent injury. Possible posterior wall MI of indeterminate age.

TEST ANSWERS: 3, 26, 58, 91, (94), 100, (106).

Comment: This is an excellent example of the concealed retrograde conduction that interpolated VPCs may manifest. Interpolated VPCs most often occur when the sinus mechanism is slow. The ventricular beat conducts retrograde into the AV junction and renders it partially refractory to the next impulse. When the next sinus beat occurs, the impulse is slowed and conducts to the ventricles with a prolonged PR interval. The retrograde conduction of the VPC is "concealed" in the sense that it cannot be actually seen electrocardiographically but is inferred by its effect on the next impulse. A probably recent, evolving inferior wall MI is present, although the true duration cannot be determined from a single tracing. The reader might also consider a posterior MI in view of the tall R wave in lead V2.

REFERENCE: Marriott and Conover p 125.

B-17

Clinical History

An 83-year-old woman who is being treated for hypertension. A year ago her electrocardiogram demonstrated LVH.

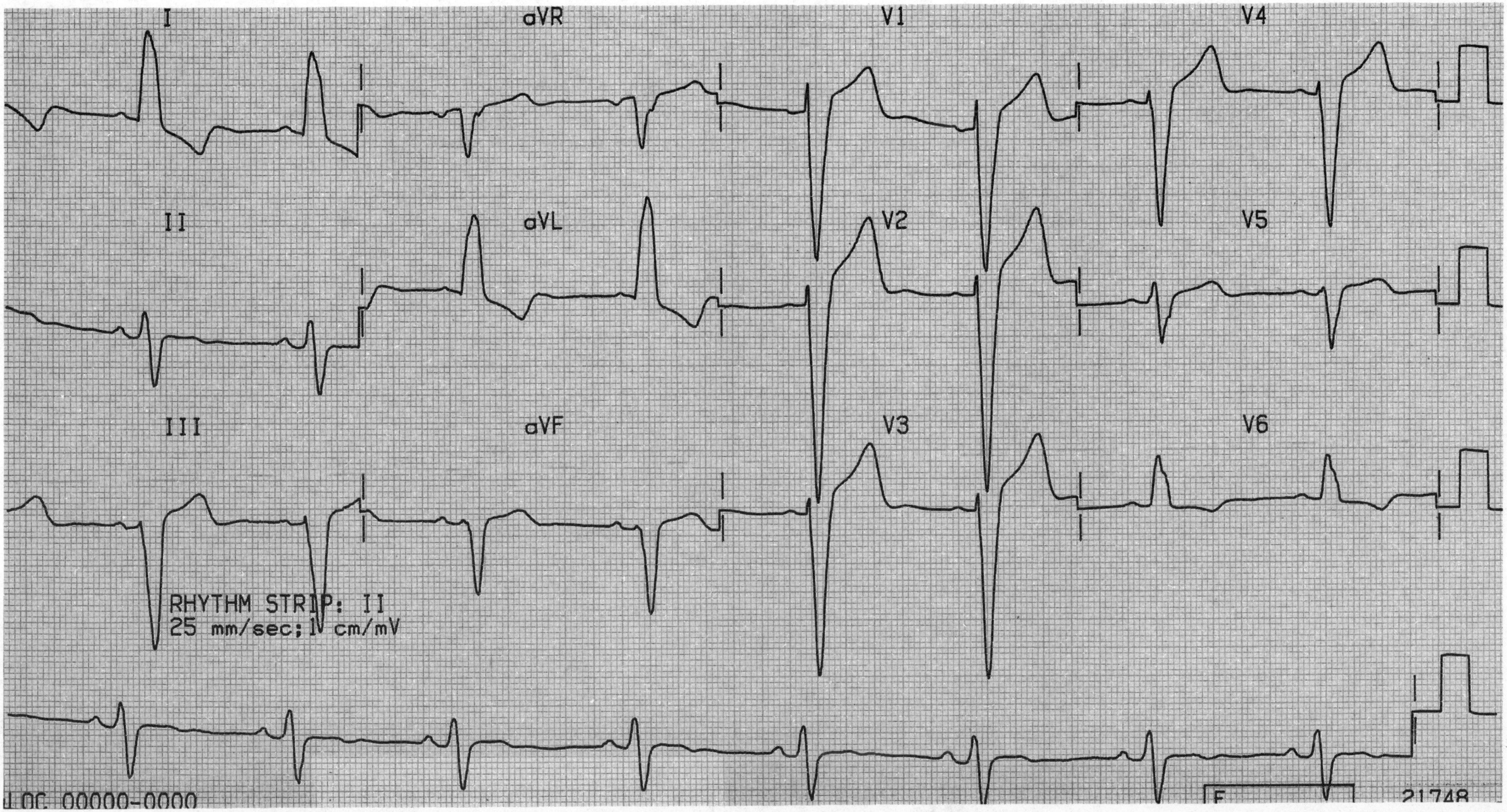

B-17

NARRATIVE INTERPRETATION

Rhythm:	**Sinus bradycardia**
Rate:	**47**
Intervals:	**PR 0.18, QRS 0.16, QT 0.52**
Axis:	**−45 degrees**

Abnormalities

Slow heart rate. Broad notched QRS leads I, aVL, V6 with associated ST depression and T-wave inversion leads I, aVL, V6. Axis leftward of −30 degrees.

Synthesis

Sinus bradycardia. LBBB with associated ST-T-wave abnormalities. Left axis deviation.

TEST ANSWERS: 3, 64, 74, 104.

Comment: The development of a "new" LBBB is an important marker for significant underlying heart disease. The Framingham study found that newly acquired LBBB signified a high-risk population with advanced hypertensive or atherosclerotic heart disease. Within 10 years of follow-up, 50 percent of those with new onset of LBBB were dead from cardiovascular disease. Importantly, progression to complete heart block is infrequent, and permanent pacemaker insertion is not indicated. Remember that standard criteria for LVH cannot be used in patients with LBBB. Some authors have suggested that if SV2 + RV6 is greater than 45 mm, then LVH may still be diagnosed. This criterion is not quite met in this example.

REFERENCES: Schneider (1979). Klein RC.

B-18

Clinical History

A 52-year-old asymptomatic man seen after a recent hospitalization.

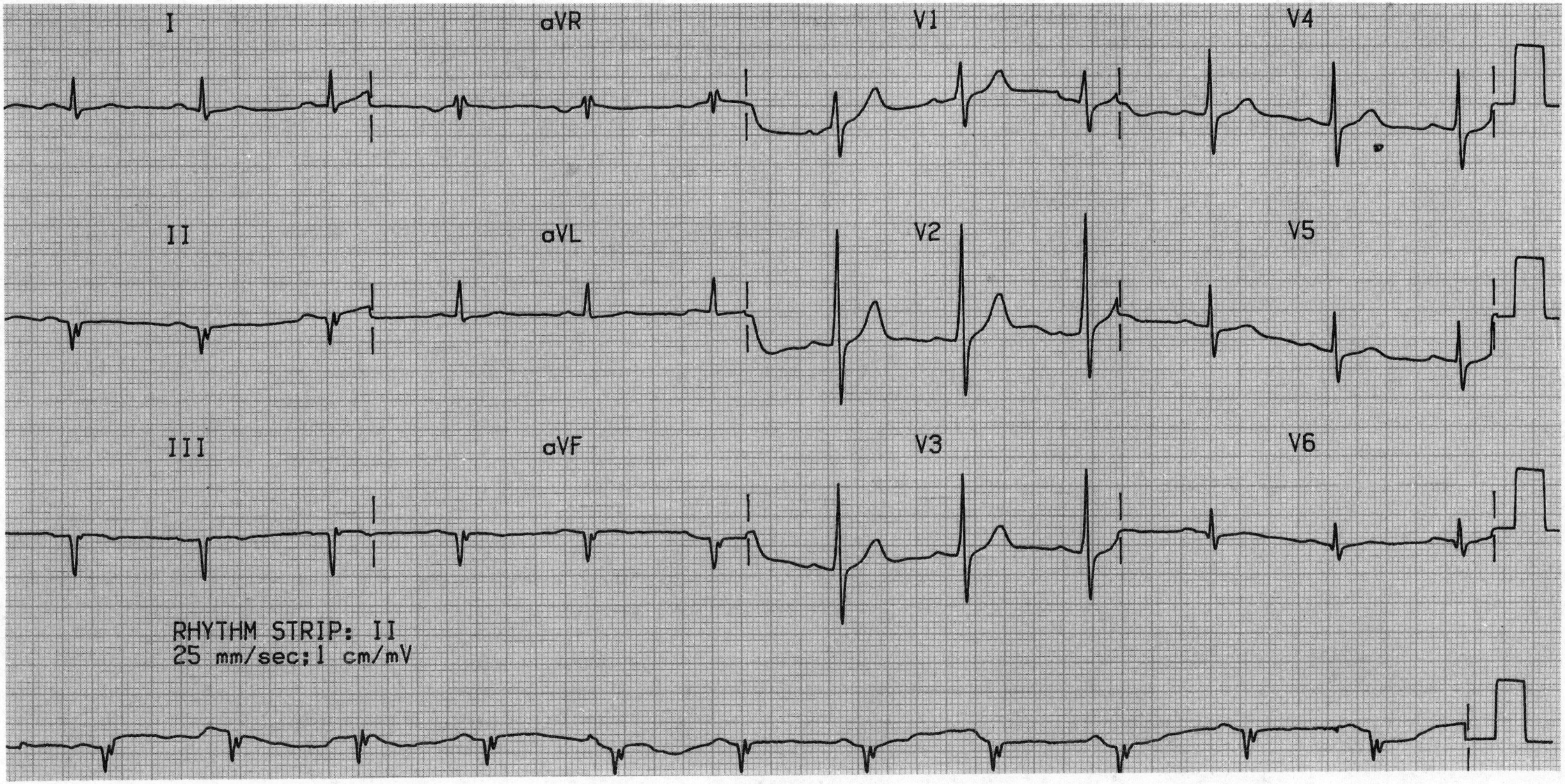

B-18

NARRATIVE INTERPRETATION

Rhythm: **Sinus**
Rate: **70**
Intervals: **PR 0.18, QRS 0.08, QT 0.40**
Axis: **−45 degrees**

Abnormalities

Axis leftward of −30 degrees. Q waves leads II, III, aVF. R wave greater than S wave with upright T wave leads V1–V2.

Synthesis

Sinus rhythm. Inferior and posterior wall MI of indeterminate duration. Left axis deviation. Left anterior fascicular block.

TEST ANSWERS: 1, 64, 72, 92, 94.

Comment: Interpretation of this electrocardiogram is not as easy as it might initially seem. There is an old inferior wall MI. There is also evidence of a posterior wall infarction on the basis of a broad, tall R wave in lead V1 (and V2), with an upright T wave in lead V1. This is a very reliable finding in combination with evidence of an inferior wall MI. This tracing also illustrates the difficulty in determining whether left anterior fascicular block (LAFB) coexists with inferior wall MI. These entities may induce left axis deviation singly or together. Note, however, that there is a terminal conduction delay in aVR that occurs after the R wave in aVL, which is indicative of a counterclockwise vector loop in the frontal plane. This is characteristic of LAFB. The "notch" in lead II and aVF is also suggestive of LAFB with inferior wall MI.

REFERENCES: Fisher. Warner (*Am Heart J*).

B-19

Clinical History

A 63-year-old hypertensive man with chest pressure for 2 h.

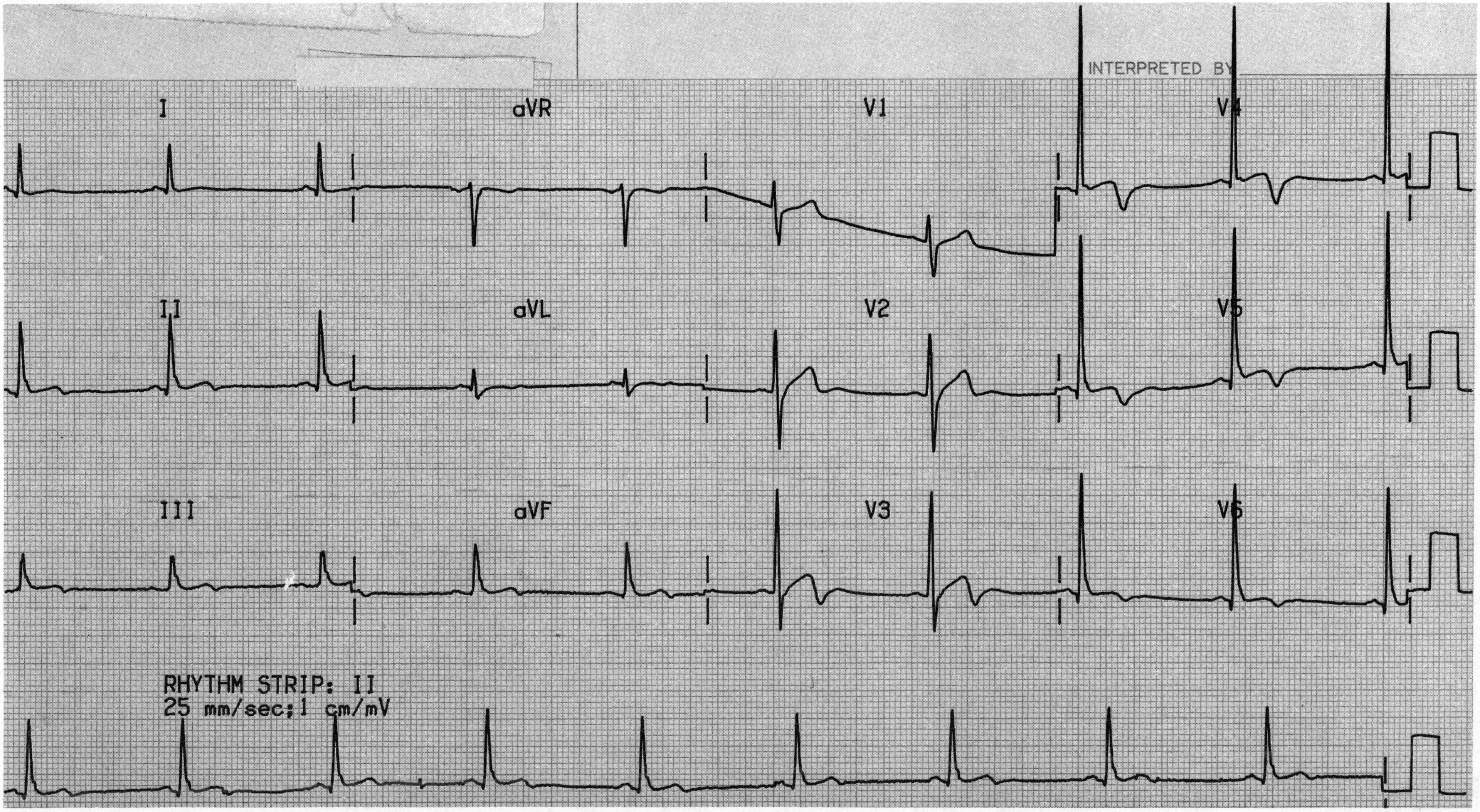

B-19

NARRATIVE INTERPRETATION

Rhythm: **Sinus bradycardia**
Rate: **54**
Intervals: **PR 0.16, QRS 0.08, QT 0.40**
Axis: **+60 degrees**

Abnormalities

Slow heart rate. ST elevation leads II, III, aVF, V2–V6. Biphasic T waves leads II, III, aVF, V2. T-wave inversion leads V3–V6. SV2 + RV5 greater than 35.

Synthesis

Sinus bradycardia. ST-T-segment changes suggesting acute myocardial injury. LVH by voltage criteria.

TEST ANSWERS: 3, 78, 100.

Comment: This patient eventually sustained an anterior, apical, non-Q-wave MI. This ST-T-wave pattern has been shown to be indicative of a high-grade stenosis of the left anterior descending coronary artery. This patient subsequently underwent cardiac catheterization and angioplasty of a proximal 95 percent stenosis of the left anterior descending coronary artery.

REFERENCE: de Zwaan.

B-20

Clinical History

An 89-year-old asymptomatic man.

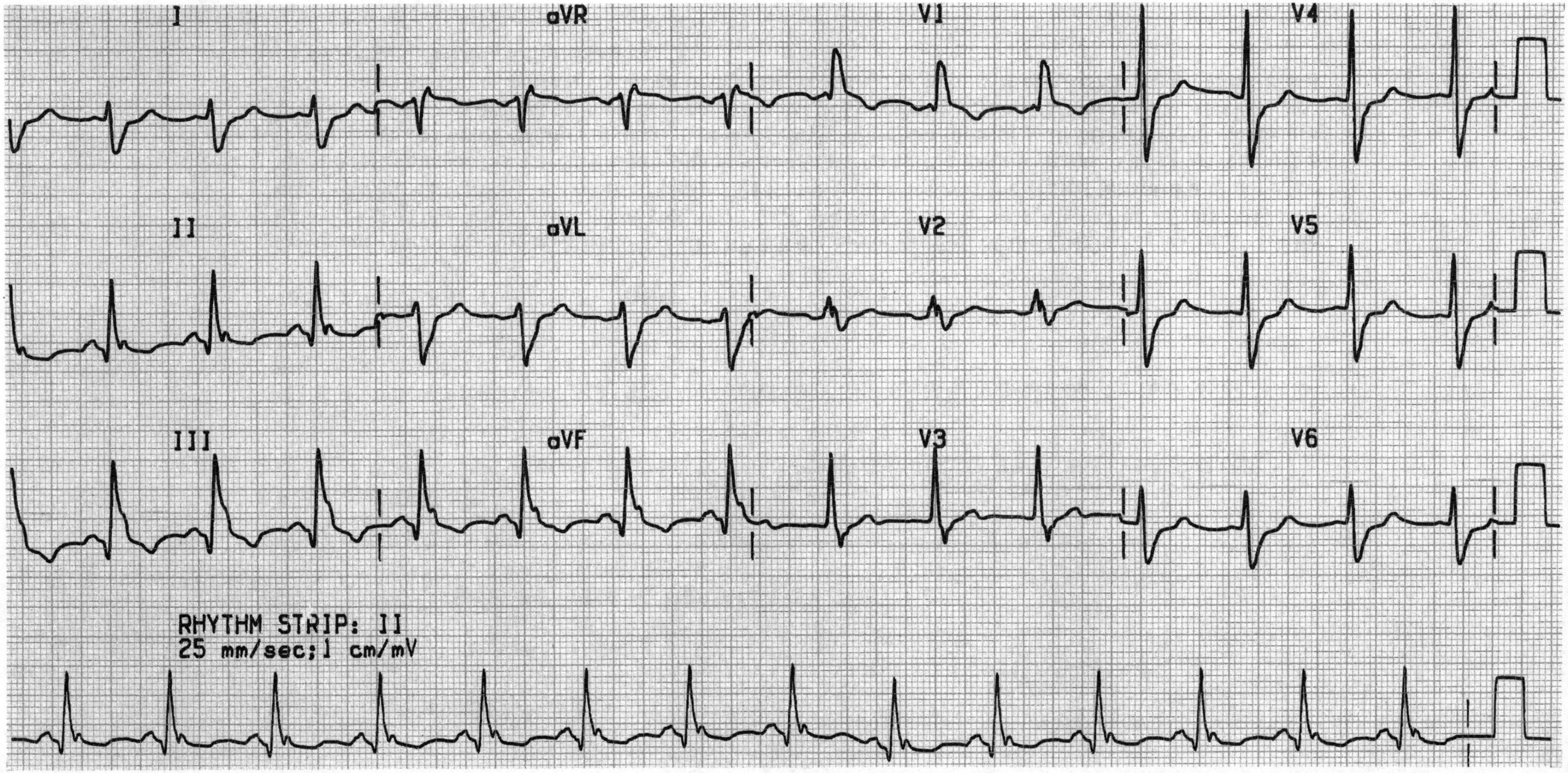

B-20

NARRATIVE INTERPRETATION

Rhythm: Sinus
Rate: 82
Intervals: PR 0.16, QRS 0.14, QT 0.38
Axis: +105 degrees

Abnormalities

Axis rightward of +90 degrees. Broad notched QRS with rSR′ pattern and T-wave inversion lead V1.

Synthesis

Sinus rhythm. RBBB. Associated ST-T-wave abnormalities. Right axis deviation. Left posterior fascicular block.

TEST ANSWERS: 1, 65, 70, 73, 104.

Comment: Remember that in patients with RBBB the initial portion of the QRS complex may still be interpreted in the usual fashion. A rightward axis is clearly evident and suggestive of left posterior fascicular block (LPFB). Also note that in LPFB, the initial forces are directed leftward and superior via the left anterior fascicle, which results in small Q waves in the inferior leads. The Q waves in this example are the result of the conduction abnormality and not an inferior wall MI. These Q waves are less than 0.04 s and are not at least 25 percent of the QRS complex. The ST findings in the inferior leads may raise suspicion of acute myocardial injury but are still consistent with the RBBB alone. The clinical history supported this interpretation.

B-21

Clinical History

A 78-year-old woman seen on routine examination.

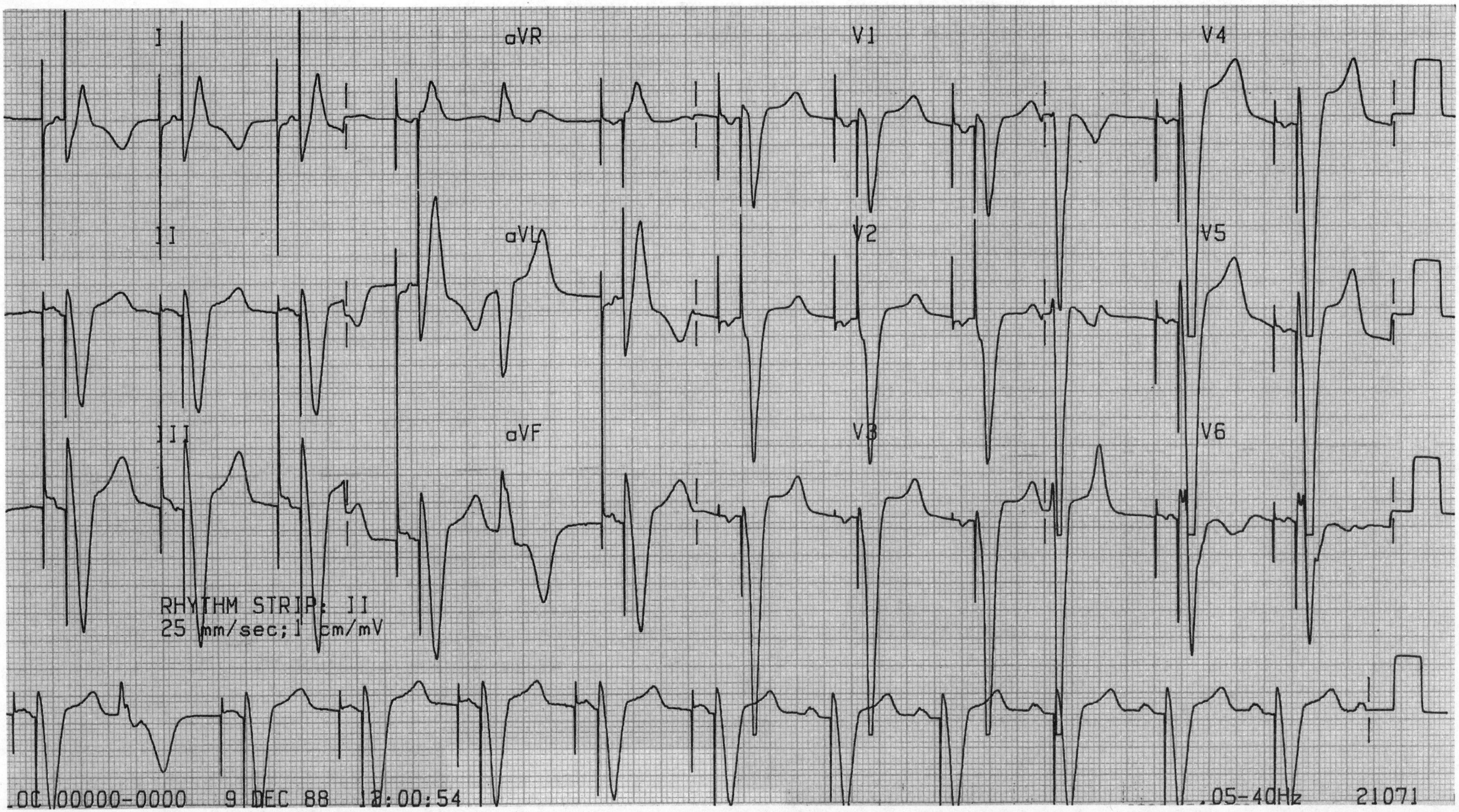

B-21

NARRATIVE INTERPRETATION

Rhythm: Sinus
Rate: 75
Intervals: PR –, QRS –, QT –
Axis: –

Abnormalities

Dual-chamber pacemaker with appropriate atrial sensing and pacing and appropriate ventricular sensing and pacing. DDD mode. VPC.

Synthesis

Sinus rhythm. VPC. Dual-chamber pacemaker functioning in DDD mode with appropriate atrial and ventricular sensing and capture.

TEST ANSWERS: 1, 26, 38.

Comment: This tracing illustrates all the functions of a dual-chamber pacemaker programmed to the DDD mode. The first three letters of the pacemaker code indicate which chamber is paced, which chamber is sensed, and what is the mode of response to sensing. The DDD pacemaker operates in an AV sequential manner; it paces the ventricle as required after either sensing an atrial depolarization or following a paced atrial beat. Note that until the intrinsic P waves appeared in the eighth complex on the rhythm strip, one could not differentiate this DDD pacemaker from one programmed to DVI because there was not yet an indicator of atrial sensing. If possible, one should first analyze the underlying rhythm. Then one should determine which chambers are paced, which are sensed, and the relationship of these factors to each other. Remember, that not all dual-chamber pacemakers are programmed to DDD.

REFERENCE: Garson.

B-22

Clinical History

A 70-year-old man admitted to the CCU.

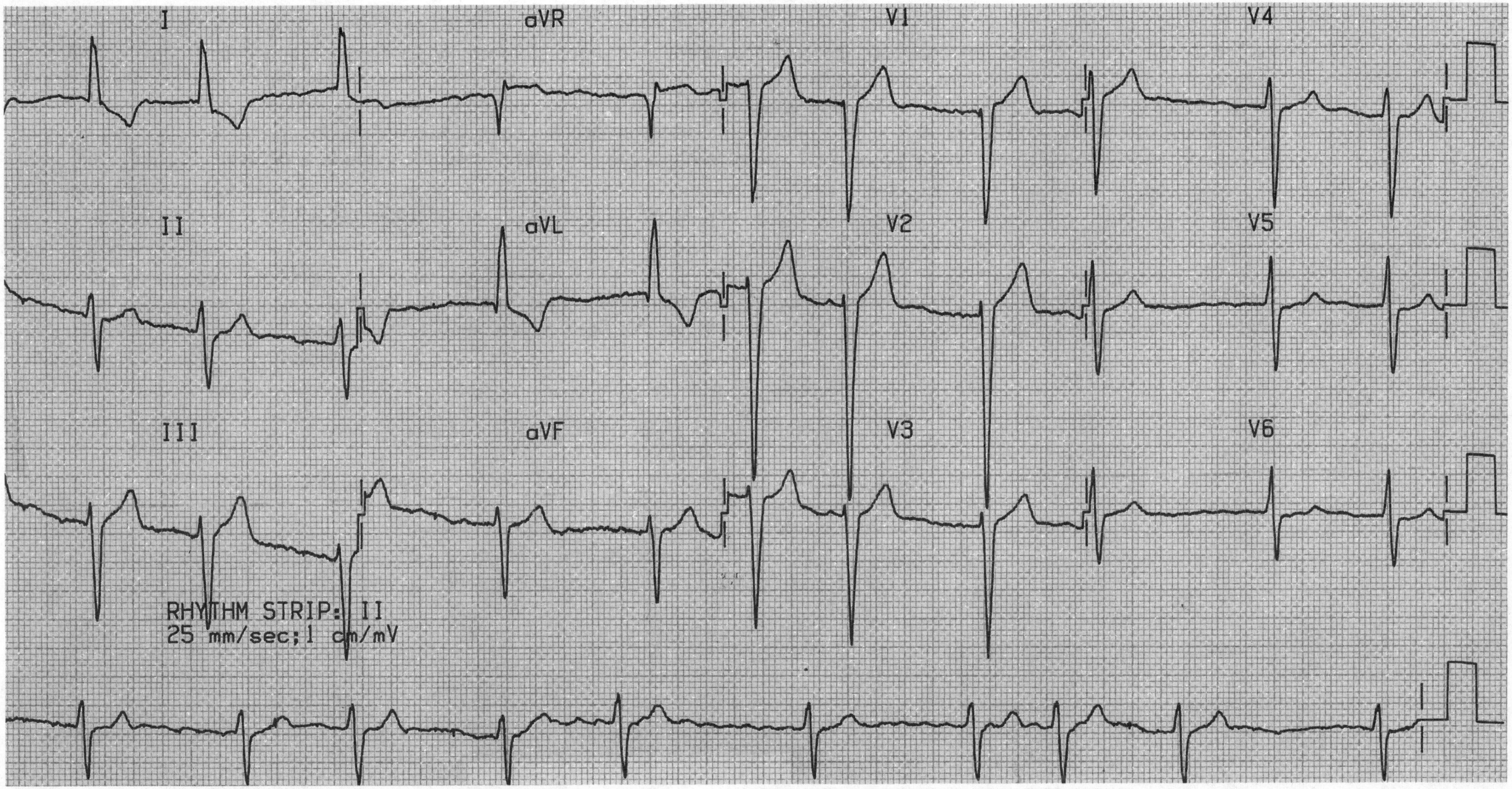

B-22

NARRATIVE INTERPRETATION

Rhythm: Atrial fibrillation
Rate: 60 (average)
Intervals: PR –, QRS 0.11, QT 0.42
Axis: −45 degrees

Abnormalities

Axis leftward of −30 degrees. ST depression leads I, aVL, V5–V6. T-wave inversion leads I, aVL. S wave lead III and R-wave voltage lead V2 greater than 30. R wave V1–V3 less than 3 mm. Prolonged QRS duration.

Synthesis

Atrial fibrillation with a controlled ventricular response. Left axis deviation. Left anterior fascicular block (LAFB). Intraventricular conduction delay. LVH. Associated nonspecific ST-T-wave abnormalities. Poor R-wave progression.

TEST ANSWERS: 20, 51, 64, 66, 72, 76, 78, 103.

Comment: This patient illustrates the combination of LVH and LAFB. The R wave in aVL is 13 mm, which is at the upper limits of normal for a patient with LAFB. The sum of the S wave in lead III and precordial voltage also suggests this finding. The intraventricular conduction delay and ST-T-wave abnormalities are likely to be related to the LVH. This patient demonstrated on echocardiography a marked increase in left ventricular wall thickness secondary to long-standing hypertension. (Also see next two tracings.)

REFERENCES: Gertsch. Willems.

B-23

Clinical History

A 70-year-old man admitted to the CCU.

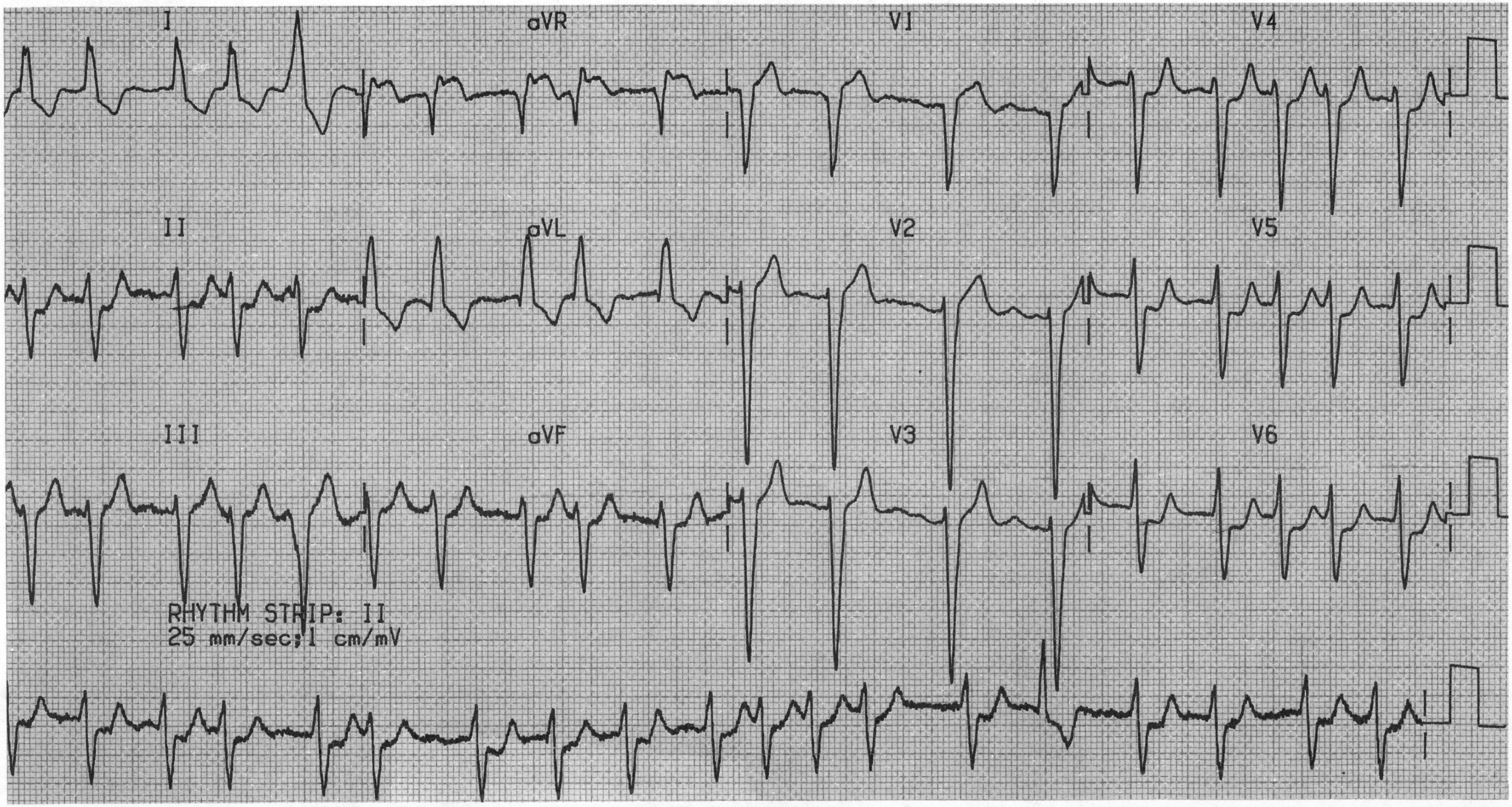

B-23

NARRATIVE INTERPRETATION

Rhythm: **Atrial fibrillation**
Rate: **118 (average)**
Intervals: **PR –, QRS 0.11, QT 0.36**
Axis: **−45 degrees**

Abnormalities

Rapid heart rate. ST depression leads I, II, aVL, aVF, V4–V6. T-wave inversion leads I, aVL. Axis leftward of −30 degrees. R wave V1–V3 less than 3 mm. Prolonged QRS duration. Wide complex beats on rhythm strip, probably ventricular in origin. S lead III + QRS voltage lead V2 greater than 30.

Synthesis

Atrial fibrillation with a rapid ventricular response. VPCs. Left axis deviation. Left anterior fascicular block. Left ventricular hypertrophy. ST-T-wave abnormalities suggestive of myocardial ischemia. Poor R-wave progression. Intraventricular conduction delay.

TEST ANSWERS: 20, 26, 50, 64, 66, 72, 76, 78, 102, (103).

Comment: This is a follow-up to the previous tracing. Compared with the earlier tracing, there are additional ST abnormalities reflective of myocardial ischemia. The ST depression is more prominent in leads I and aVL and is now much more characteristic of myocardial ischemia in leads II and V4–V6 than of LVH. The increase in the heart rate allows the interpreter to consider the AV response as "physiologic." (Also see next tracing.)

B-24

Clinical History

A 70-year-old man admitted to the CCU. He has been administered anti-ischemic agents.

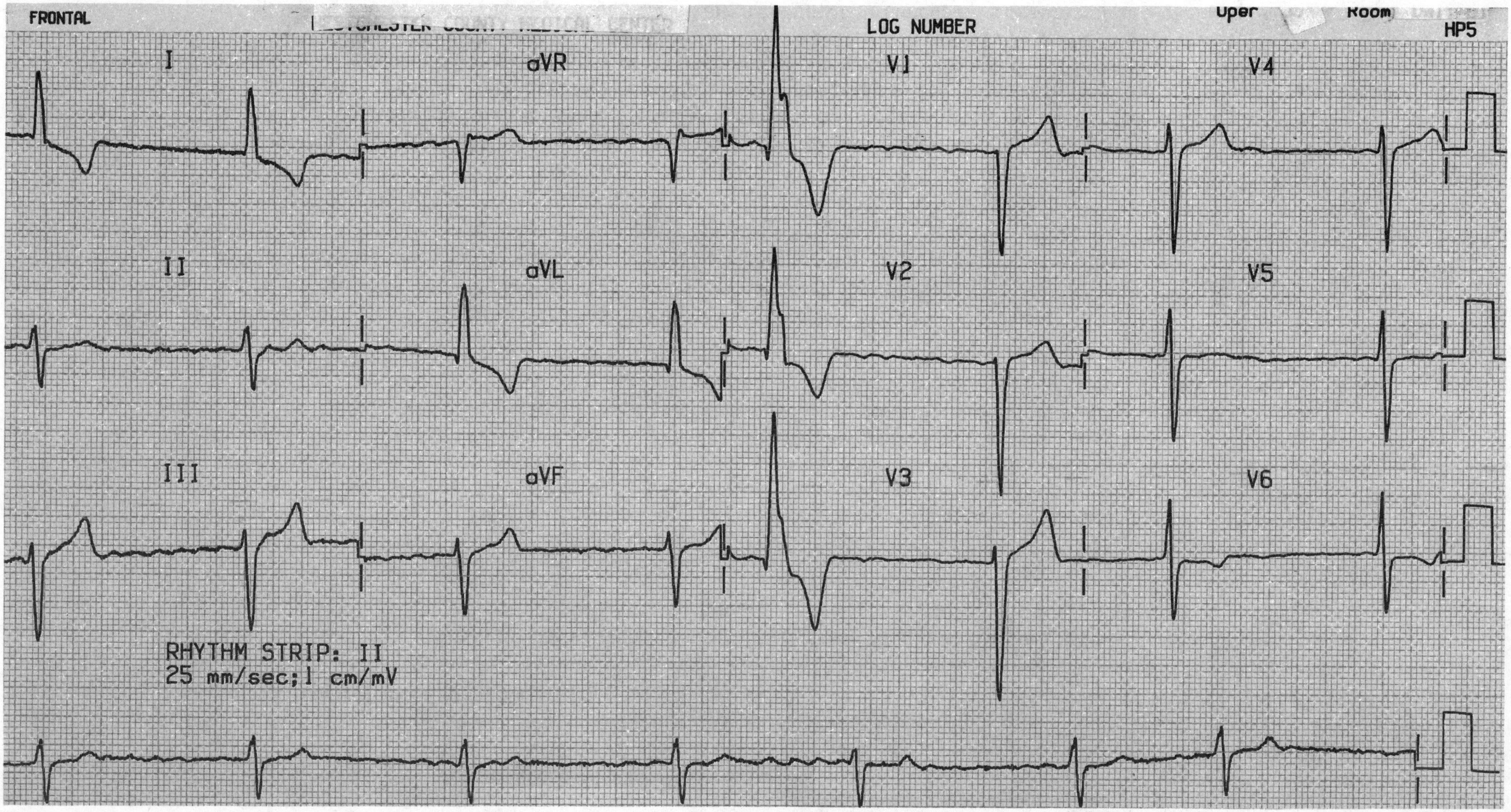

B-24

NARRATIVE INTERPRETATION

Rhythm:	**Atrial fibrillation with high-grade AV block; AV junctional escape rhythm**
Rate:	**40**
Intervals:	**PR –, QRS 0.11, QT 0.46**
Axis:	**−45 degrees**

Abnormalities

Slow heart rate. ST depression leads I, aVL, V6. T-wave inversion leads I, aVL, V6. Axis leftward of −30 degrees. R-wave voltage V1–V3 less than 3 mm. Intraventricular conduction delay. S lead III + QRS voltage lead V3 greater than 30. Prolonged QRS duration. Nonspecific ST-T-wave abnormalities associated with LVH. VPC.

Synthesis

Atrial fibrillation with high-degree AV block. AV junctional escape rhythm. VPC. Left axis deviation. Left anterior fascicular block. LVH. Poor R-wave progression. Intraventricular conduction delay.

TEST ANSWERS: 20, 22, 26, 46, (51), 64, 66, 72, 76, 78, 103, (106).

Comment: This example represents the third tracing in this series. This patient required the combination of beta blockers and diltiazem to control myocardial ischemia. The result on the cardiac conduction system was high-grade AV block with an AV junctional escape rhythm. The majority of the complexes have the identical RR interval and indicate a junctional escape focus. Complete AV block is not evident as the fifth and seventh complexes occur earlier than expected and reflect AV conduction of the atrial impulses. It is important to remember that this rhythm disturbance, often characteristic of digitalis toxicity, is not limited to patients treated with digoxin.

B-25

Clinical History

A 76-year-old man with valvular heart disease.

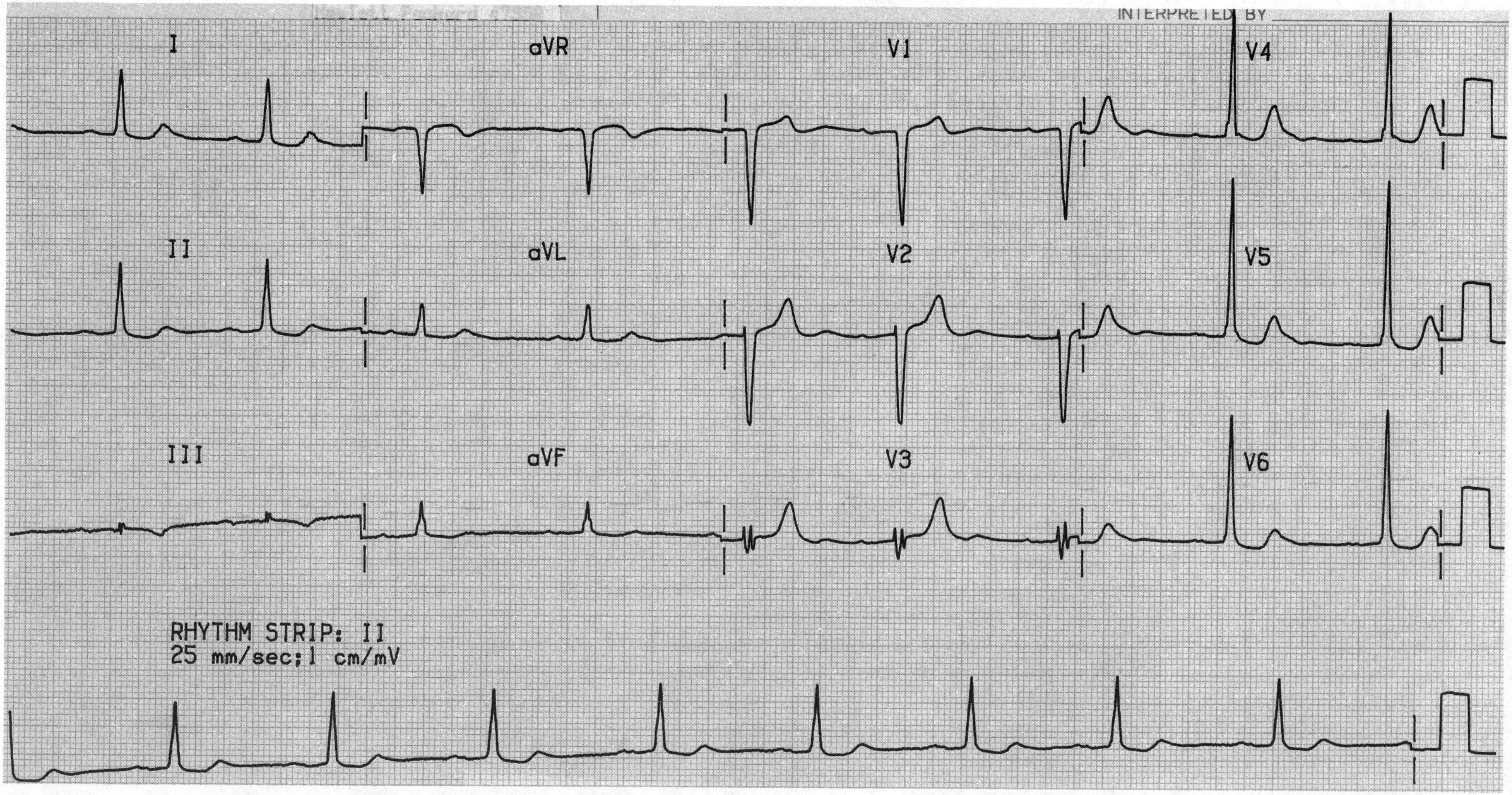

B-25

NARRATIVE INTERPRETATION

Rhythm: **Sinus bradycardia with first-degree AV block**
Rate: **55**
Intervals: **PR 0.26, QRS 0.10, QT 0.44**
Axis: **+30 degrees**

Abnormalities
Slow heart rate. Prolonged PR interval. Absent septal Q waves with slightly prolonged QRS interval and slurred initial upstroke in leads V4–V6. ST depression leads I, II, aVL, aVF, V4–V6. SV2 + RV5 greater than 35. P-wave duration greater than 0.12 s.

Synthesis
Sinus bradycardia. First-degree AV block. Nonspecific atrial abnormality. Incomplete LBBB. LVH by voltage criteria. ST-T-wave abnormalities associated with ventricular hypertrophy and/or conduction abnormality.

TEST ANSWERS: 3, 42, 62, 75, 78, 103, 104.

Comment: This patient demonstrates the frequent association of LVH and incomplete LBBB. Standard voltage criteria for LVH may be used in the presence of incomplete LBBB. The concomitant conduction abnormality is suggested most by absent septal Q waves and a slurred upstroke in the left precordial leads. Both incomplete LBBB and LVH may result in prolongation of the QRS complex and ST-T-wave abnormalities. An additional finding in this tracing is nonspecific atrial abnormality. This may be diagnosed when there is a prolongation of the P wave without specific criteria for left or right atrial abnormality.

REFERENCES: Schamroth. Barold.

B-26

Clinical History

A 76-year-old man with valvular heart disease.

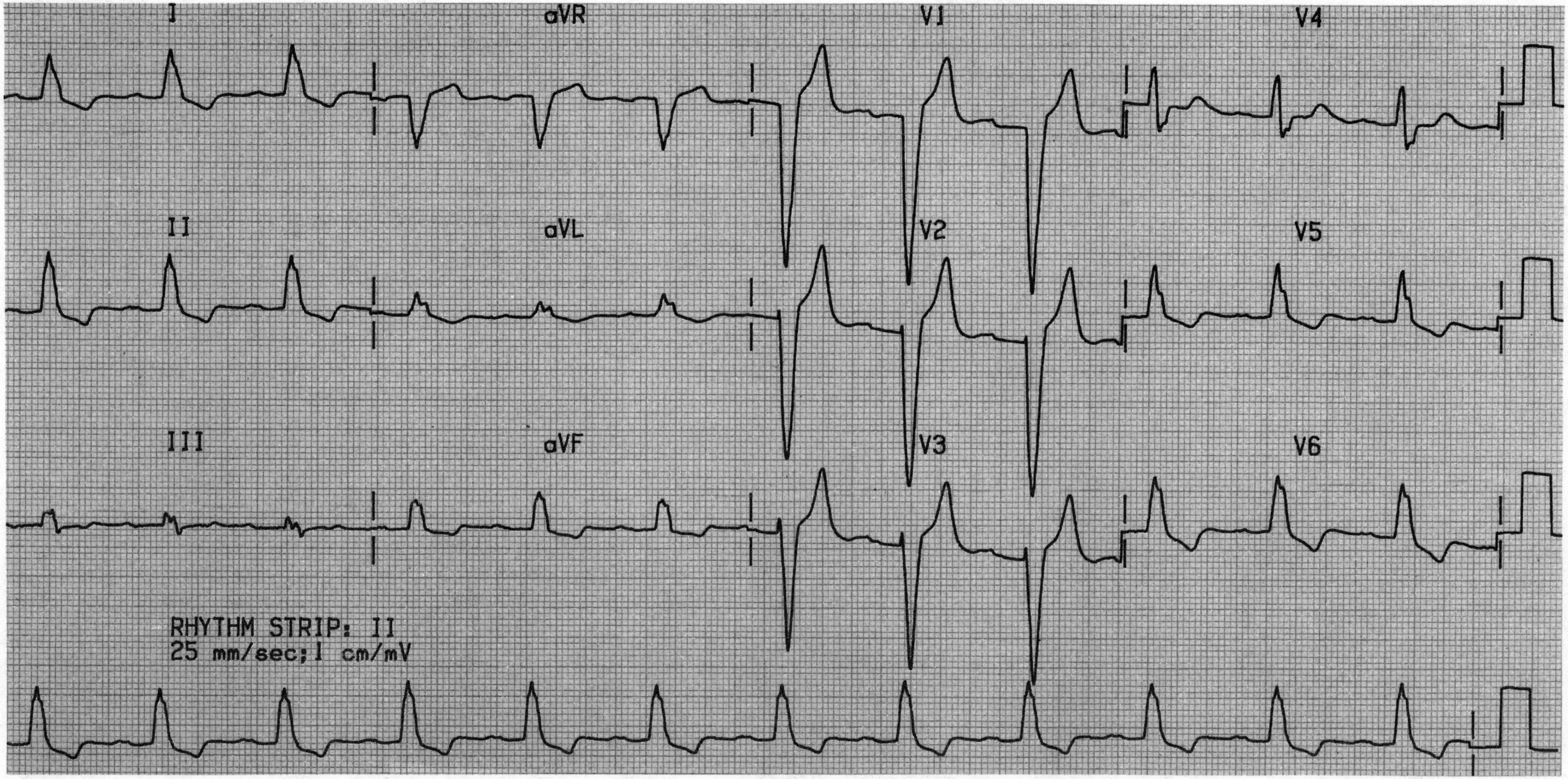

B-26

NARRATIVE INTERPRETATION

Rhythm: **Sinus with first-degree AV block**
Rate: **72**
Intervals: **PR 0.26, QRS 0.14, QT 0.36**
Axis: **+30 degrees**

Abnormalities

Prolonged PR interval. P-wave duration greater than 0.12 s. Broad, notched QRS with ST depression and T-wave inversion leads I, aVL, V5–V6.

Synthesis

Sinus rhythm. First-degree AV block. Nonspecific atrial abnormality. LBBB with associated ST-T-wave abnormalities.

TEST ANSWERS: 1, 42, 62, 74, 104.

Comment: This tracing may be compared with the previous example from the same patient. The incomplete LBBB has now become complete. Standard voltage criteria for LVH, which may be used with incomplete LBBB, are now invalid. Some authors have suggested that LVH may still be diagnosed with complete LBBB if the sum of the voltage of the S wave in lead V2 and the R wave in lead V5 is greater than 45 mm. In this example, the precordial voltage actually decreases when complete LBBB develops.

REFERENCES: Friedman p 196. Klein, RC. Kafka. Vandenberg.

B-27

Clinical History

A 61-year-old obese man with dyspnea.

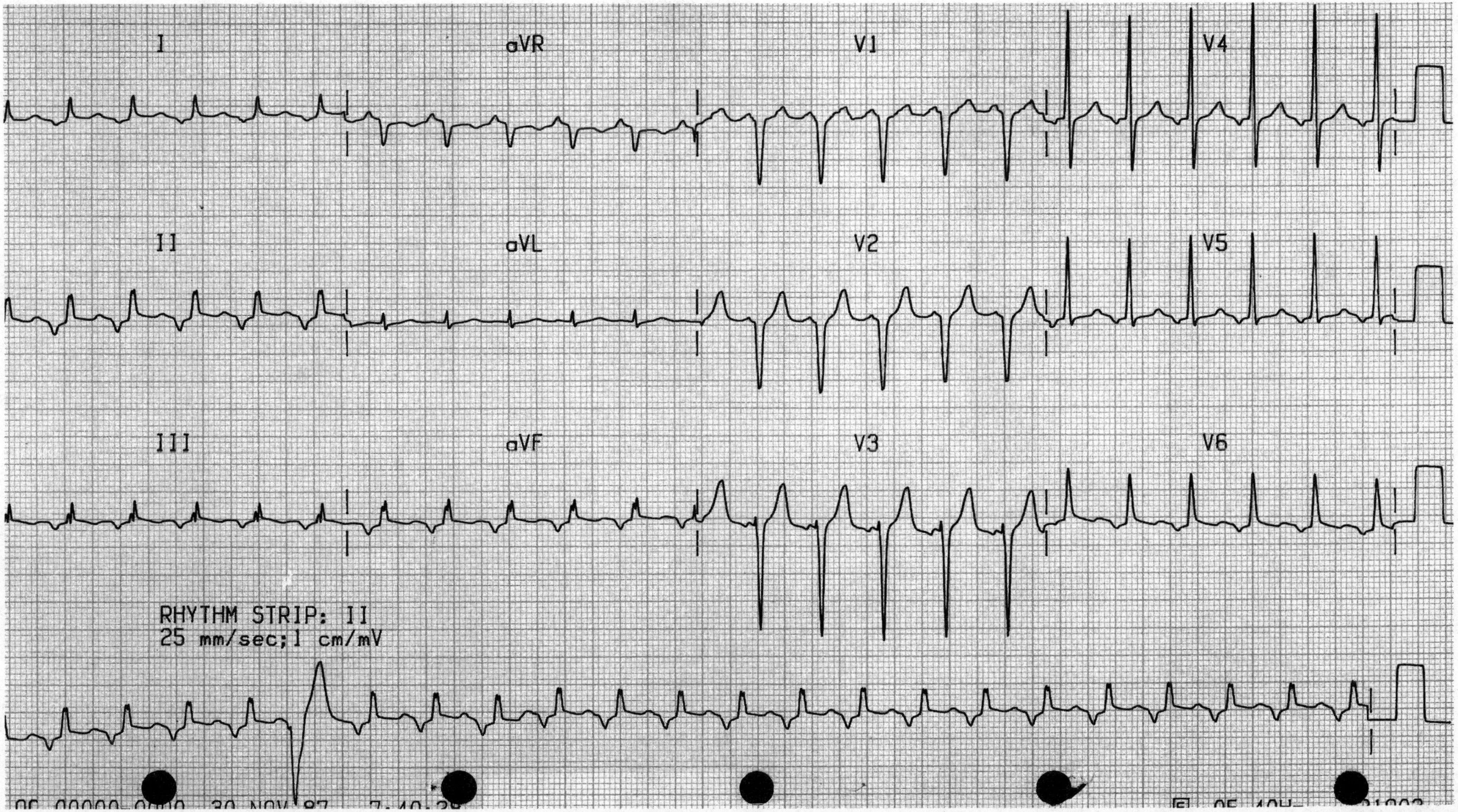

B-27

NARRATIVE INTERPRETATION

Rhythm:	**Accelerated AV junctional rhythm**
Rate:	**130**
Intervals:	**PR 0.12, QRS 0.08, QT 0.28**
Axis:	**+45 degrees**

Abnormalities

Inverted P waves II, III, aVF with PR interval at lower limit of normal. QRS voltage in limb leads less than 6 mm. ST elevation leads I, II, III, aVF, V6. R-wave voltage less than 3 mm leads V1–V3. VPC.

Synthesis

Accelerated AV junctional rhythm. VPC. Low-voltage limb leads. Poor R-wave progression. ST abnormalities suggestive of myocardial injury.

TEST ANSWERS: (9), 23, 26, 66, 67, 100.

Comment: Accelerated AV junctional rhythm, otherwise known as *nonparoxysmal junctional tachycardia,* is characterized by an increase in the rate of discharge of the AV junction to 70 to 130 beats per minute. It is usually seen in patients with underlying cardiac disease such as acute MI, COPD, myocarditis, or after cardiac surgery. This patient was hypoxic on the basis of COPD and marked obesity. In addition to the rhythm disturbance, other findings secondary to these conditions were low voltage in the limb leads and poor R-wave progression. Obesity and pulmonary disease can cause these findings alone or in concert. The ST-segment abnormalities are suggestive of early myocardial injury of the inferior and lateral walls but are not yet diagnostic of acute Q-wave MI. Note in this example that the PR interval is 0.12 s; therefore, an accelerated ectopic atrial, rather than AV junctional, rhythm cannot be excluded.

B-28

Clinical History

A 68-year-old asymptomatic man.

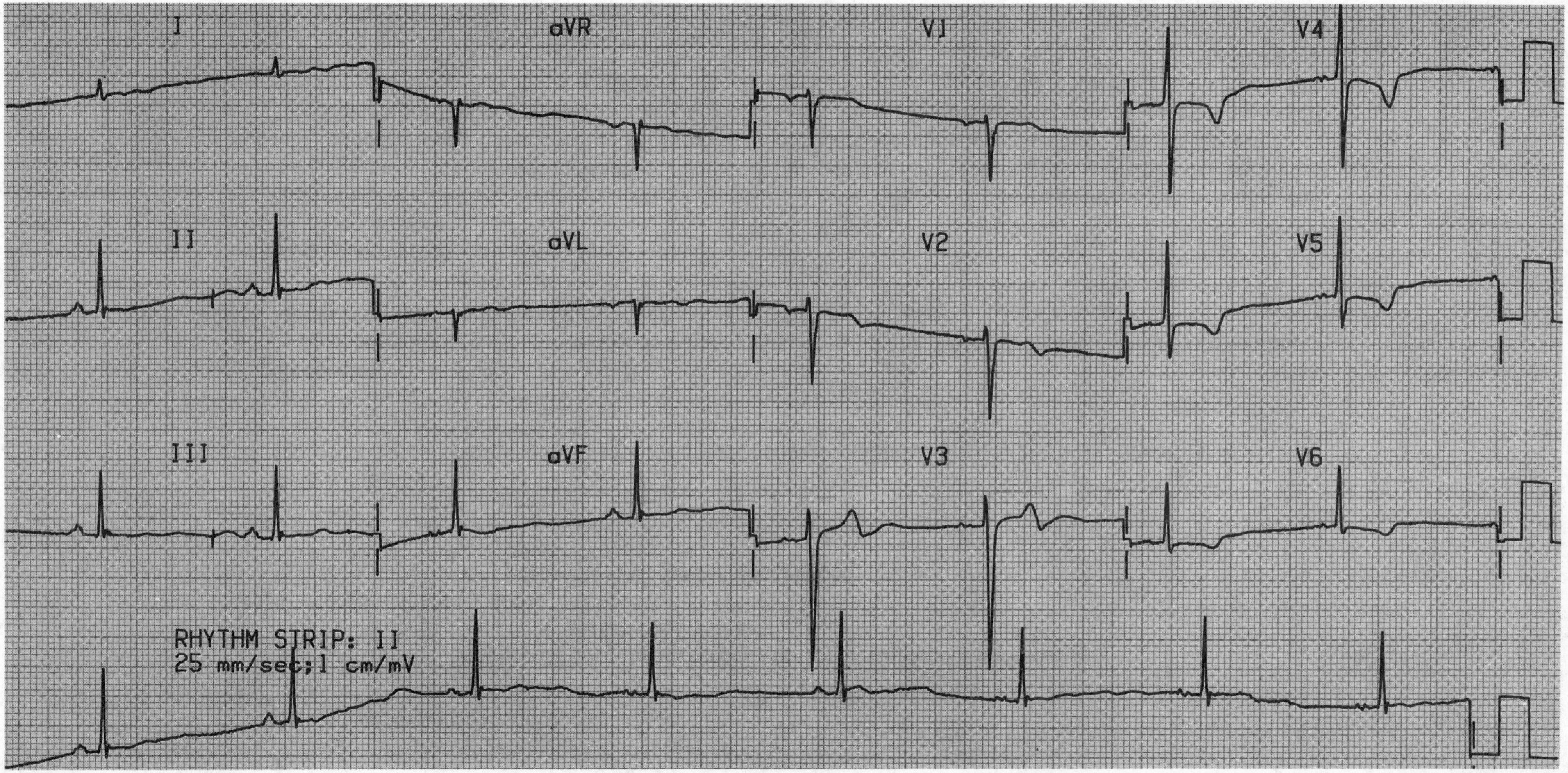

B-28

NARRATIVE INTERPRETATION

Rhythm:	**Sinus bradycardia with wandering atrial pacemaker within the SA node**
Rate:	**47**
Intervals:	**PR 0.16, QRS 0.08, QT 0.40**
Axis:	**+75 degrees**

Abnormalities

Slow heart rate. Changing P-wave morphology. T-wave inversion leads V2–V6. Prominent U wave lead V3.

Synthesis

Sinus bradycardia with wandering atrial pacemaker within the SA node. Nonspecific T-wave abnormalities. Prominent U waves.

TEST ANSWERS: 3, 5, 106, 110.

Comment: Wandering atrial pacemaker within the SA node refers to a change in the origin of conduction while a sinus mechanism is maintained. This is diagnosed when there are differing P-wave morphologies and minimal, if any change in the PR interval. The pacemaker may also "wander" to the AV junction, which would produce inverted P waves in leads II, III, and aVF with a shortening of the PR interval. It is important to search for an artifactual change in the P wave caused by respiratory variation. In this example, the abrupt change in P-wave morphology in the fourth through sixth beats on the rhythm strip indicates that true wandering atrial pacemaker is likely.

REFERENCE: Friedman p 455.

B-29

Clinical History

A 44-year-old man with palpitations.

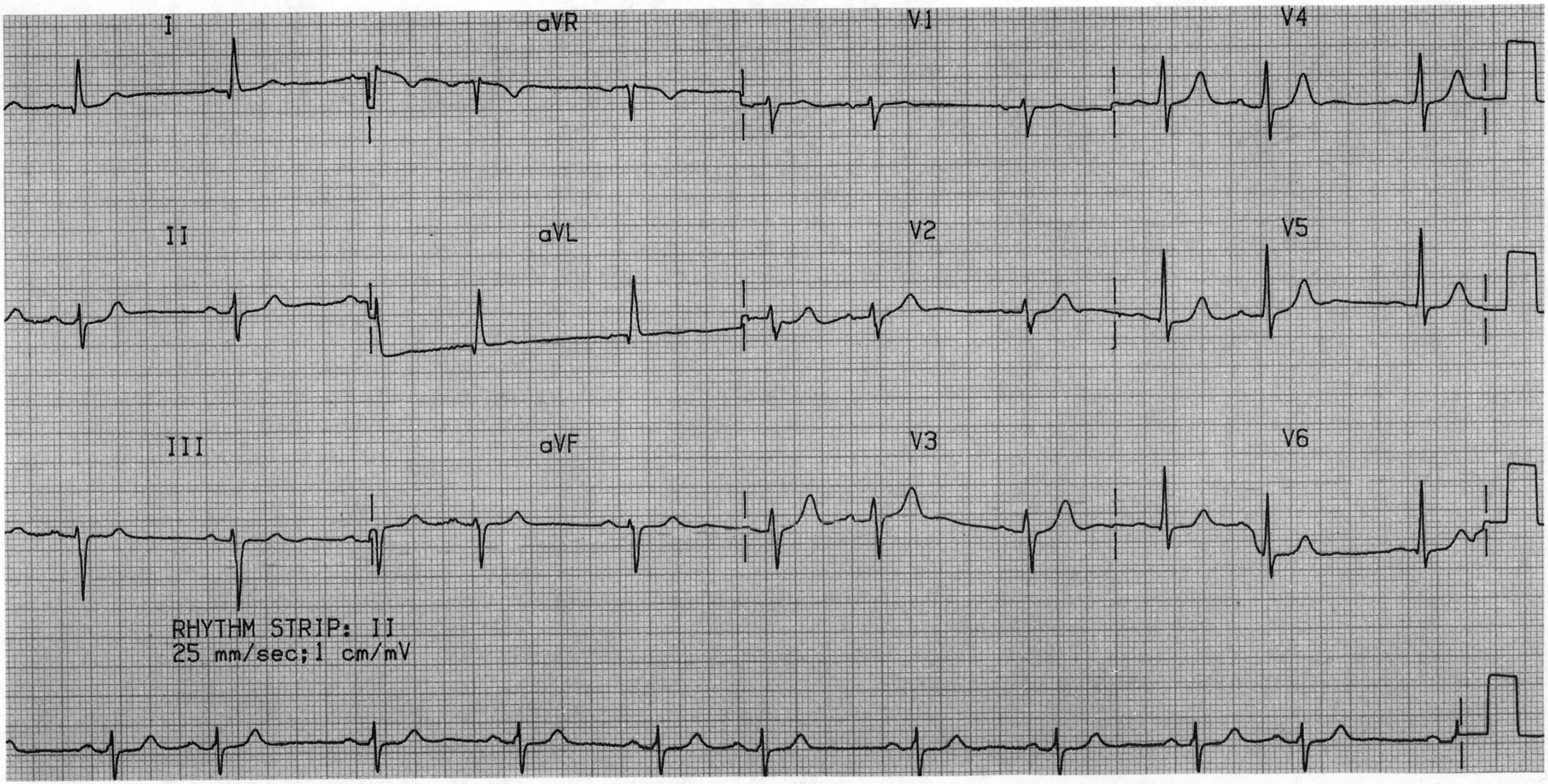

B-29

NARRATIVE INTERPRETATION

Rhythm: **Sinus**
Rate: **64**
Intervals: **PR 0.16, QRS 0.09, QT 0.40**
Axis: **−45 degrees**

Abnormalities
APCs. Axis leftward of −30 degrees.

Synthesis
Sinus rhythm. APCs. Left axis deviation. Left anterior fascicular block.

TEST ANSWERS: 1, 10, 64, 72.

Comment: Atrial premature complexes (APCs) are frequently observed in normal persons. Studies of healthy airmen found that 0.7 to 3 percent had atrial premature complexes on routine 12-lead electrocardiograms. One study using 24 h Holter monitoring of 50 male medical students found that 56 percent had APCs. Frequent atrial extrasystoles may also be related to excessive fatigue, alcohol, or caffeine. They may also be related to COPD, valvular heart disease, or thyrotoxicosis.

REFERENCE: Barrett.

B-30

Clinical History

A 62-year-old man with lightheadedness.

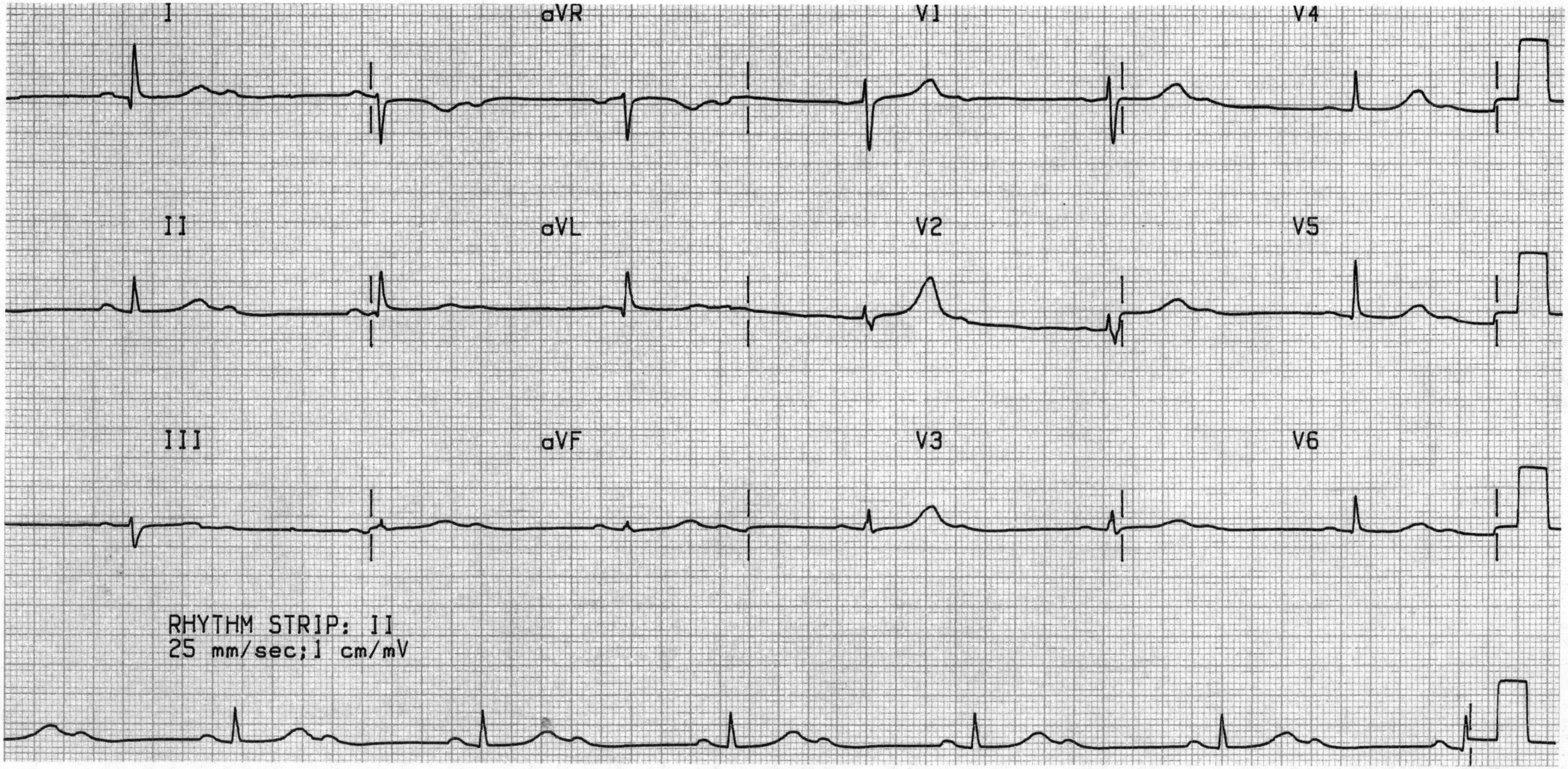

B-30

NARRATIVE INTERPRETATION

Rhythm:	**Sinus with 2:1 AV block**
Rate:	**Atrial rate 72, ventricular rate 36**
Intervals:	**PR 0.20 (in conducted beats), QRS 0.08, QT 0.52**
Axis:	**+15 degrees**

Abnormalities
2:1 AV conduction.

Synthesis
Sinus rhythm with second-degree AV block, 2:1. Otherwise within normal limits.

TEST ANSWERS: 1, 45.

Comment: The reader should note that it is not possible from the surface electrocardiogram to distinguish between Mobitz type I (Wenckebach) and Mobitz type II, 2:1 AV block. Type I block is most often located in the AV node, whereas type II block with a narrow QRS complex is most likely to be in the His bundle. In order to confirm a Wenckebach sequence, at least two cycles of PR prolongation are required to demonstrate the progressively prolonged PR interval before the dropped beat occurs. When every other beat is nonconducted, as in the current example, the opportunity to observe gradual prolongation of the PR interval simply does not exist. A number of clues can help the clinician to distinguish these two entities. In type I (intranodal) block, atropine will generally improve and carotid sinus pressure worsen conduction. In type II (intra-His) block, the opposite effects will generally occur.

REFERENCES: Zipes. Langendorf. Mangiardi.

B-31

Clinical History

A 50-year-old man with chest discomfort.

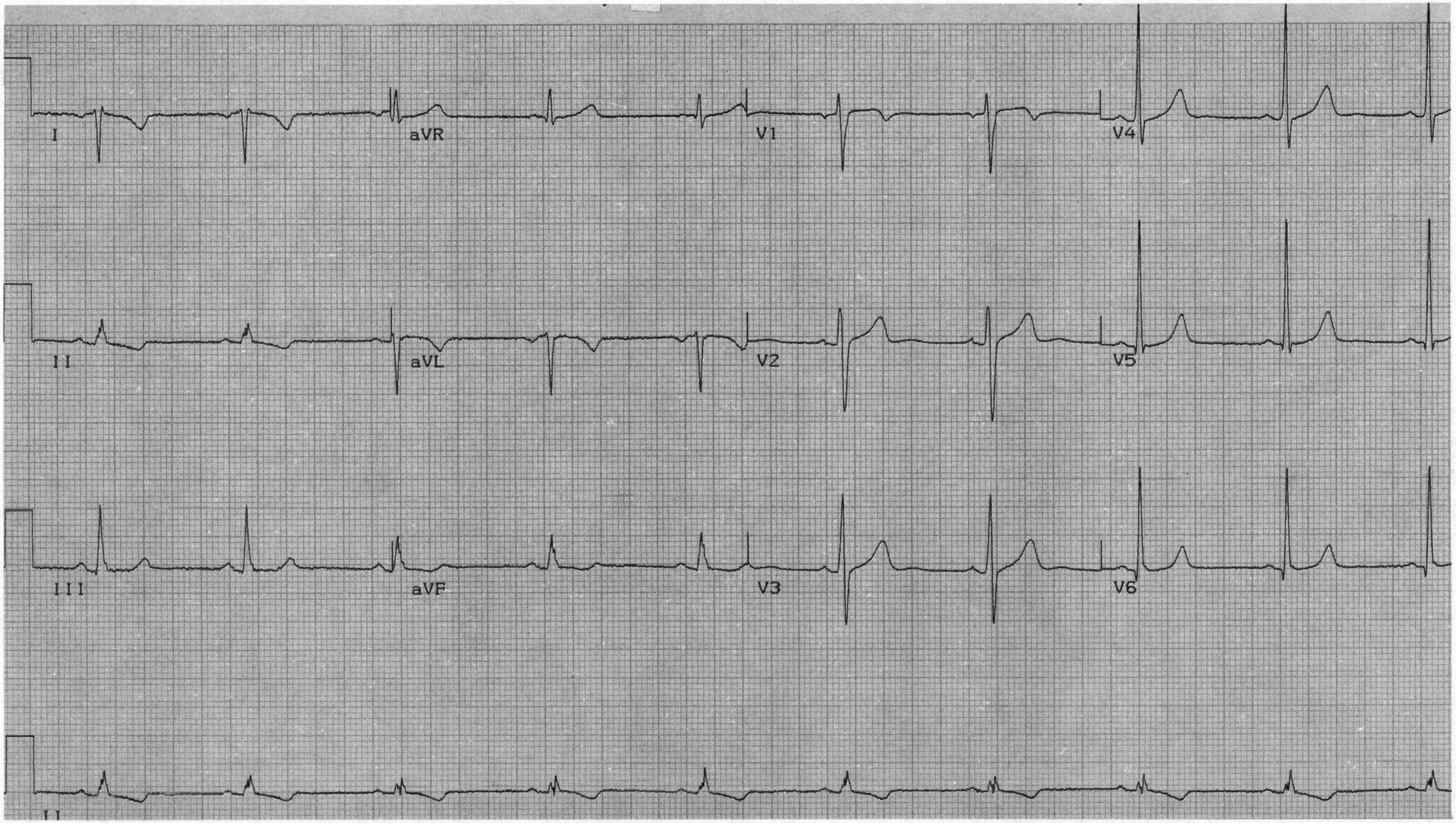

B-31

NARRATIVE INTERPRETATION

Rhythm:	**Sinus bradycardia**
Rate:	**57**
Intervals:	**PR 0.16, QRS 0.08, QT 0.40**
Axis:	**+45 degrees (corrected)**

Abnormalities
Slow heart rate. Right-left arm electrode reversal. Slight ST depression lead II (actual lead III). T-wave inversion lead II (actual lead III). T biphasic lead aVF.

Synthesis
Incorrect electrode placement (right-left arm reversal). Sinus bradycardia. Nonspecific ST-T-wave abnormalities.

TEST ANSWERS: 3, 106, 112.

Comment: This tracing demonstrates a common misplacement of the recording electrodes. The right and left arm electrodes have been reversed. Accordingly, lead I is recorded with reversed polarity. Lead II appears as lead III normally would and vice versa. Similarly, the configuration of leads aVL and aVR is reversed. Lead aVF is unaffected and may be interpreted normally. The precordial leads are unaltered, which helps to distinguish arm electrode reversal from dextrocardia. Patients with dextrocardia demonstrate a reversed configuration in both the limb and chest leads.

B-32

Clinical History

An 88-year-old woman in the CCU. Medications include digoxin.

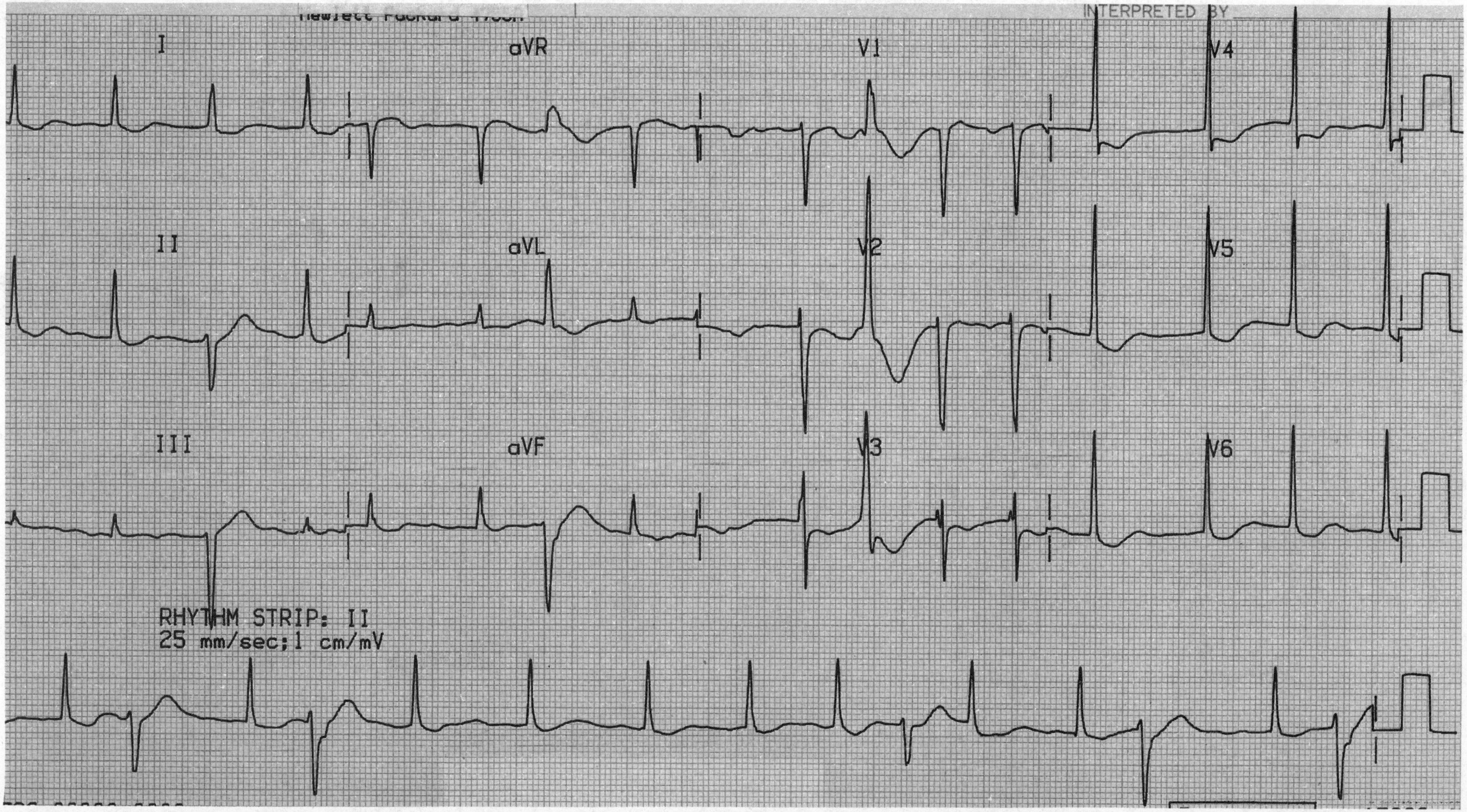

B-32

NARRATIVE INTERPRETATION

Rhythm: **Atrial fibrillation**
Rate: **86 (average)**
Intervals: **PR –, QRS 0.08, QT 0.38**
Axis: **+45 degrees**

Abnormalities

Multiform VPCs. ST depression leads I, II, aVL, aVF, V3–V6. SV2 + RV5 greater than 35.

Synthesis

Atrial fibrillation with a controlled ventricular response. Multiform VPCs. LVH by voltage criteria. Associated, diffuse ST-T-wave abnormalities.

TEST ANSWERS: 20, 27, 51, 78, 103.

Comment: Various criteria have been proposed to differentiate wide complex beats of ventricular origin from those of supraventricular origin with aberrant conduction in patients with atrial fibrillation. Most have been found lacking in sensitivity and specificity. A number of criteria for analysis are present in this example and demonstrate their pitfalls. This patient had an underlying rhythm of atrial fibrillation with wide complex ectopic beats. In this patient, a ventricular origin for these wide beats was confirmed by observing identical complexes when the patient was in sinus rhythm. The wide beats demonstrate a right bundle branch pattern with an rR′ configuration in lead V1. This particular pattern does not allow a firm prediction of the origin of the beats. It has been suggested that fixed coupling of the ectopic beats favors ventricular ectopy, whereas variable coupling favors aberrancy. Fixed coupling is present in this example; however, this has been shown to be unreliable. It has also been suggested that a long pause after the wide complex beat favors ventricular ectopy. As seen in this example, ventricular premature complexes may occur with or without a subsequent pause.

REFERENCES: Marriott. Wellens. Gulamhusein.

B-33

Clinical History

An 88-year-old woman in the CCU. Medications include digoxin and quinidine sulfate.

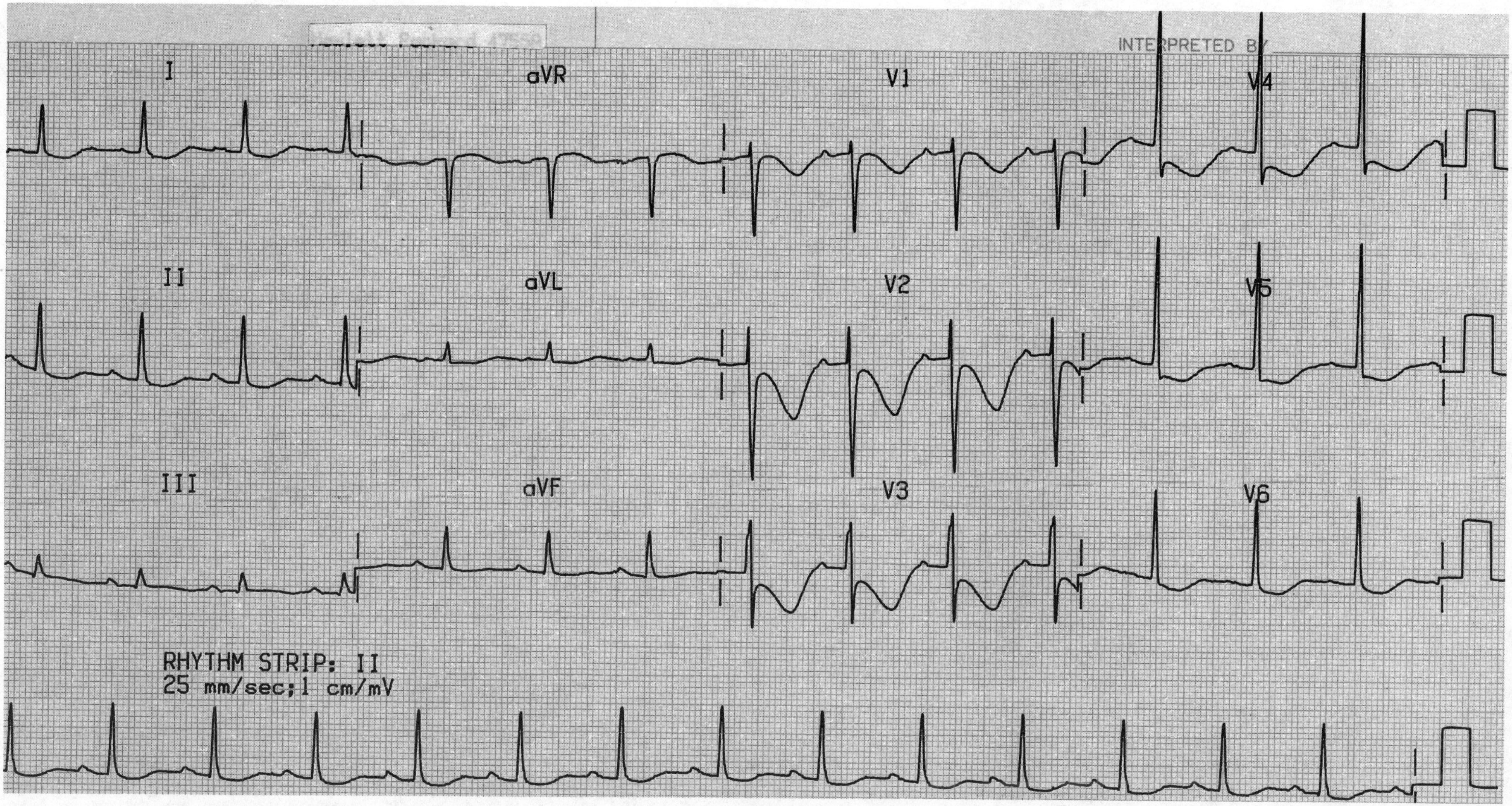

B-33

NARRATIVE INTERPRETATION

Rhythm:	**Sinus**
Rate:	**84**
Intervals	**PR 0.20, QRS 0.08, QT 0.50**
Axis:	**+45 degrees**

Abnormalities

ST depression leads I, II, aVL, aVF, V2–V6. T-wave inversion leads V1–V6. SV2 + RV5 greater than 35. Prolonged QT interval for heart rate.

Synthesis

Sinus rhythm. Prolonged QTc. LVH by voltage criteria. Diffuse, nonspecific ST-T-wave abnormalities.

TEST ANSWERS: 1, 78, (103), 106, 109.

Comment: The patient from the previous example has been treated with digoxin and quinidine, with conversion of atrial fibrillation to sinus rhythm. There is evidence of quinidine toxicity by virtue of marked prolongation of the QT interval. One cannot be certain that some of the QT interval prolongation is not secondary to measurement of the U wave. Nevertheless, the clinician must be alerted to quinidine toxicity in such patients.

REFERENCE: Chou p 470.

B-34

Clinical History

A 64-year-old man seen in preoperative evaluation.

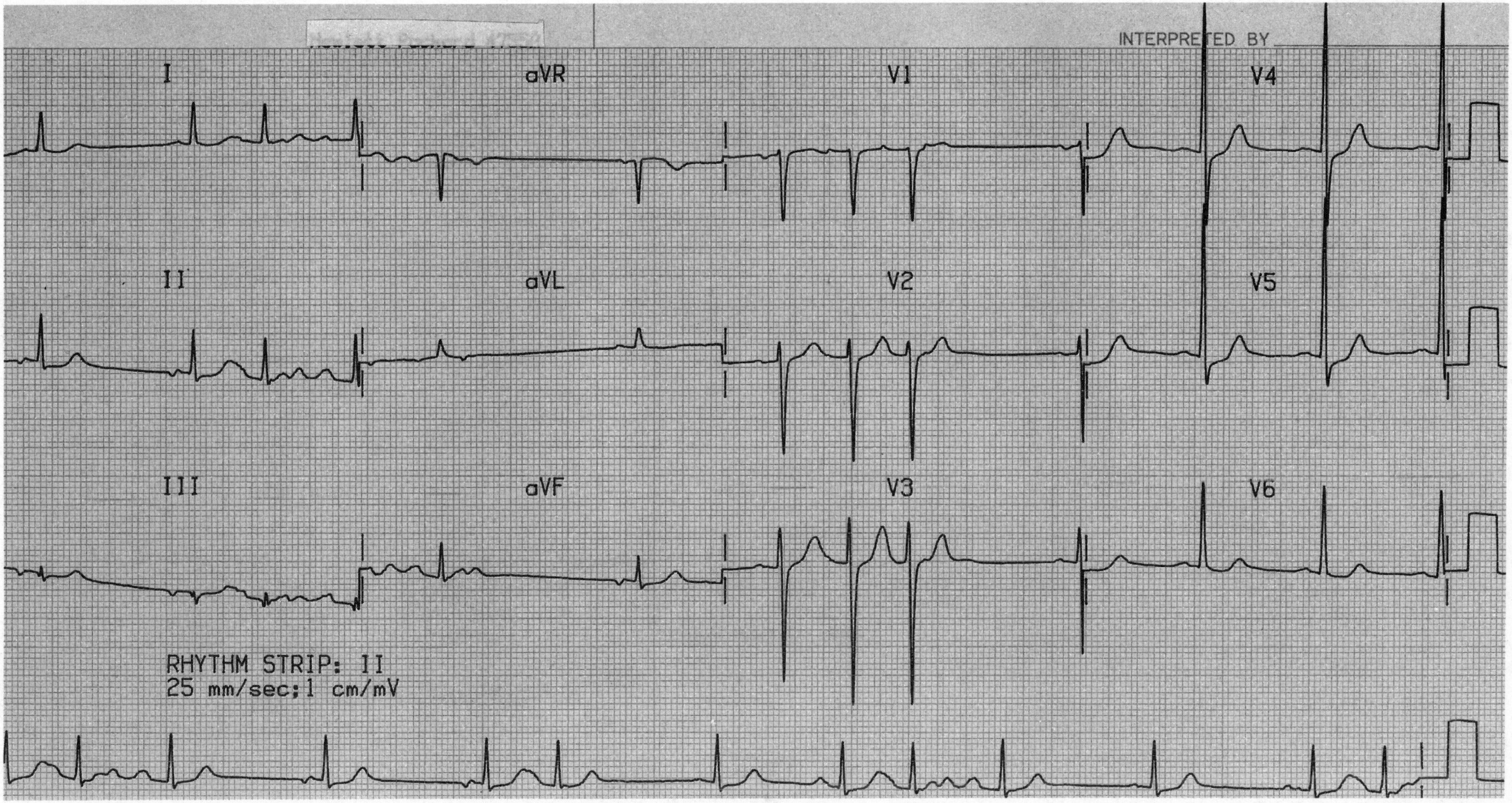

B-34

NARRATIVE INTERPRETATION

Rhythm: **Sinus with multifocal atrial rhythm**
Rate: **70**
Intervals: **PR 0.16, QRS 0.08, QT 0.36**
Axis: **+30 degrees**

Abnormalities

Frequent APCs, normally conducted. Nonconducted APC. ST depression leads I, II, aVL, aVF, V4–V6. SV2 + RV5 greater than 35.

Synthesis

Sinus rhythm with multifocal atrial rhythm. LVH by voltage criteria. Associated ST-T-wave abnormalities.

TEST ANSWERS: 1, (10), (12), 13, 78, 103.

Comment: This tracing demonstrates sinus rhythm in only the last four complexes (the fourth complex from the end is obscured but is likely to be a sinus beat). In the remainder of the tracing, and the entire rhythm strip, there is no discernible sinus mechanism. Multiple atrial foci are evident. Accordingly, the rhythm may be classified as a multifocal, or chaotic, atrial rhythm. Sinus rhythm with frequent APCs is an alternative. The fifth complex of the 12-lead tracing shows an ectopic beat that is nonconducted. The complexes with inverted P waves in leads II, III, and aVF are most likely low atrial rather than junctional in origin because the PR interval is at least 0.12 s or more. One cannot completely exclude the possibility that these beats are junctional with antegrade block.

REFERENCE: Chou p 325.

B-35

Clinical History

A 71-year-old woman in the CCU.

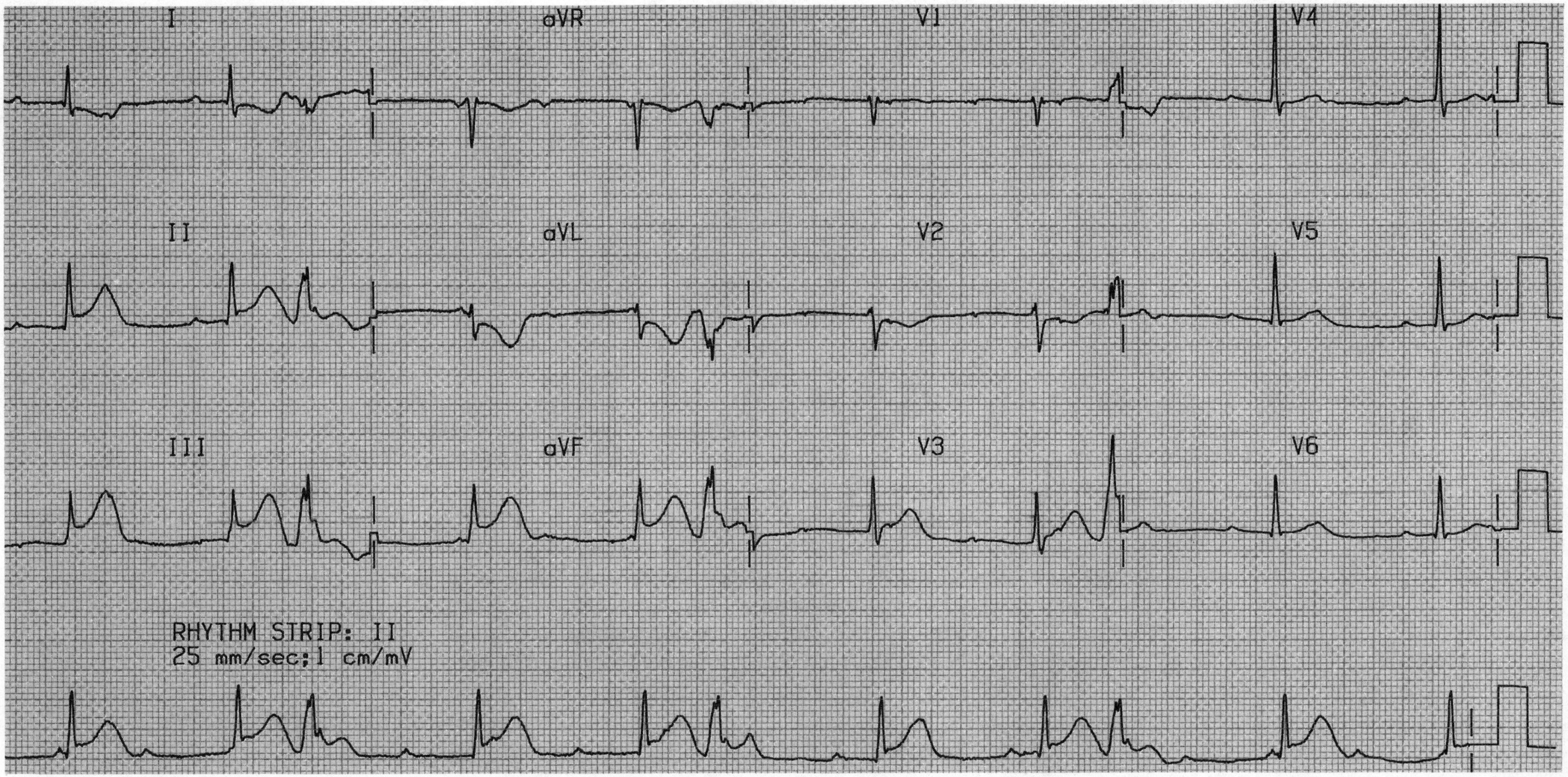

B-35

NARRATIVE INTERPRETATION

Rhythm:	**Sinus with third-degree AV block; AV junctional escape rhythm**
Rate:	**Sinus rate 100; AV junctional rate 53**
Intervals:	**PR –, QRS 0.08, QT 0.38**
Axis:	**+60 degrees**

Abnormalities
P waves fail to conduct to ventricles. VPCs. ST elevation leads II, III, aVF. ST depression leads I, aVL, V2. T-wave inversion leads I, aVL.

Synthesis
Sinus rhythm with complete (third-degree) AV block. AV junctional escape rhythm. VPCs. Acute inferior wall MI with ST-T-wave abnormalities of acute myocardial injury. Nonspecific ST-T-wave abnormalities consistent with MI or reciprocal change.

TEST ANSWERS: 1, 22, 26, 47, 91, 100, 101.

Comment: Various degrees of AV block may accompany acute inferior wall MI. Complete AV block is seen in 3 to 7 percent of patients who have not been treated with thrombolytic therapy. In patients with inferior wall MI, the conduction abnormality is a result of profound vagal influences. If the escape rhythm is satisfactory and there is no hemodynamic compromise, most patients will not require temporary pacemaker therapy. The rhythm disturbance generally resolves within a number of days, although an occasional patient may require 2 weeks to regain normal conduction.

REFERENCE: Nicod.

B-36

Clinical History

A 70-year-old man admitted with chest pain.

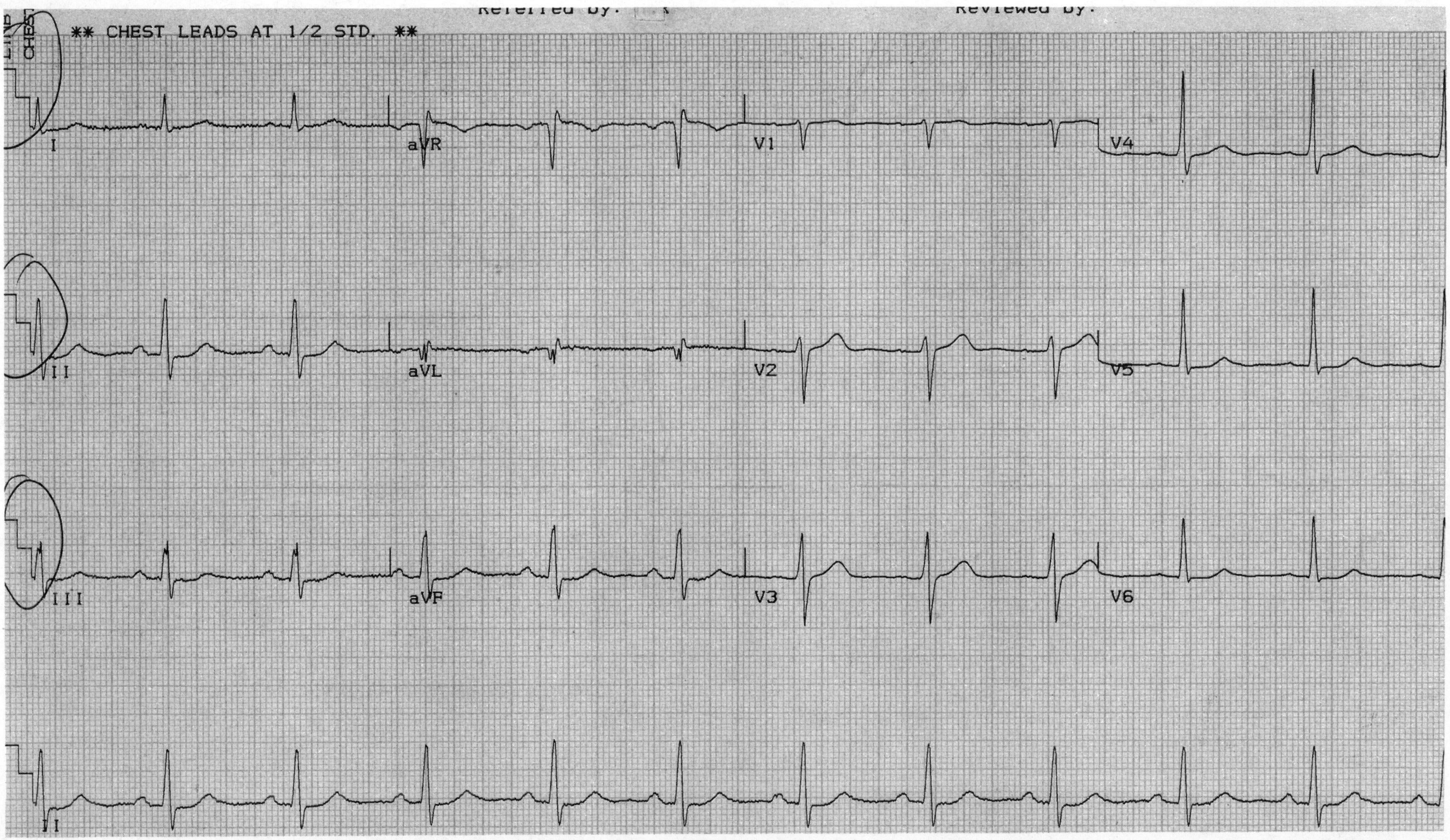

B-36

NARRATIVE INTERPRETATION

Rhythm: **Sinus**
Rate: **66**
Intervals: **PR 0.18, QRS 0.10, QT 0.40**
Axis: **+60 degrees**

Abnormalities

ST depression leads II, III, aVF, V5, V6. SV2 + RV5 greater than 35.

Synthesis

Sinus rhythm. LVH by voltage criteria. Nonspecific ST abnormalities.

TEST ANSWERS: 1, 78, (103), 106.

Comment: This tracing serves as a reminder that the interpreter should always make note of the standardization. The reader would mistakenly overlook the increased voltage for LVH if one failed to notice that the chest leads are recorded at half standard. An isolated, broad, notched Q wave is noted in lead aVL; however, the absence of a Q wave in lead I precludes the diagnosis of a lateral wall MI. The minor ST abnormalities are not characteristic of those usually associated with LVH and are best considered nonspecific.

B-37

Clinical History

A 71-year-old man with congestive heart failure.

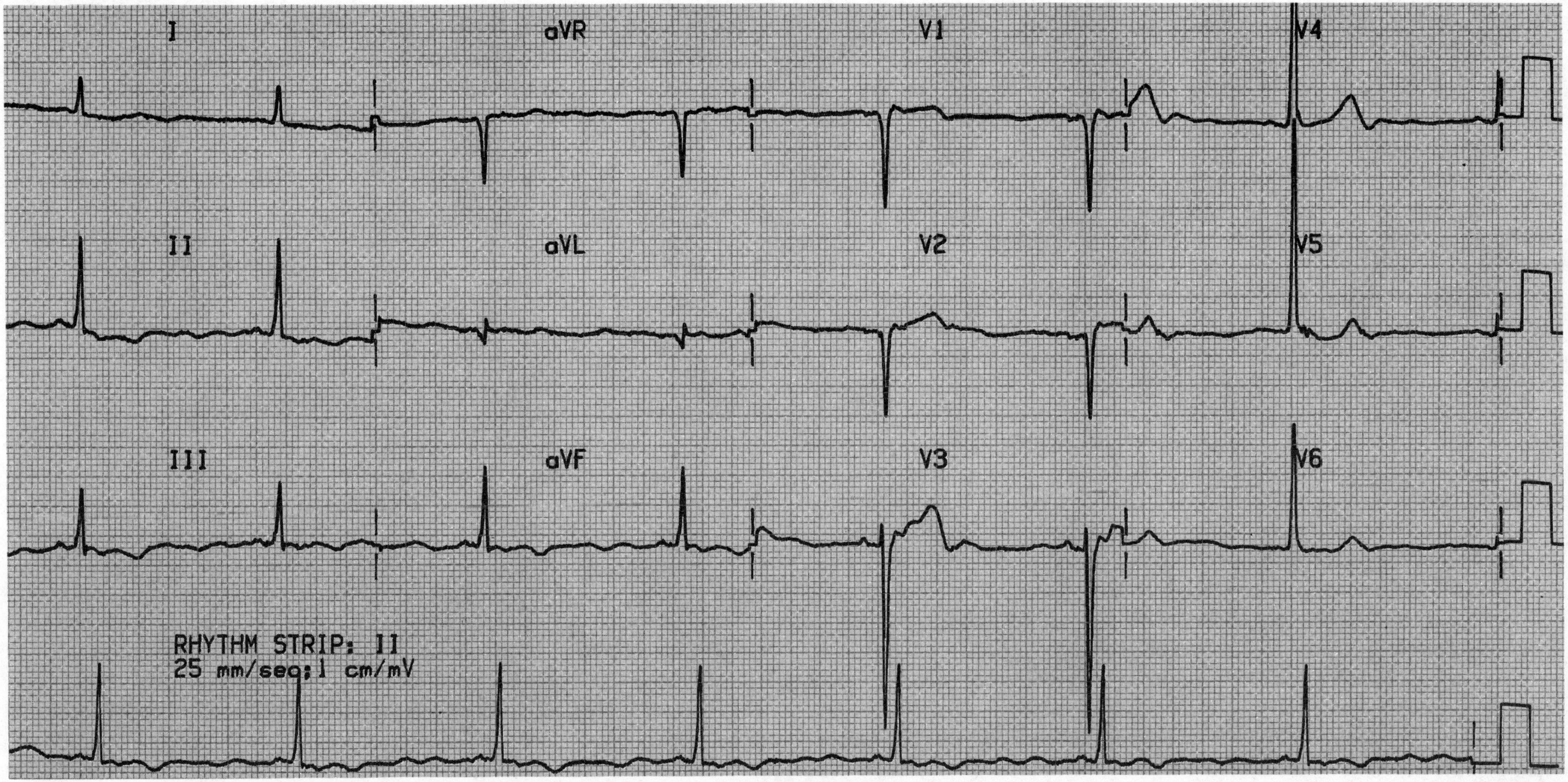

B-37

NARRATIVE INTERPRETATION

Rhythm:	**Sinus bradycardia**
Rate:	**44**
Intervals:	**PR 0.14, QRS 0.08, QT 0.52**
Axis:	**+60 degrees**

Abnormalities
Slow heart rate. Somatic tremor artifact. ST depression leads I, II, V4–V6. T-wave inversion leads II, III, aVF. SV2 + RV5 greater than 35. Prominent U waves. Inverted U wave leads V4–V6.

Synthesis
Sinus bradycardia. LVH by voltage criteria. Associated ST-T-wave abnormalities. Prominent U waves. Inverted U waves. Somatic tremor with baseline artifact.

TEST ANSWERS: 3, 78, 103, 110, 111, 113.

Comment: On first inspection, the reader might misinterpret this electrocardiogram as atrial fibrillation because of the irregular baseline. Moreover, the slow regular rhythm might suggest atrial fibrillation with complete AV block and an AV junctional escape rhythm. On closer review, note the discrete P waves in the right precordial leads, particularly in lead V3. This slow, regular rhythm is sinus bradycardia with a somatic tremor—the result of Parkinson's disease. LVH is present in this electrocardiogram with increased precordial voltage and ST-T-wave abnormalities. A prominent U wave is best appreciated in lead V3, a finding that may be seen in LVH. Negative U waves are pathologic and are evident in leads V4–V6.

REFERENCES: Kishida. Lepeschkin.

B-38

Clinical History

A 48-year-old man 18 h after hospital admission for chest discomfort.

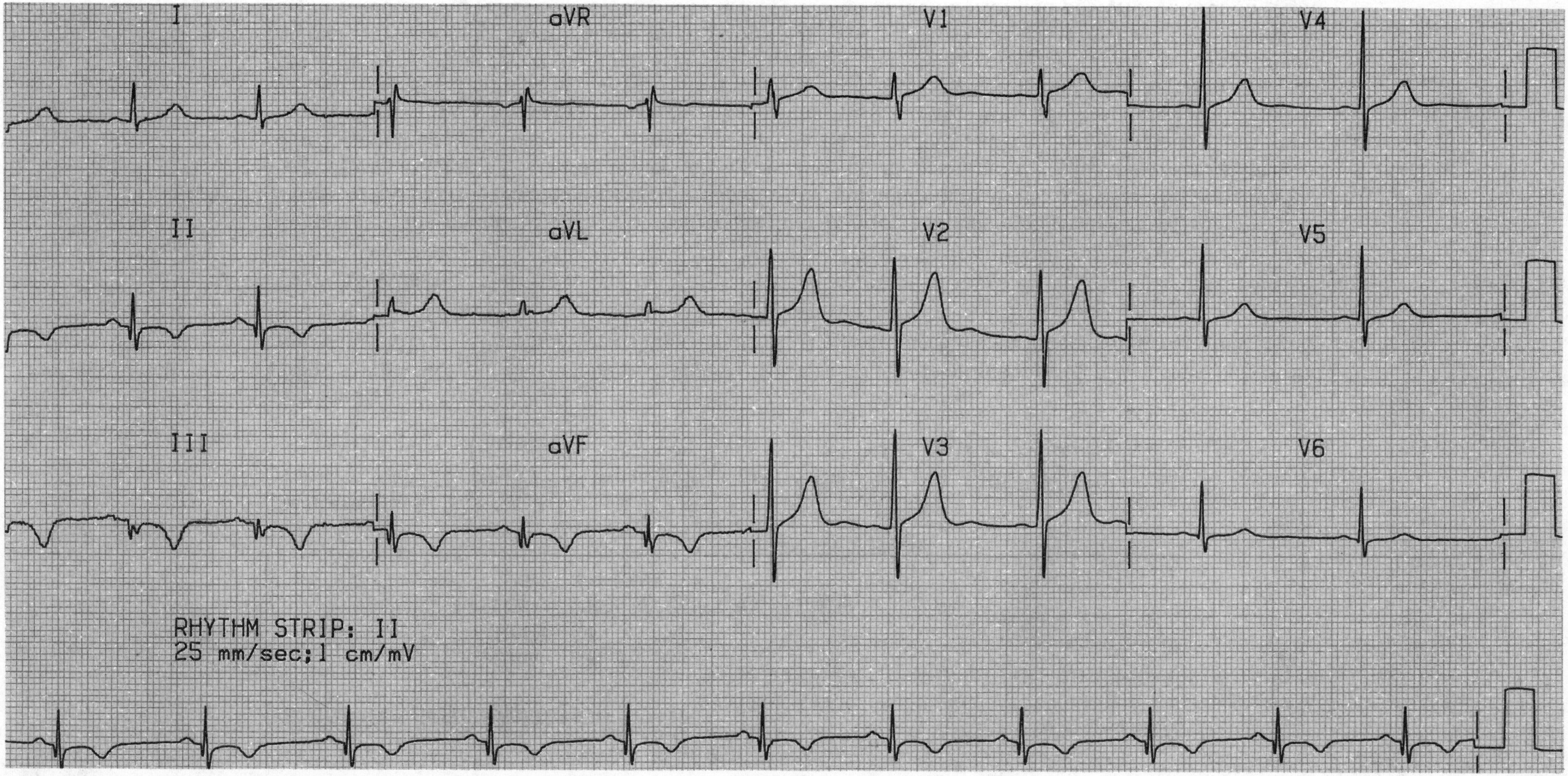

B-38

NARRATIVE INTERPRETATION

Rhythm: **Sinus**
Rate: **64**
Intervals: **PR 0.16, QRS 0.08, QT 0.40**
Axis: **0 degrees**

Abnormalities

Q waves leads II, III, aVF. R wave greater than S leads V1, V2, with upright T wave. "Coved" ST segments leads II, III, aVF. ST elevation leads aVL, V1–V3. T-wave inversion leads II, III, aVF.

Synthesis

Sinus rhythm. Recent (acute) inferior wall MI. Posterior wall MI of indeterminate age. Possible lateral wall acute MI. ST-T-wave abnormalities in leads II, III, aVL, aVF, suggesting acute myocardial injury.

TEST ANSWERS: 1, 91, (93), 94, 100.

Comment: This patient sustained a relatively minor inferior and posterolateral wall MI with new Q waves in the inferior leads and an increase in R-wave amplitude in leads V1 and V2. This tracing illustrates that pathologic Q waves may not always be 0.04 ms in duration. They are, however, 25 percent of the amplitude of the associated R wave in leads II, III, and aVF. The ST-T-wave abnormalities in the inferior leads represent recent infarction. The prominent R waves in the right precordial leads with an upright T wave reflects involvement of the posterior wall. It must be classified as of indeterminate age because there are no corresponding acute ST changes in those leads or prior tracings for comparison. In reality, it was part of the acute inferior wall MI. The slight ST elevation in lead aVL should be commented on and reflects involvement of the lateral wall in the inferior and posterior infarction. Nonpathologic U waves are also noted in leads V1–V3.

B-39

Clinical History

A 90-year-old woman with congestive heart failure.

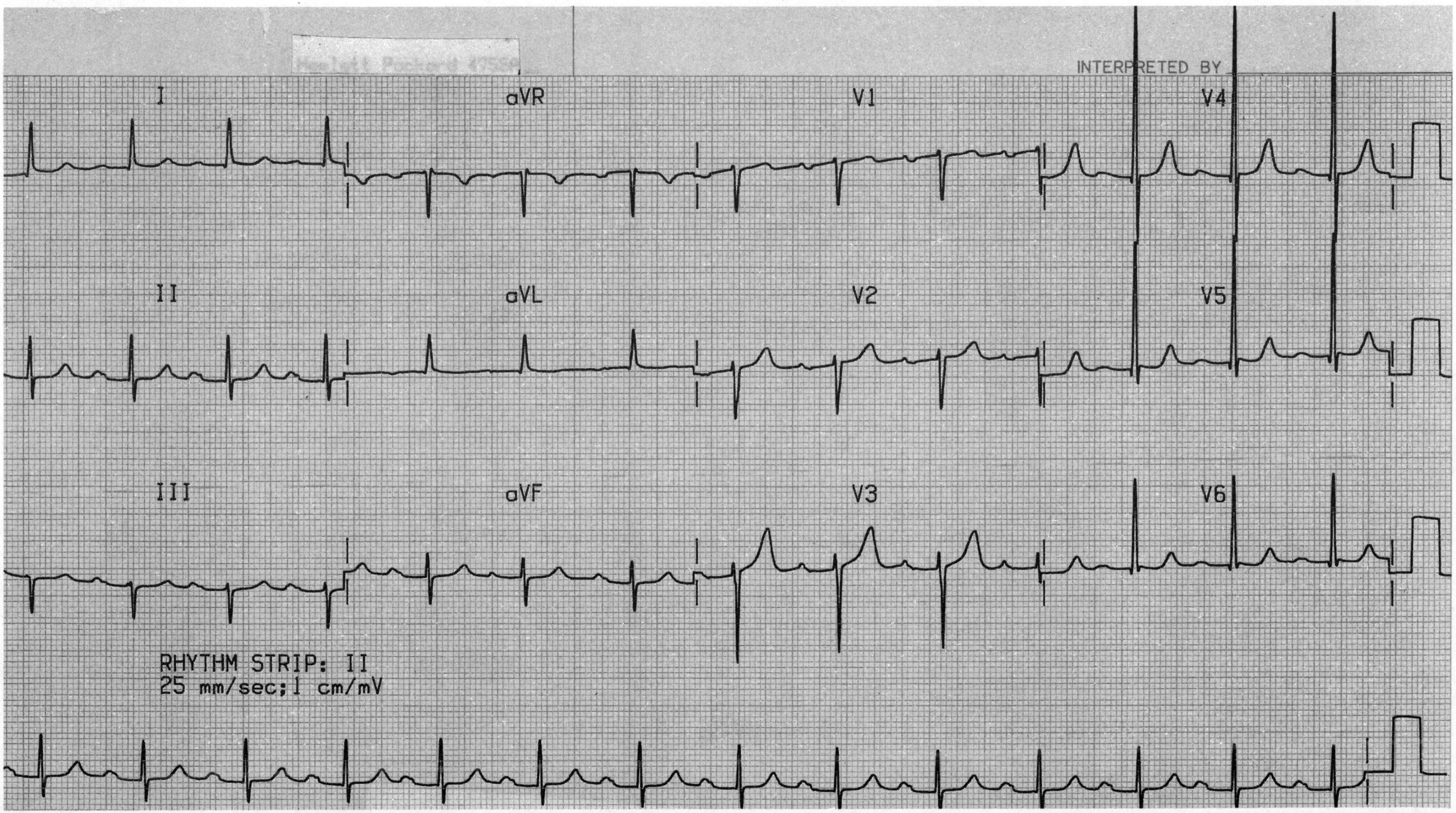

B-39

NARRATIVE INTERPRETATION

Rhythm:	**Sinus with first-degree AV block**
Rate:	**80**
Intervals:	**PR 0.24, QRS 0.08, QT 0.36**
Axis:	**−15 degrees**

Abnormalities
Prolonged PR interval. ST flat lead II, aVF. Slight ST depression leads V5–V6.

Synthesis
Sinus rhythm. First-degree AV block. Nonspecific ST abnormalities.

TEST ANSWERS: 1, 42, 106.

Comment: First-degree AV block is a common manifestation of relative digitalis toxicity. Prolongation of the PR interval is secondary to an increase in the AH interval, which reflects delay in AV conduction. In this patient the serum digoxin level was in the "therapeutic" range. However, in this elderly female with underlying conduction system disease, the therapeutic blood level was "toxic." The ST flattening and depression are nonspecific findings, secondary either to a normal variant or to medication effects.

REFERENCE: Chou p 459.

B-40

Clinical History

A 78-year-old woman with hypotension.

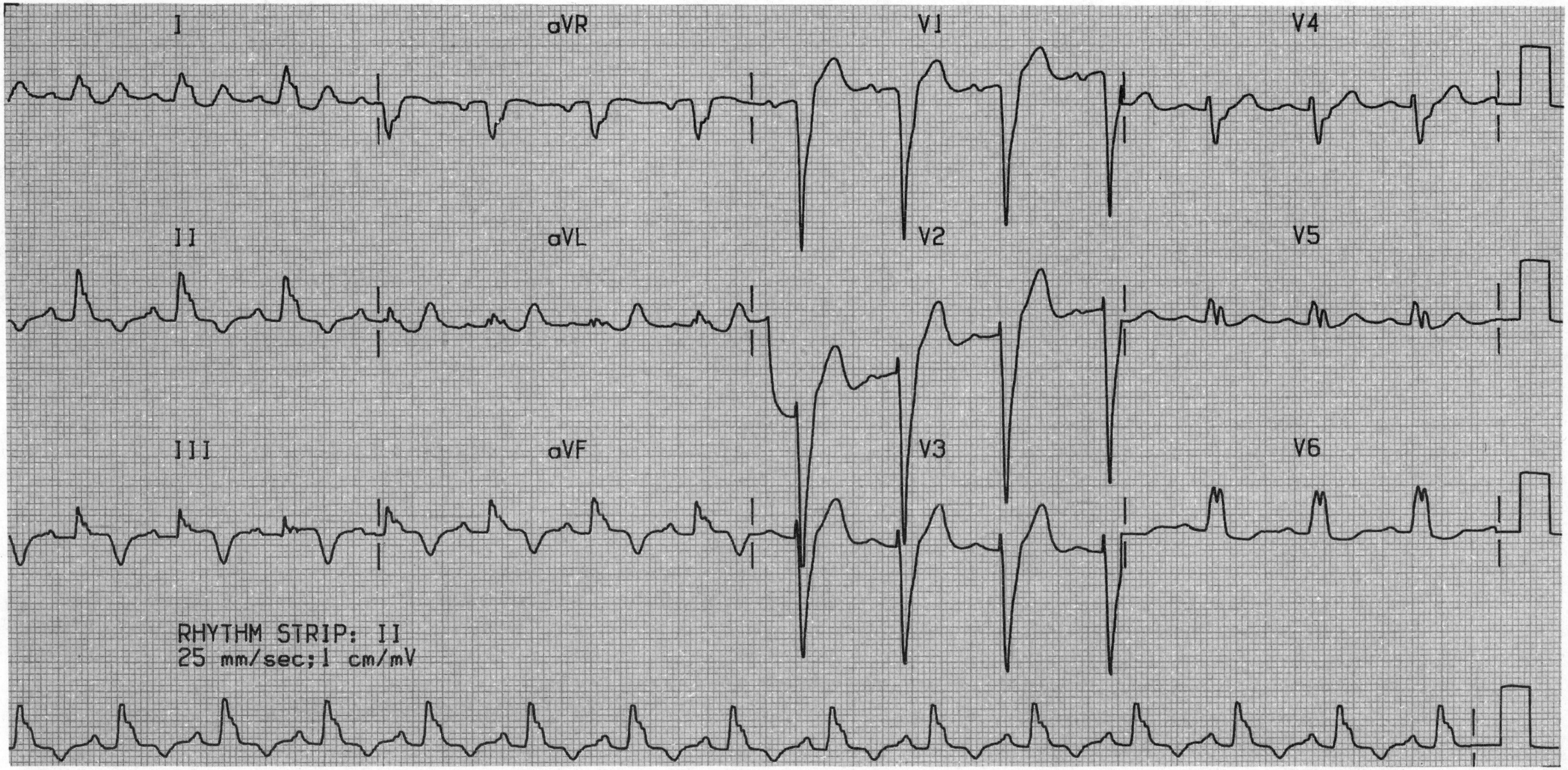

B-40

NARRATIVE INTERPRETATION

Rhythm: **Sinus**
Rate: **88**
Intervals: **PR 0.20, QRS 0.14, QT 0.40**
Axis: **+60 degrees**

Abnormalities

Broad, notched QRS in I, aVL, V5–V6. ST elevation leads II, III, aVF. Symmetric T-wave inversion leads II, III, aVF. T wave upright leads I, aVL.

Synthesis

Sinus rhythm. LBBB with associated ST-T-wave abnormalities. ST-T-wave abnormalities suggestive of acute inferior wall myocardial injury. Nonspecific ST-T-wave abnormalities in leads I, aVL.

TEST ANSWERS: 1, 74, 100, 104, 106.

Comment: This tracing demonstrates early, acute inferior wall myocardial injury in the presence of an underlying LBBB. Normally the diagnosis of MI is very difficult in patients with LBBB. In this example, the inferior ST-T-wave abnormalities are quite pronounced. Note, in addition, the upright T waves in leads I and aVL suggestive of lateral wall involvement, although these features must be categorized as nonspecific. In uncomplicated LBBB the T-wave vectors are directed in the opposite direction of the mean QRS vector and should be negative in leads I and aVL. In this example, the abnormal T waves are upright in these leads.

REFERENCE: Timmis.

TEST C

C-1

Clinical History

A 55-year-old woman with palpitations.

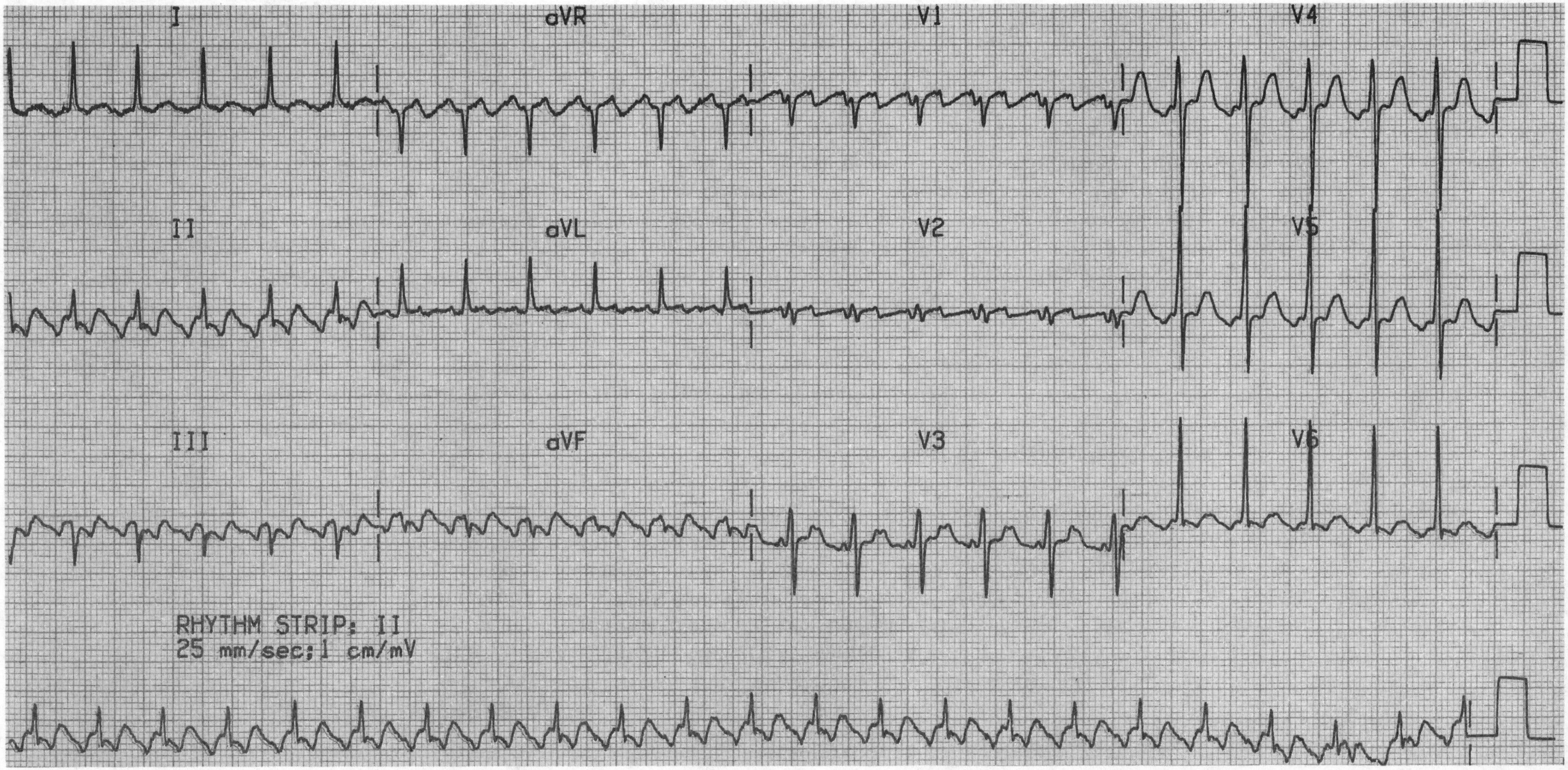

C-1

NARRATIVE INTERPRETATION

Rhythm:	**Atrial flutter with 2:1 AV conduction**
Rate:	**Atrial rate 280, ventricular rate 140**
Intervals:	**PR –, QRS 0.06, QT 0.28**
Axis:	**0 degrees**

Abnormalities

ST depression leads I, II, III, aVF, V5, V6.

Synthesis

Atrial flutter with 2:1 AV conduction. Nonspecific ST abnormalities.

TEST ANSWERS: 19, 50, 106.

Comment: Atrial flutter may be divided into type I (classic) or type II (very rapid). This tracing demonstrates classic atrial flutter with characteristic saw-toothed flutter waves in leads II, III, and aVF. In type I flutter, the atrial rate is between 240 and 340 beats per minute and may be interrupted with rapid atrial pacing. Type II atrial flutter is characterized by very rapid atrial rates of 340 to 433 beats per minute and cannot be controlled by atrial pacing. It is appropriate to describe the 2:1 ratio of atrial to ventricular impulses as 2:1 AV "conduction" rather than "block." The 2:1 conduction is a physiologic response of the AV node and should not imply a pathologic state, or "heart block." Atrial flutter with 1:1 conduction can rarely occur with sympathetic stimulation or when antiarrhythmic agents slow the intrinsic atrial rate. Atrial flutter with 1:1 conduction may represent a cardiac emergency because the resulting extremely rapid ventricular rate prevents physiologic cardiac filling and contraction.

REFERENCE: Horowitz pp 58–63.

C-2

Clinical History

A 79-year-old hypertensive woman who presents to the emergency department with severe dyspnea.

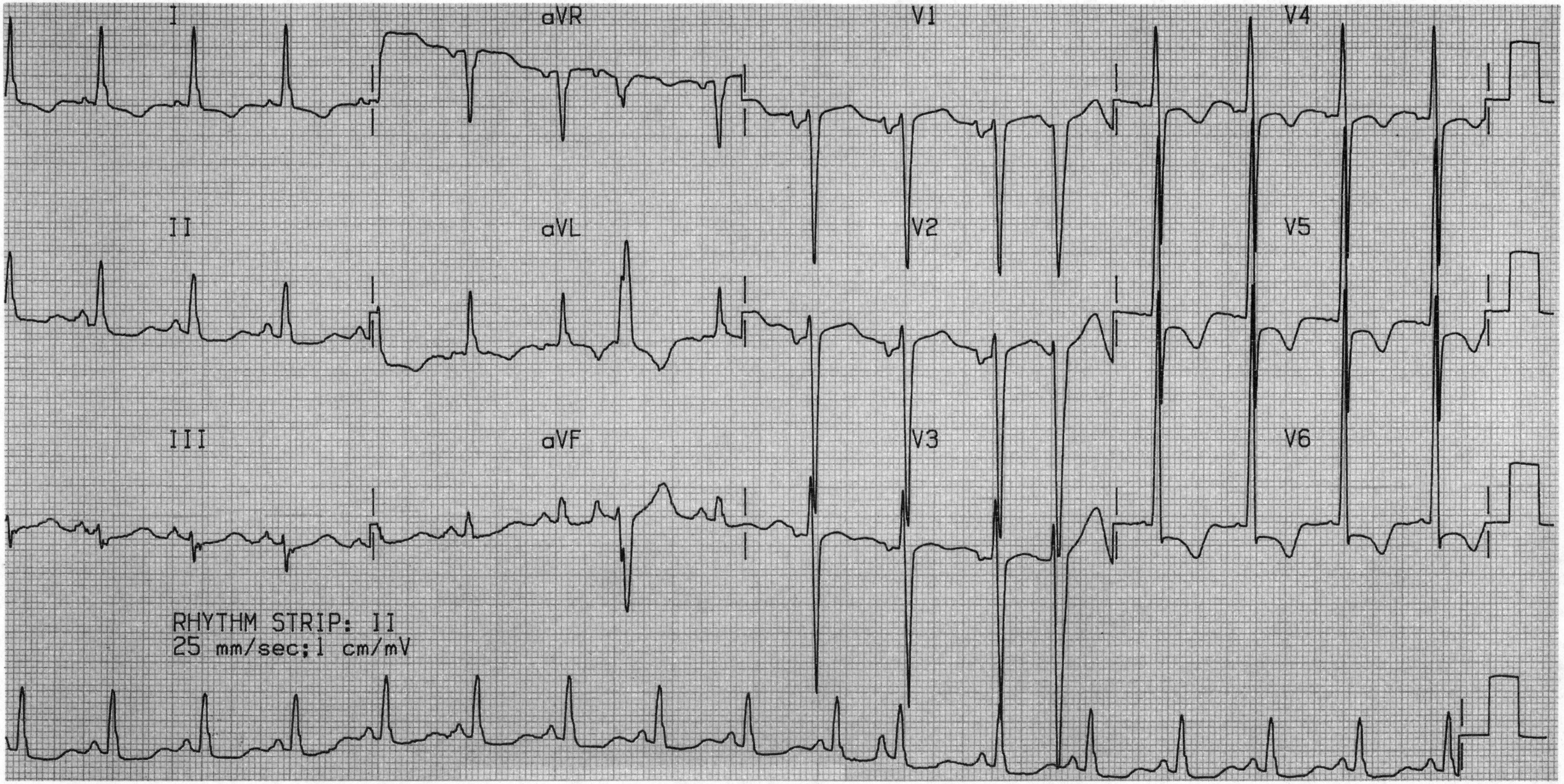

C-2

NARRATIVE INTERPRETATION

Rhythm: **Sinus**
Rate: **96**
Intervals: **PR 0.16, QRS 0.08, QT 0.38**
Axis: **+15 degrees**

Abnormalities
APC. APC conducted aberrantly. ST depression leads I, II, III, aVL, aVF, V4–V6. T-wave inversion leads I, aVL, V4–V6. SV2 + RV5 greater than 35. Abnormal P terminal force V1.

Synthesis
Sinus rhythm. APCs with normal and aberrant conduction. LVH by voltage criteria. Associated ST-T-wave abnormalities. Left atrial abnormality.

TEST ANSWERS: 1, 10, 11, 60, 78, 103.

Comment: This tracing demonstrates a number of findings, most of them related to LVH. A potential incorrect interpretation would be in considering the wide complex as ventricular in origin rather than as an aberrantly conducted atrial complex. On close examination, a P wave is clearly seen to be deforming the preceding T wave, which indicates that the complex is supraventricular. An APC that is also aberrantly conducted is seen subsequently, and a normally conducted atrial complex is evident on the rhythm strip. Although the ST-T-wave abnormalities were most likely on the basis of LVH, one cannot completely exclude the presence of MI.

C-3

Clinical History

A 59-year-old asymptomatic man on his fifth hospital day.

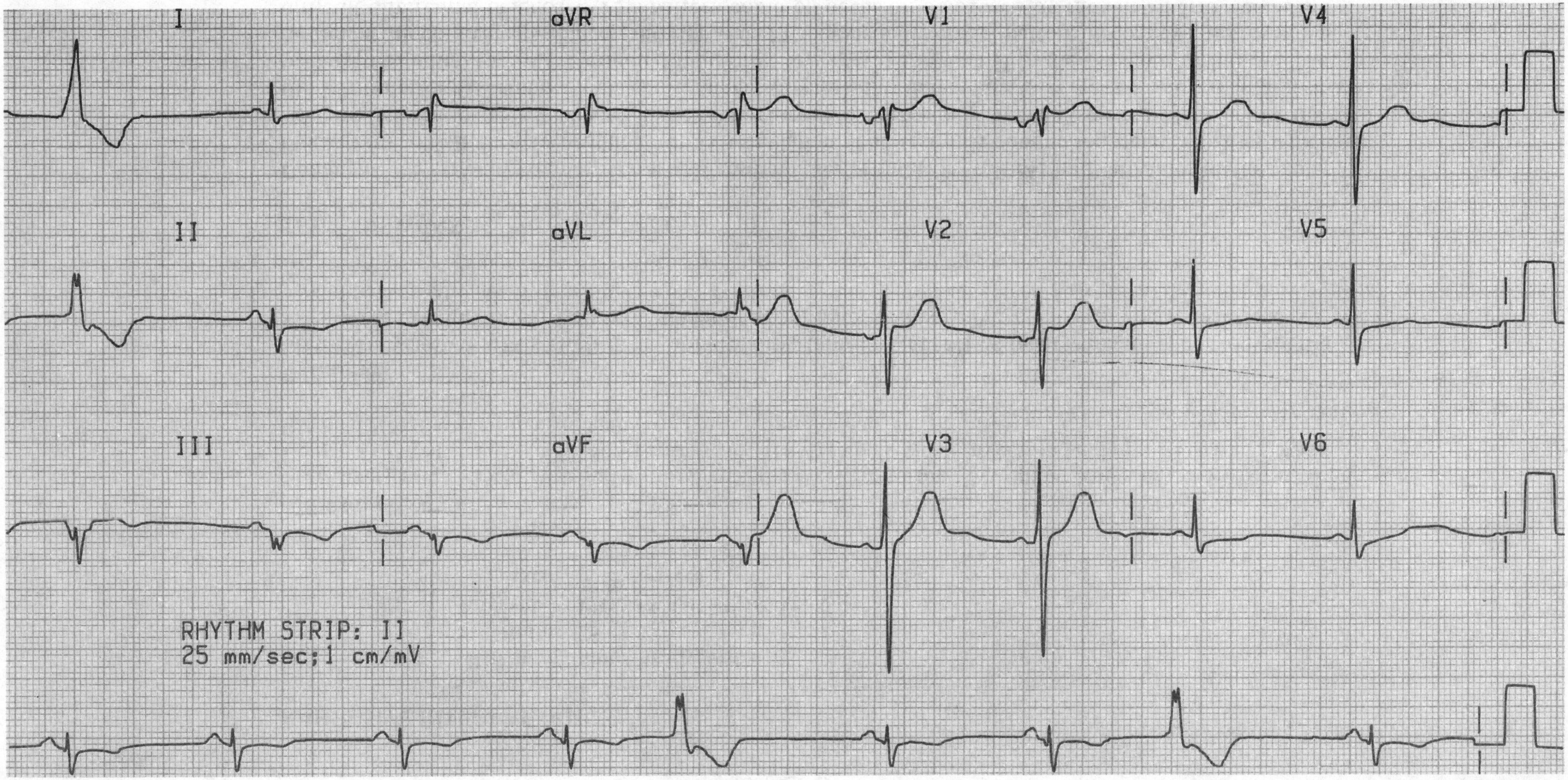

C-3

NARRATIVE INTERPRETATION

Rhythm: **Sinus bradycardia**
Rate: **55**
Intervals: **PR 0.14, QRS 0.10, QT 0.44**
Axis: **−45 degrees**

Abnormalities

Slow heart rate. VPCs. Axis leftward of −30 degrees. Abnormal P terminal force V1. Q waves leads II, III, aVF. rSr′ lead V1. ST depression leads II, V5, V6. T-wave inversion leads II, III, aVF. T wave flat lead V5. T wave biphasic lead V6. T wave upright lead V1.

Synthesis

Sinus bradycardia. VPCs. Left atrial abnormality. Inferior wall MI of indeterminate age. Nonspecific ST-T-wave abnormalities. Left axis deviation. Left anterior fascicular block. rSr′ pattern in lead V1, probably normal variant.

TEST ANSWERS: 3, 26, 60, 64, 72, 92, 98, 106.

Comment: This tracing demonstrates the combination of inferior wall MI and left anterior fascicular block, both of which may produce left axis deviation. The terminal conduction delay in aVR, which occurs after that of aVL, suggests the counterclockwise vector loop of the fascicular block. Note that the left anterior fascicular block can diminish or mask the diagnostic Q waves of inferior infarction because the initial forces are directed inferiorly. The Q wave in lead II in the presence of left anterior fascicular block suggests that an inferior wall MI coexists. The rSr′ pattern in lead V1 represents a difficult differential diagnosis. This pattern could on occasion be caused by the left anterior fascicular block, or it may represent a normal variant. Alternatively it could represent an incomplete RBBB. In this example, the r and r′ are of low amplitude, are less than the amplitude of the S wave, and occur only in lead V1, and therefore are likely to represent a normal variant.

REFERENCES: Fisher. Warner (*Am Heart J*). Friedman p 164. Marriott p 79. Chou p 93.

C-4

Clinical History

A 57-year-old man with chest discomfort.

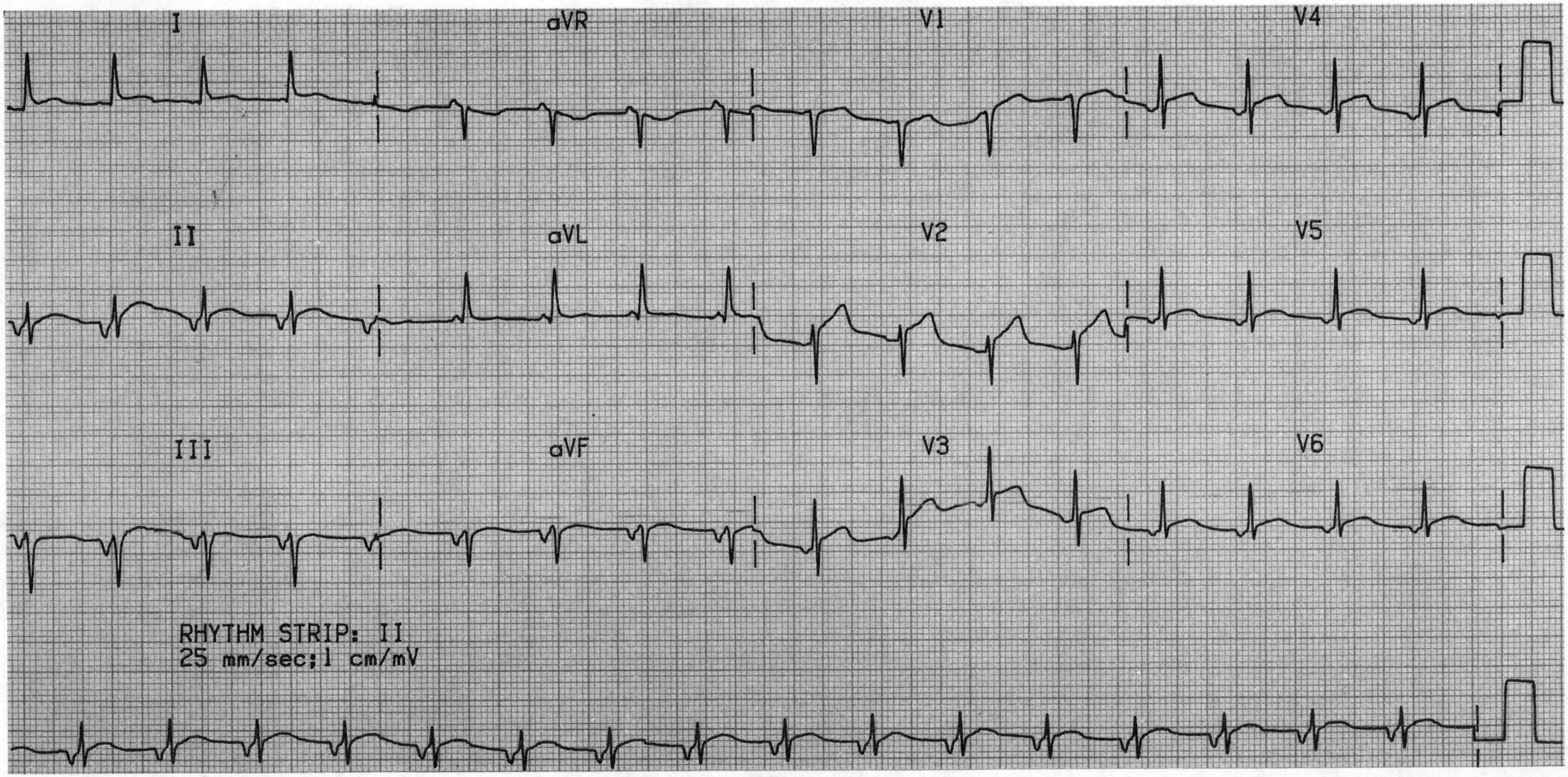

C-4

NARRATIVE INTERPRETATION

Rhythm: **Accelerated AV junctional rhythm**
Rate: **100**
Intervals: **PR 0.10, QRS 0.08, QT 0.32**
Axis: **−30 degrees**

Abnormalities

Inverted P waves II, III, aVF, with short PR interval. ST elevation leads I, II, III, aVL, aVF, V2–V6.

Synthesis

Accelerated AV junctional rhythm. ST-segment elevation suggestive of acute myocardial injury of inferior, lateral, and anterior walls.

TEST ANSWERS: 23, 100.

Comment: Accelerated AV junctional rhythm is most often seen in patients with underlying cardiac disease. The rhythm may also be called *nonparoxysmal junctional tachycardia*, which distinguishes it from paroxysmal junctional tachycardia, a common form of reentrant supraventricular tachycardia. It may be the result of acute MI, COPD, or myocarditis or it may be seen after cardiac surgery. In this example, note the subtle but clear ST elevation in leads I and aVL, in the inferior leads, and across the precordium. This patient went on to develop an anteroapical and lateral wall MI. Q waves have not yet appeared; therefore, the best characterization of this example is to comment on the ST abnormalities without a definitive diagnosis of MI. The ST elevation is generally concave downward and suggests myocardial injury. However, the generalized nature of the abnormalities might also raise the suspicion of pericarditis.

C-5

Clinical History

A 68-year-old asymptomatic man seen in preoperative evaluation.

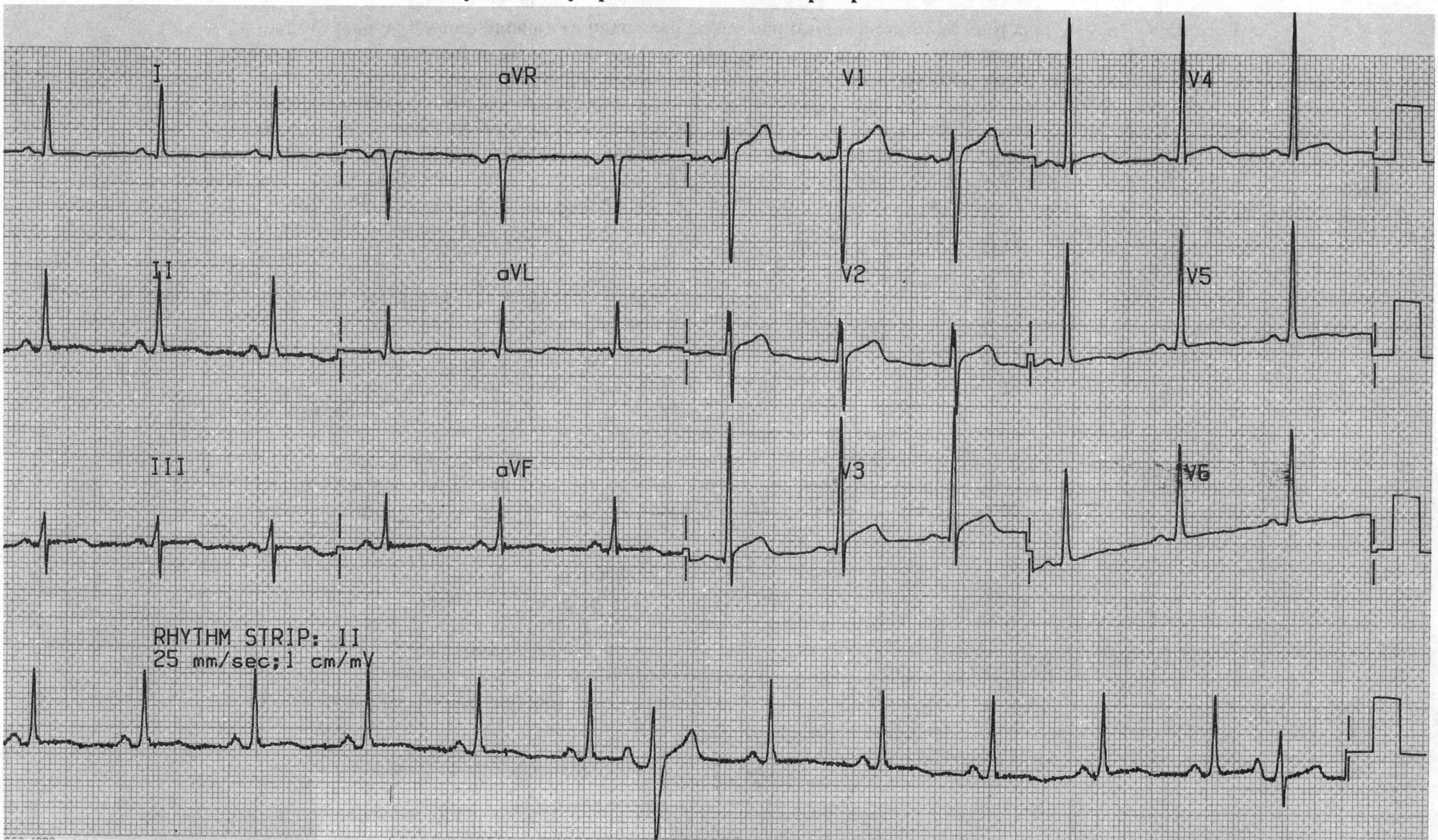

C-5

NARRATIVE INTERPRETATION

Rhythm: **Sinus**
Rate: **75**
Intervals: **PR 0.16, QRS 0.08, QT 0.36**
Axis: **+30 degrees**

Abnormalities

APCs with aberrant conduction. ST elevation at J point leads II, III, aVF, V1–V4. T-wave inversion leads I, aVL. T wave flat leads V5–V6. SV1 + RV5 greater than 35.

Synthesis

Sinus rhythm. APCs with aberrant conduction. Nonspecific T-wave abnormalities. Normal variant J-point elevation. LVH by voltage criteria.

TEST ANSWERS: 1, 11, 78, 96, (103), 106, (112).

Comment: The T wave represents ventricular repolarization and generally has the same direction as QRS depolarization. In normal persons, the T-wave vector is directed leftward and inferiorly and is therefore upright in leads I, II, and V3–V6. T waves may be variable in leads III, aVL, aVF, V1, and V2. In this example there is also a slight ST elevation at the J point, which is probably within normal limits. Without clinical correlation, it would be difficult to completely exclude early myocardial injury. APCs with variable degrees of aberrant conduction are noted on the rhythm strip. In the absence of underlying cardiac disease or tachyarrhythmias, these would generally require no preoperative treatment. It would be important for the surgical staff to be aware of the aberrant conduction of these complexes to avoid mistaking them for ventricular arrhythmias. One minor additional point is the lead placement of lead V3, which appears to have been positioned too far laterally toward lead V4.

REFERENCE: Marriott p 24.

C-6

Clinical History

A 72-year-old woman admitted to the CCU.

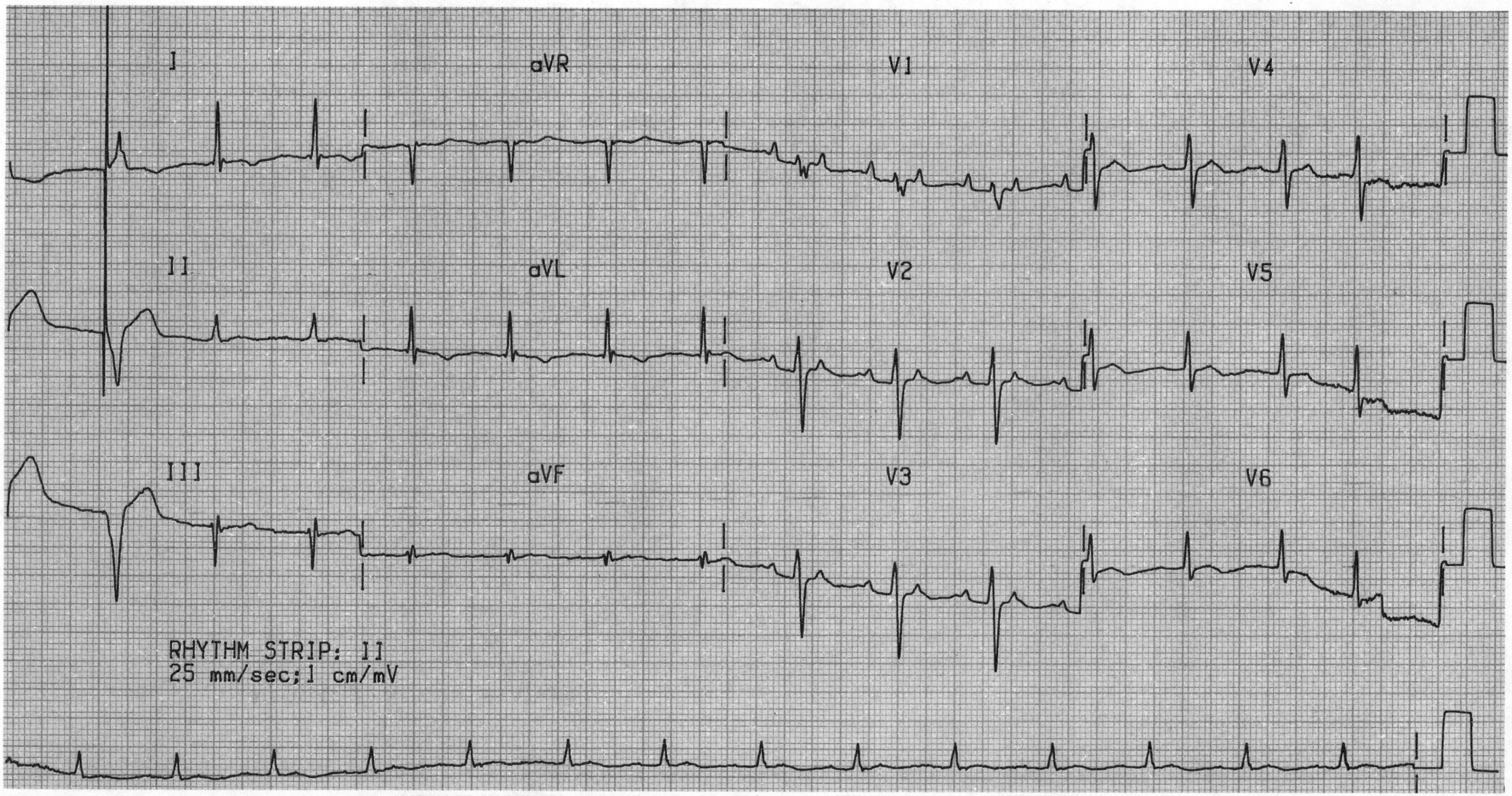

C-6

NARRATIVE INTERPRETATION

Rhythm: **Atrial tachycardia with 2:1 AV conduction**
Rate: **Atrial 170, ventricular 85**
Intervals: **PR 0.20, QRS 0.10, QT 0.36**
Axis: **0 degrees**

Abnormalities

T wave inverted leads I, aVL, V5–V6. Ventricular pacemaker complex with capture.

Synthesis

Atrial tachycardia with 2:1 AV conduction. Nonspecific T-wave abnormalities. Ventricular pacemaker complex with appropriate capture.

TEST ANSWERS: 17, 35, (50), 51, 106.

Comment: This patient was being treated with digoxin for sick sinus syndrome. The arrhythmia demonstrated here is characteristic of digitalis toxicity. PAT with 2:1 AV conduction (block) usually presents with an atrial rate of 200 to 250 beats per minute. In this example, the atrial rate is a bit slower. The 2:1 conduction ratio at this atrial rate is probably "nonphysiologic" secondary to the effect of digoxin but is difficult to confirm on the surface electrocardiogram. Note the prominent P waves in leads V1 and V2. The P wave following the QRS complex should not be mistaken for a T wave, which would normally occur further beyond the R wave. A ventricular pacemaker capture is seen in the first complex. This is likely to be normal function, but it is impossible to determine the demand function without visualizing the preceding beat.

C-7

Clinical History

A 78-year-old man treated with a calcium channel blocker and digoxin.

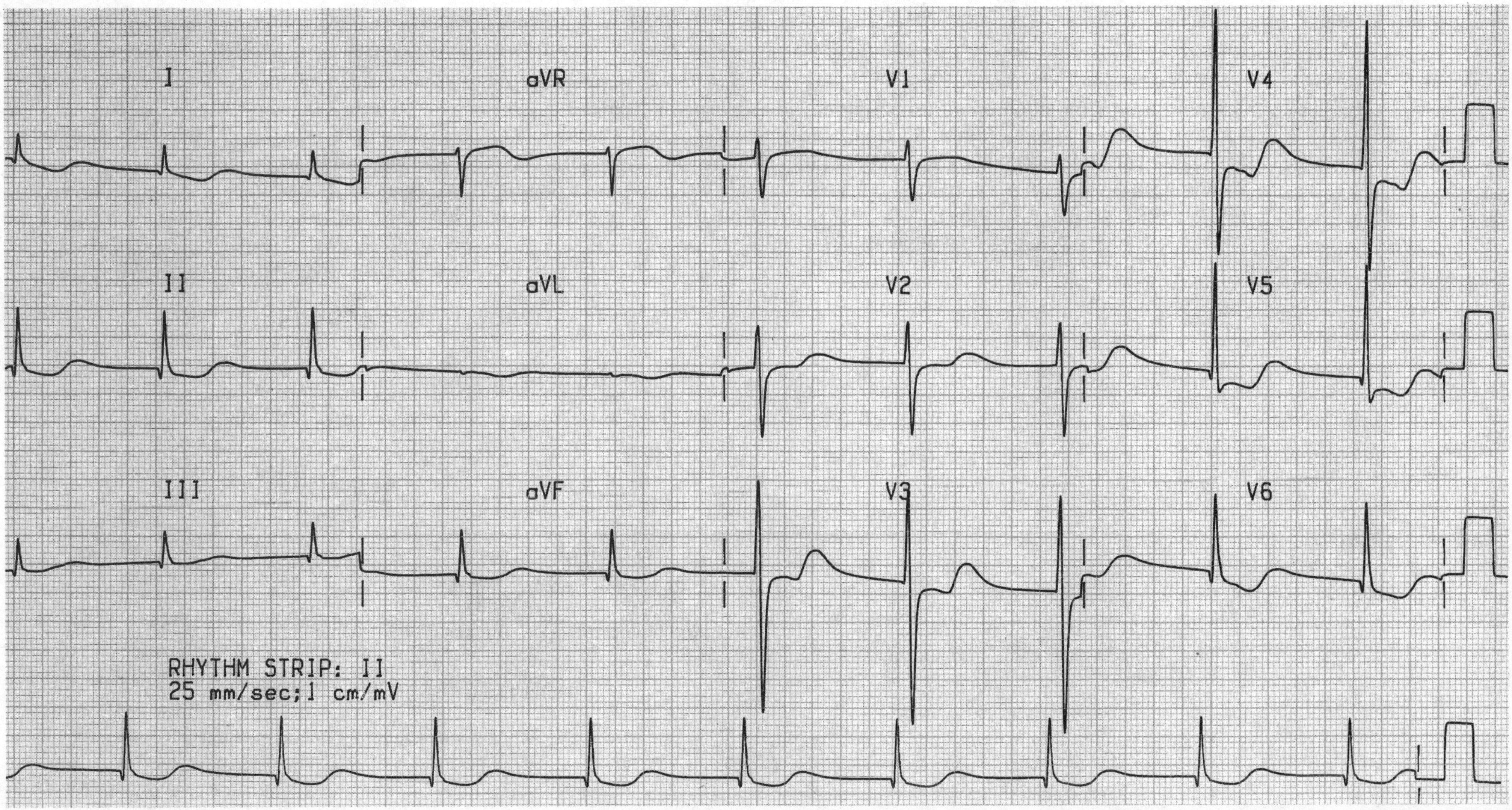

C-7

NARRATIVE INTERPRETATION

Rhythm: **AV junctional rhythm**
Rate: **55**
Intervals: **PR –, QRS 0.10, QT –**
Axis: **+60 degrees**

Abnormalities

Absent P waves. ST depression leads I, II, aVF, V3–V6. T-wave inversion leads I, II, aVL, V3–V6.

Synthesis

AV junctional rhythm. Diffuse nonspecific ST-T-wave abnormalities. Prominent U waves suggested.

TEST ANSWERS: 21, 106, (110).

Comment: This patient had suppression of sinus node function induced by high doses of verapamil prescribed with digoxin. This yielded an AV junctional rhythm. No inverted P waves from the AV junction are evident because they are "buried" in the QRS complex. Remember that the inverted, retrograde P wave of AV junctional complexes can appear either before, within, or after the QRS complex; its position depends on the relative rates of antegrade and retrograde conduction. The QT interval is difficult to determine in this example as there is considerable blurring of the T and U waves. Prominent U waves may be present as the primary abnormality of repolarization in conjunction with a relatively short QT interval secondary to digoxin.

C-8

Clinical History

A 77-year-old woman with 6 h of chest discomfort. She has been told of a "blockage" on her prior electrocardiogram.

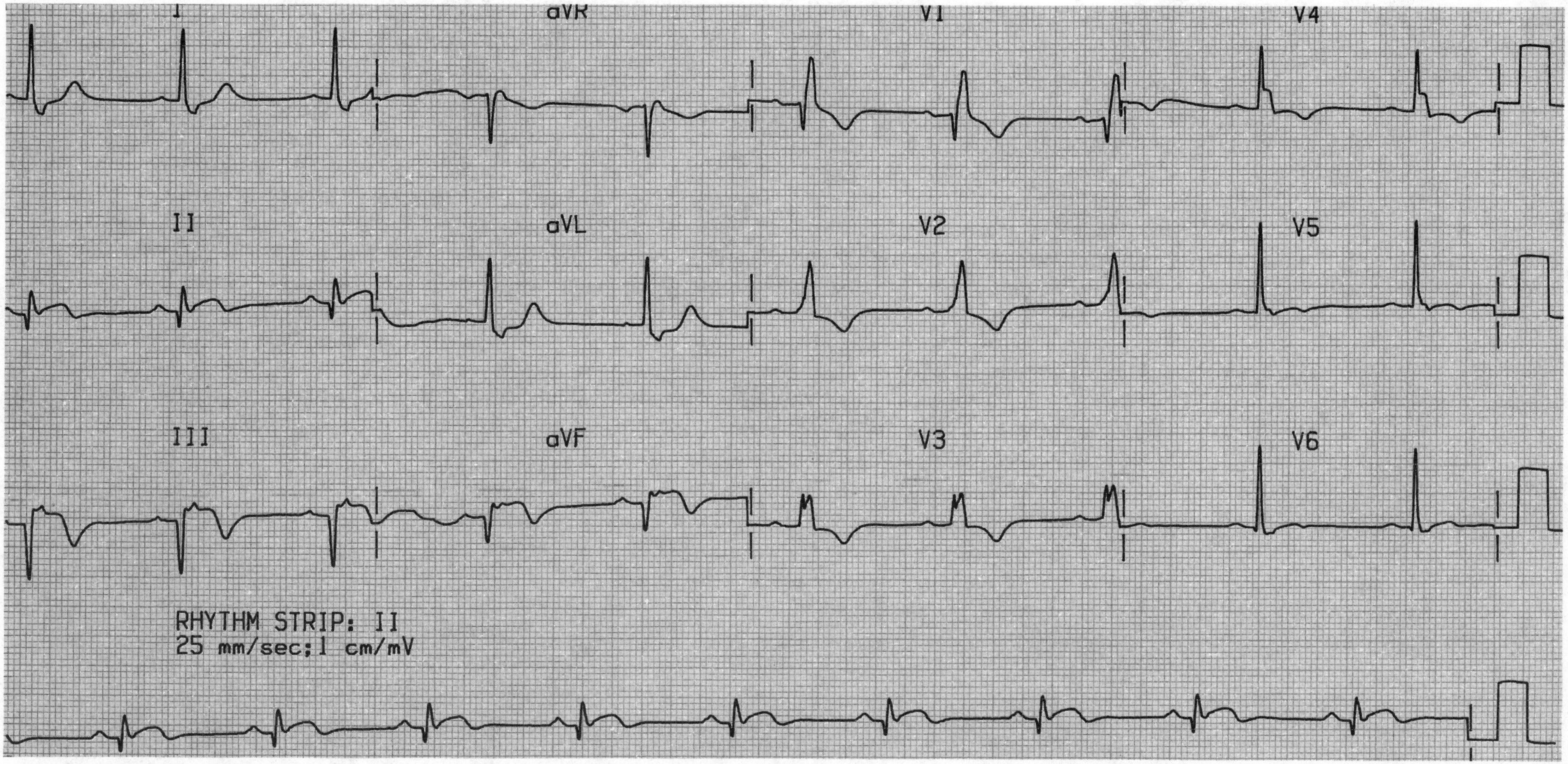

C-8

NARRATIVE INTERPRETATION

Rhythm:	**Sinus bradycardia**
Rate:	**56**
Intervals:	**PR 0.18, QRS 0.12, QT 0.44**
Axis:	**−15 degrees**

Abnormalities

Slow heart rate. Q waves leads II, III, aVF. ST elevation leads II, III aVF. ST depression leads I, aVL. Slight ST elevation leads V5, V6. ST depression leads I, aVL. T wave inverted leads III, aVF. T wave biphasic lead II. Prolonged QRS with rSR′ pattern leads V1–V3 with T-wave inversion.

Synthesis

Sinus bradycardia. Inferior wall and possible inferolateral wall MI with ST-T-wave abnormalities that suggest acute myocardial injury. RBBB with associated ST-T-wave abnormalities. ST-T-wave abnormalities in leads I and aVL, which suggest either reciprocal changes or lateral wall myocardial ischemia.

TEST ANSWERS: 3, 70, 91, 100, 101, 104.

Comment: This patient was suffering from an acute inferior wall MI. Extension laterally is also suggested by coved ST-segment elevation in the lateral precordial leads. In this patient, the RBBB was noted previously and T-wave inversion in leads V1–V3 would be expected; therefore, these findings are secondary rather than primary abnormalities. However, the acute ST-T-wave abnormalities in the inferior and lateral leads may be interpreted even in the presence of complete RBBB. Remember also that the presence of a preexisting RBBB in a patient with an acute MI does not suggest a higher likelihood of progression to complete heart block, and temporary pacemaker insertion is not indicated.

REFERENCES: Hindman I. Hindman II.

C-9

Clinical History

A 70-year-old woman with a history of congestive heart failure who has been admitted for abdominal surgery.

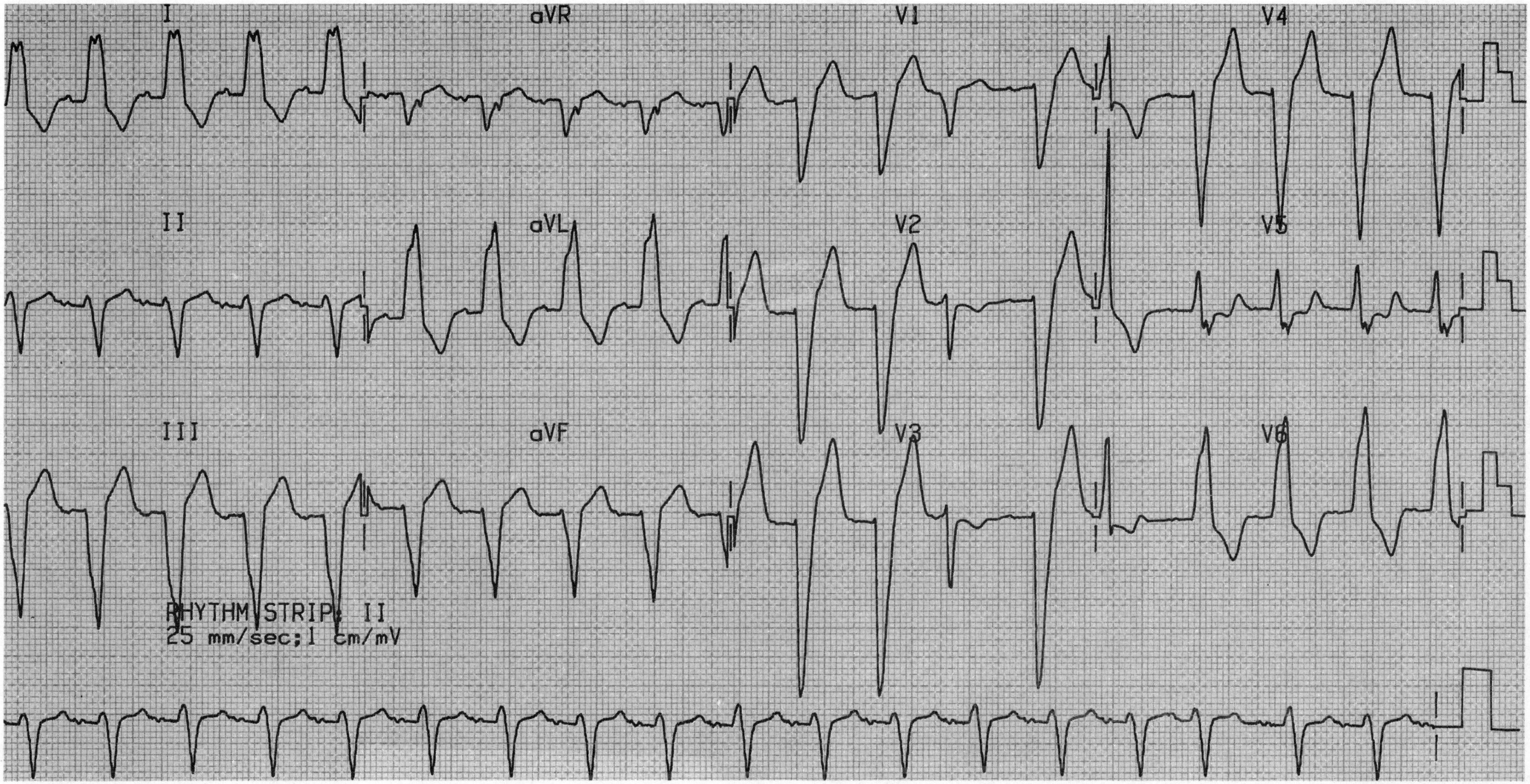

C-9

NARRATIVE INTERPRETATION

Rhythm:	**Sinus tachycardia**
Rate:	**106**
Intervals:	**PR 0.18, QRS 0.14, QT 0.36**
Axis:	**−45 degrees**

Abnormalities

Rapid heart rate. Broad, notched QRS complex with T-wave inversion leads I, aVL, V6. Axis leftward of −30 degrees. SV2 + RV5 greater than 45. VPC. APC.

Synthesis

Sinus tachycardia. LBBB. Left axis deviation. Possible LVH. VPC. APC.

TEST ANSWERS: 4, 10, 26, 74, (78), 104.

Comment: Note that the duration of the ventricular premature contractions is less than that of the native complex. This is not an infrequent finding in patients with LBBB. It is likely that the ectopic impulse originates from a location distal to the area of conduction delay and depolarizes the ventricles more rapidly. Note that the precordial leads are recorded at one-half standard, and marked precordial voltage is present. This is suggestive of LVH, even in the presence of LBBB. A single atrial premature complex is present on the rhythm strip.

REFERENCES: Chou p 371. Klein RC. Kafka. Vandenberg. Howard.

C-10

Clinical History

A 57-year-old man with 6 h of chest discomfort.

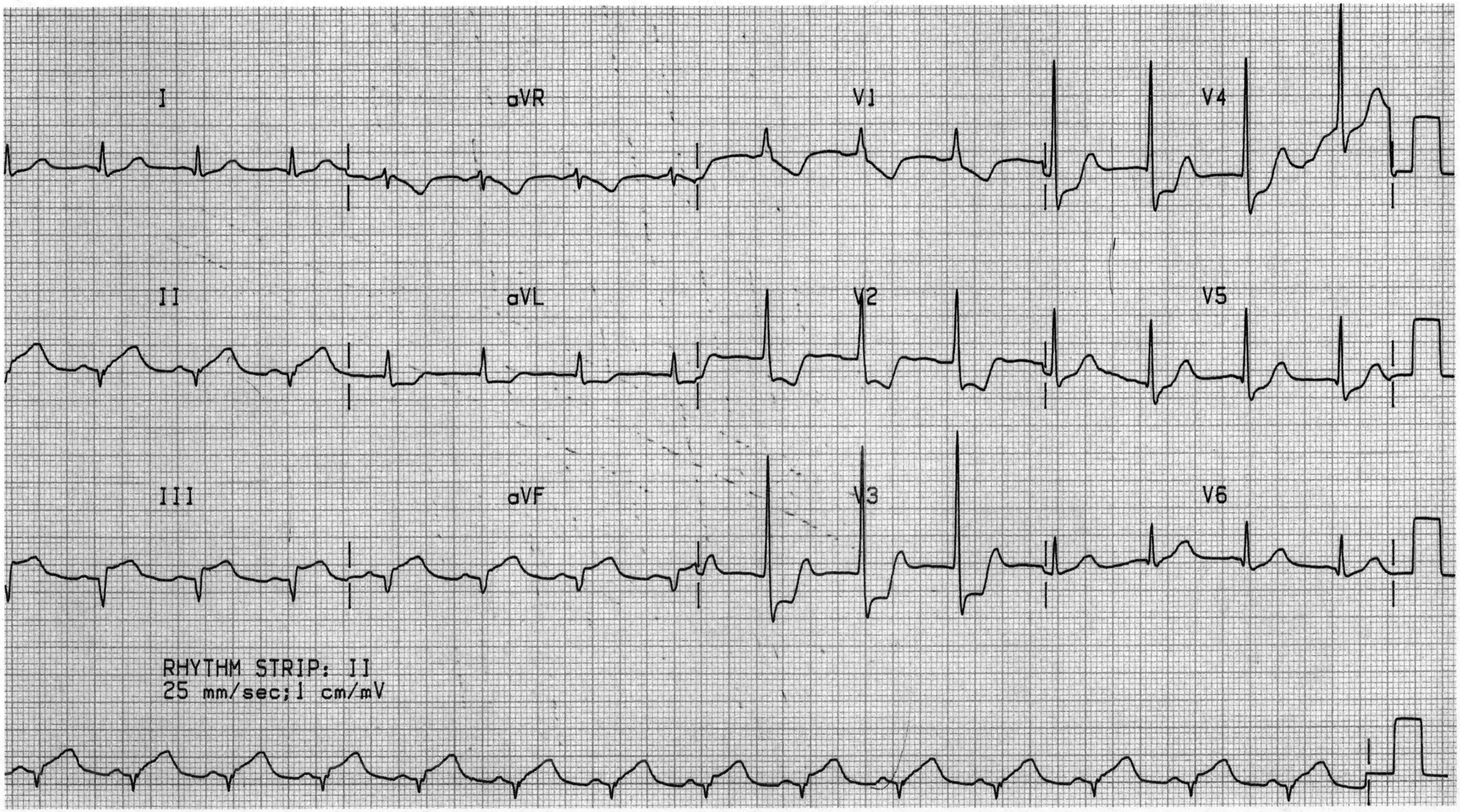

C-10

NARRATIVE INTERPRETATION

Rhythm: **Sinus**
Rate: **85**
Intervals: **PR 0.16, QRS 0.08, QT 0.36**
Axis: **−45 degrees**

Abnormalities

Left axis deviation. Q waves leads II, III, aVF. Tall R waves, with R greater than S leads V1, V2. ST elevation leads II, III, aVF. ST depression leads I, aVL, V1–V6. Deeply inverted T wave leads V1–V2.

Synthesis

Sinus rhythm. Inferior wall MI with ST abnormalities of recent infarction. Posterior wall MI with ST abnormalities of recent infarction. ST depression in lateral leads suggesting possible lateral wall ischemia. Left axis deviation.

TEST ANSWERS: 1, 64, 91, 93, 100, 101.

Comment: This tracing demonstrates an obvious recent inferior wall MI. The tall R waves with ST depression in the anterior precordial leads indicate that a posterior wall infarction is also present. The presence of significant Q waves inferiorly and tall R waves anteriorly indicates that a significant amount of myocardial necrosis has already occurred in this infarction. On angiography, this patient was shown to have occlusion of a dominant left circumflex artery with a resultant extensive posterior-inferior infarction. The ST depression in the lateral leads may be an electrical reciprocal phenomenon or may represent additional ischemia distant from the infarction. This ECG also indicates that inferior wall MI can produce left axis deviation in the absence of left anterior fascicular block (LAFB). LAFB is not suspected because a clockwise vector loop may be inferred in the frontal plane. Note the absence of a terminal R wave in lead aVR.

REFERENCES: Schweitzer (1990). Fuchs. Bush. Warner (1982). Warner (*Am Heart J*). Warner (*Am J Cardiol* 52:690–692, 1983). Fisher.

C-11

Clinical History

A 43-year-old asymptomatic man with a history of "indigestion."

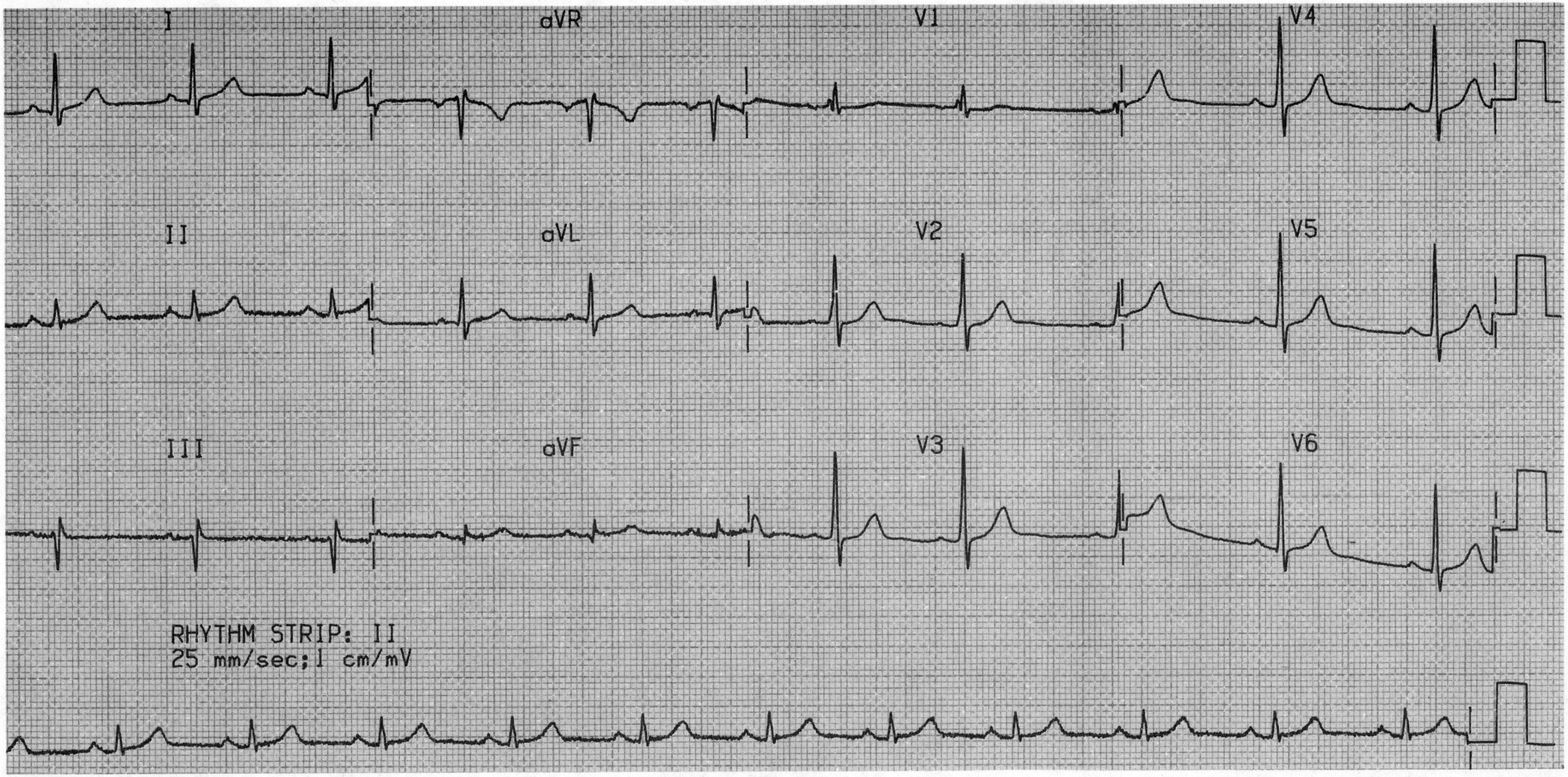

C-11

NARRATIVE INTERPRETATION

Rhythm:	**Sinus**
Rate:	**66**
Intervals:	**PR 0.16, QRS 0.08, QT 0.36**
Axis:	**+15 degrees**

Abnormalities
Tall, broad R wave with upright T wave leads V1–V2.

Synthesis
Sinus rhythm. Posterior wall MI of indeterminate age.

TEST ANSWERS: 1, 94.

Comment: This patient was found to have a previous posterior wall MI secondary to an occlusion of the left circumflex coronary artery. A diagnosis of a coexistent inferior wall MI should not be made because of the absence of significant Q waves in the inferior leads. The rR′ in lead V1 should not be mistaken for an incomplete RBBB as there are no other criteria supporting this diagnosis.

C-12

Clinical History

A 56-year-old man with dyspnea.

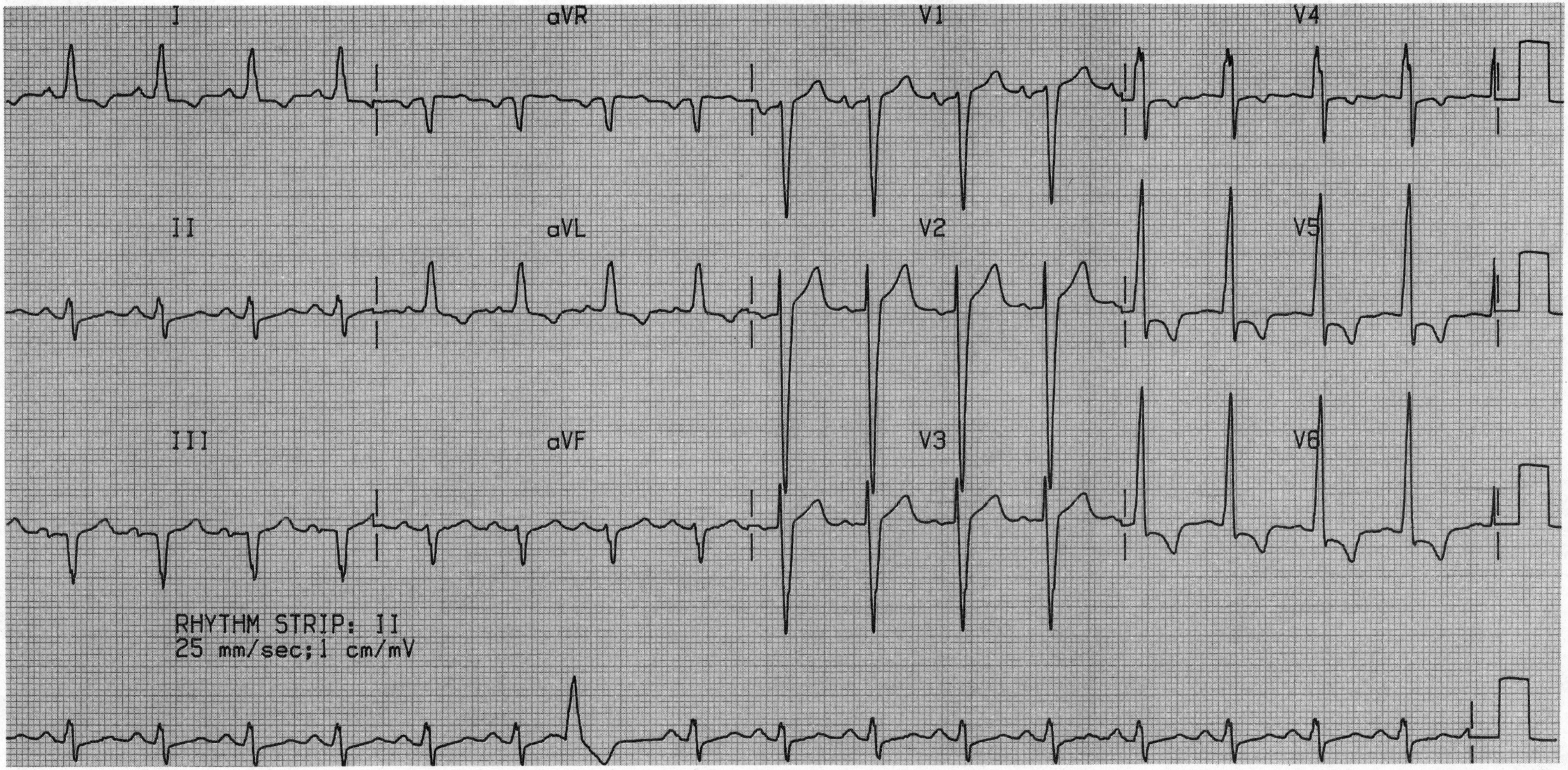

C-12

NARRATIVE INTERPRETATION

Rhythm: **Sinus**
Rate: **98**
Intervals: **PR 0.18, QRS 0.11, QT 0.34**
Axis: **−35 degrees**

Abnormalities

Axis leftward of −30 degrees. Abnormal P terminal force lead V1. SV2 + RV5 greater than 35. Broad, slurred QRS leads I, aVL, V4–V6. Notching of R wave lead V4. Absent Q waves leads I, aVL, V6. Delayed intrinsicoid deflection of 0.06 s leads V5–V6. T-wave inversion leads I, aVL, V4–V6. VPC.

Synthesis

Sinus rhythm. VPC. Left axis deviation. Left atrial abnormality. LVH. Incomplete LBBB. ST-T-wave abnormalities associated with LVH or conduction abnormality or both.

TEST ANSWERS: 1, 26, 60, 64, 75, 103, (104).

Comment: This tracing demonstrates most of the standard criteria for LVH, including increased QRS voltage, left axis deviation, left atrial abnormality, and an increased QRS duration. An often confounding issue is whether there is coexistent incomplete LBBB. Suggestive criteria for incomplete LBBB in addition to LVH in this tracing are the absent septal Q waves, delayed intrinsicoid deflection in the left precordial leads, notching in lead V4, and slurring of the QRS in leads V5–V6.

REFERENCES: Friedman p 195. Chou pp 44, 81. Schamroth. Barold.

C-13

Clinical History

A 37-year-old man with chest discomfort and dyspnea 2 h after inhaling cocaine.

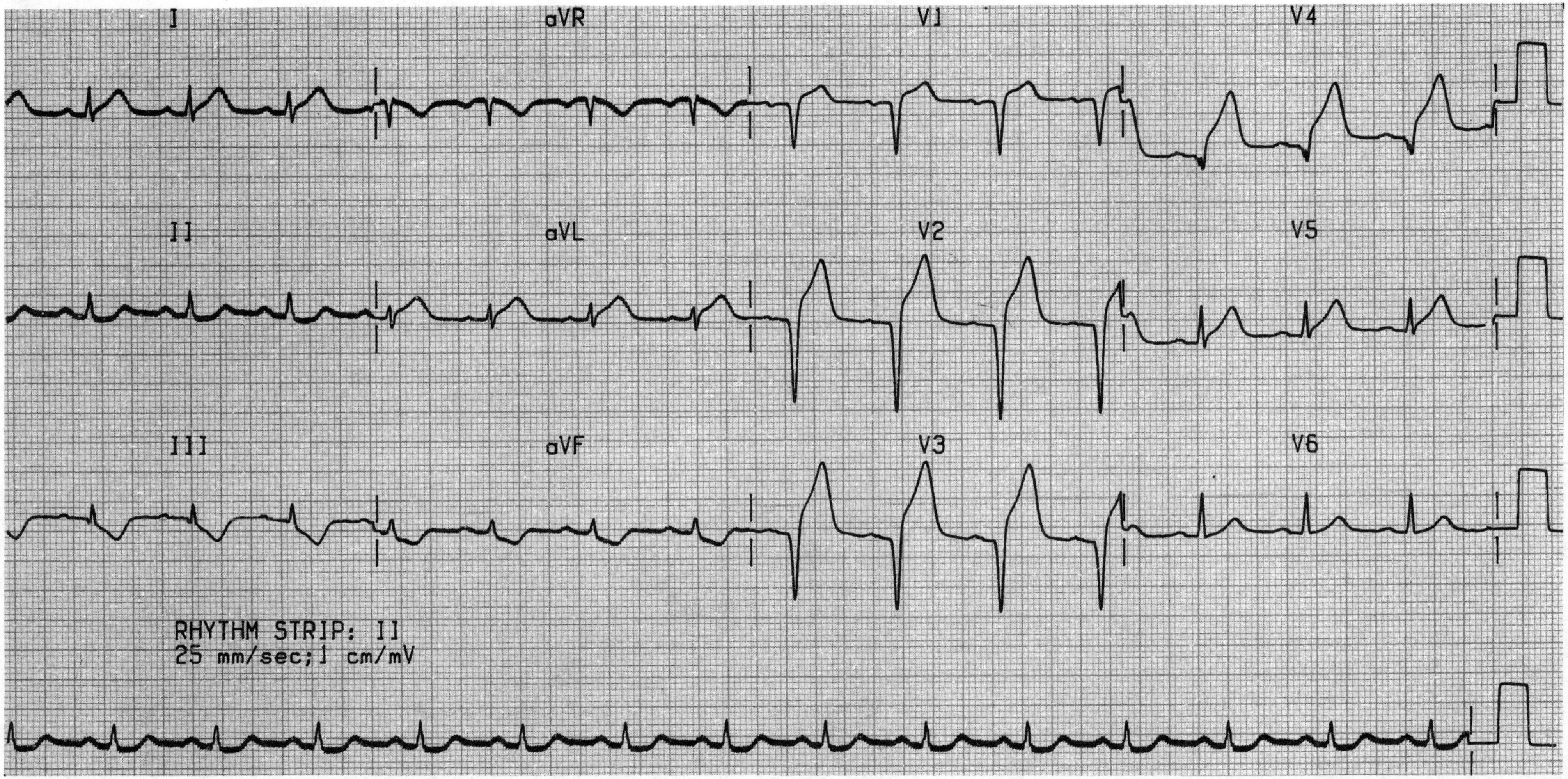

C-13

NARRATIVE INTERPRETATION

Rhythm:	**Sinus**
Rate:	**85**
Intervals:	**PR 0.16, QRS 0.08, QT 0.32**
Axis:	**+60 degrees**

Abnormalities

Q waves leads V1–V4. ST elevation leads I, aVL, V1–V5. ST depression leads II, III, aVF.

Synthesis

Sinus rhythm. Extensive anterior and lateral wall MI with ST-T-wave abnormalities of acute myocardial injury. ST-T-wave abnormalities in inferior leads suggesting either myocardial ischemia or reciprocal changes.

TEST ANSWERS: 1, 87, 89, 100, 101.

Comment: This patient sustained an extensive MI related to abuse of cocaine. On catheterization, he was found to have normal coronary arteries. This is not an unusual finding in young patients with MI secondary to cocaine use. It has been hypothesized that coronary spasm initiates formation of an intracoronary thrombus that results in an acute MI, even in patients with no underlying coronary obstruction.

REFERENCE: Zimmerman.

C-14

Clinical History

A 22-year-old man in the emergency department following a motor vehicle accident.

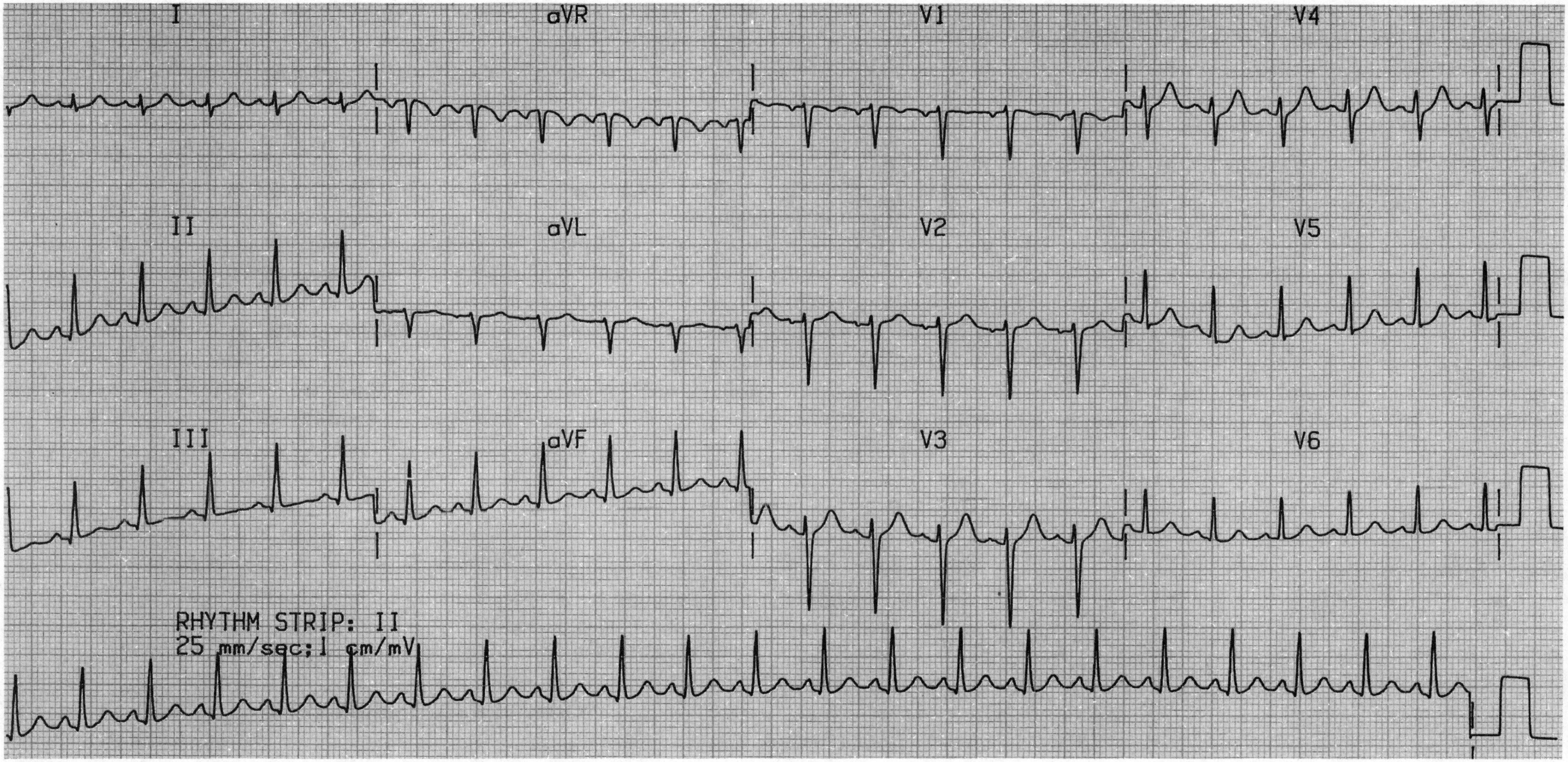

C-14

NARRATIVE INTERPRETATION

Rhythm:	**Sinus tachycardia**
Rate:	**135**
Intervals:	**PR 0.14, QRS 0.08, QT 0.26**
Axis:	**+90 degrees**

Abnormalities
Rapid heart rate.

Synthesis
Sinus tachycardia. Otherwise within normal limits.

TEST ANSWERS: 4.

Comment: Patients with blunt chest trauma may suffer cardiac contusion. A variety of electrocardiographic abnormalities may result. The most common arrhythmia is sinus tachycardia, which occurs in more than 70 percent of cases. Ventricular and atrial extrasystoles, intraventricular conduction abnormalities, and heart block are seen less frequently. Mechanical complications may also occur, including myocardial necrosis, valvular injury, coronary laceration, and hemopericardium. This patient suffered a mild cardiac contusion confirmed by elevation of CPK isoenzymes.

REFERENCES: Tenzer. Macdonald. Berk.

C-15

Clinical History

A 69-year-old man seen in the emergency department 12 h after an episode of chest discomfort.

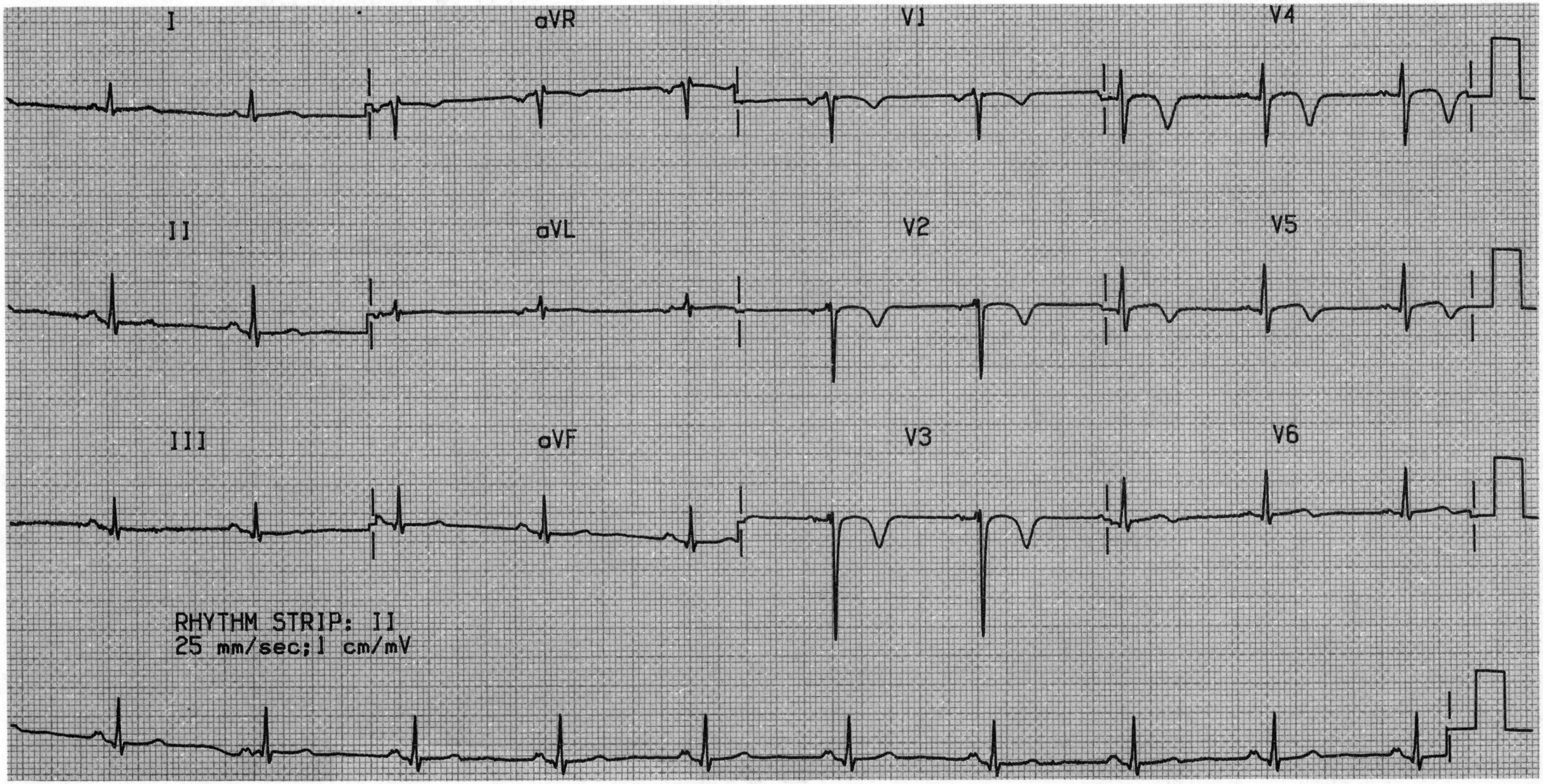

C-15

NARRATIVE INTERPRETATION

Rhythm:	**Sinus**
Rate:	**60**
Intervals:	**PR 0.16, QRS 0.08, QT 0.38**
Axis:	**+60 degrees**

Abnormalities
R waves V1–V3 less than 3 mm. Slight ST elevation with "coved" ST segment leads V2–V5. T wave inverted leads V2–V5. T wave biphasic leads I, II, III, aVF, V6.

Synthesis
Sinus rhythm. Poor R-wave progression. Probable recent anteroseptal wall MI. ST-T-wave abnormalities in leads V2–V6 suggesting recent myocardial injury. Nonspecific T-wave abnormalities leads I, II, III, aVF.

TEST ANSWERS: 1, 66, (81), 100, 106.

Comment: This patient suffered an MI a number of hours prior to presenting to the emergency department. By this time, more pronounced ST elevation has started to return toward baseline and T-wave inversion has occurred. Although profound ST elevation is no longer apparent, subtle elevation remains with downward concavity, or "coving." Myocardial necrosis has resulted in loss of anterior R forces; hence, poor R-wave progression is observed in leads V1–V3. The ST-T-wave abnormalities reflect extensive involvement although criteria for an extensive, anterior, Q wave MI are not met.

REFERENCES: Bar (*J Am Coll Cardiol*). DePace.

C-16

Clinical History

A 55-year-old asymptomatic woman on her second hospital day.

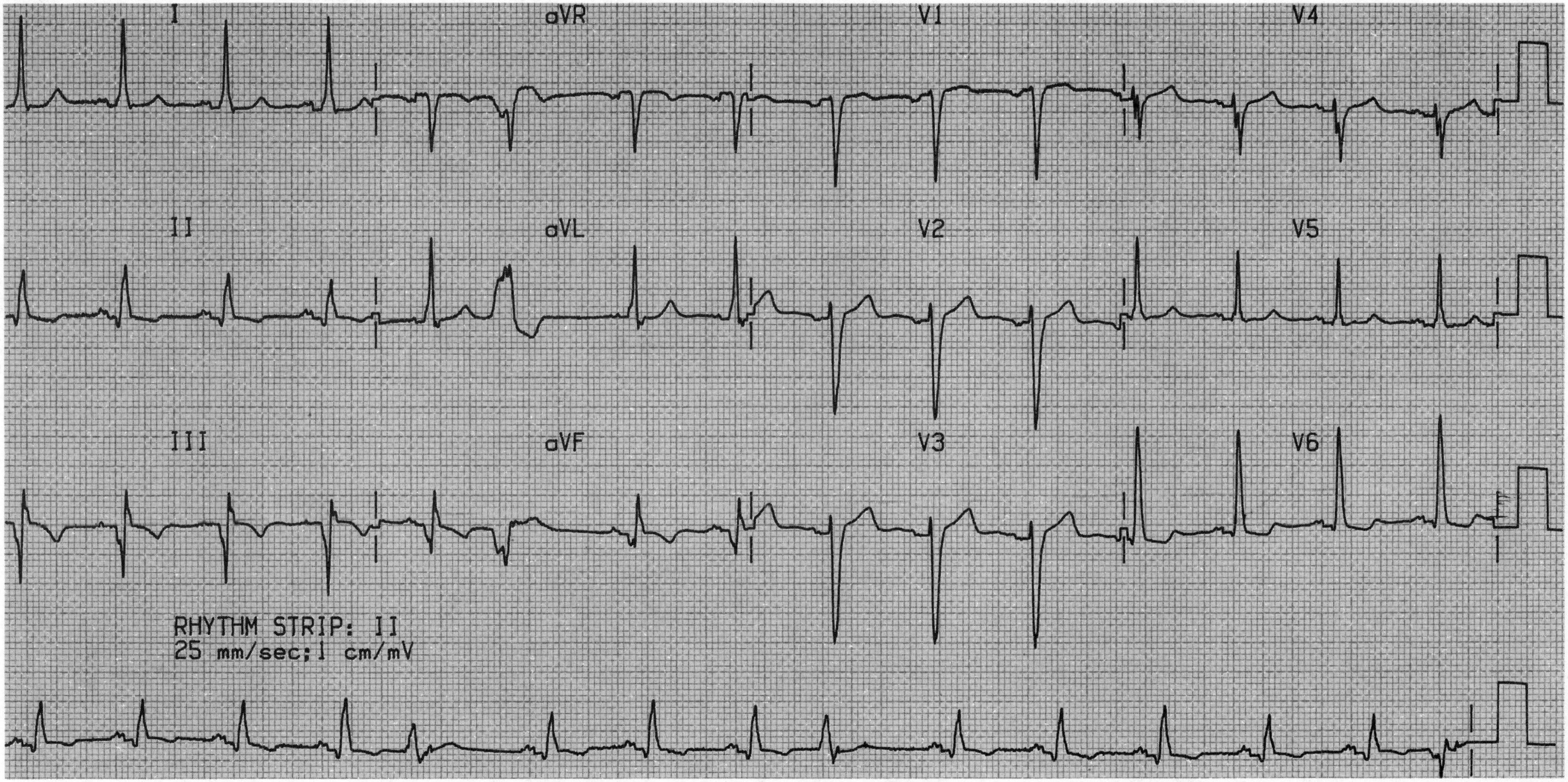

C-16

NARRATIVE INTERPRETATION

Rhythm: **Sinus**
Rate: **84**
Intervals: **PR 0.14, QRS 0.09, QT 0.36**
Axis: **+15 degrees**

Abnormalities

Q waves leads II, III, aVF. Slight ST elevation and "coving" leads II, III, aVF. ST depression leads V5–V6. T-wave inversion leads II, III, aVF, V6. R wave lead aVL >11. VPCs. Abnormal P terminal force lead V1.

Synthesis

Sinus rhythm. VPCs. Inferior wall MI with ST-T-wave abnormalities suggesting recent myocardial injury. LVH by voltage criteria. Associated ST-T-wave abnormalities. Left atrial abnormality.

TEST ANSWERS: 1, 26, 60, 78, 91, 100, 103.

Comment: The reader should not mistakenly identify the slurred upstroke seen in lead I or aVL as a delta wave and consider this tracing a "pseudoinfarction" pattern of WPW. The PR interval is not abnormally short and there are not other supporting criteria. This patient sustained an inferior wall MI. Evolving ST-T-wave abnormalities are present in the inferior limb leads. This patient also had LVH, which was likely secondary to long-standing hypertension. The limb lead voltage criteria for LVH are quite specific although they are not sensitive.

REFERENCE: Chou p 38.

C-17

Clinical History

A 56-year-old man with hypertension.

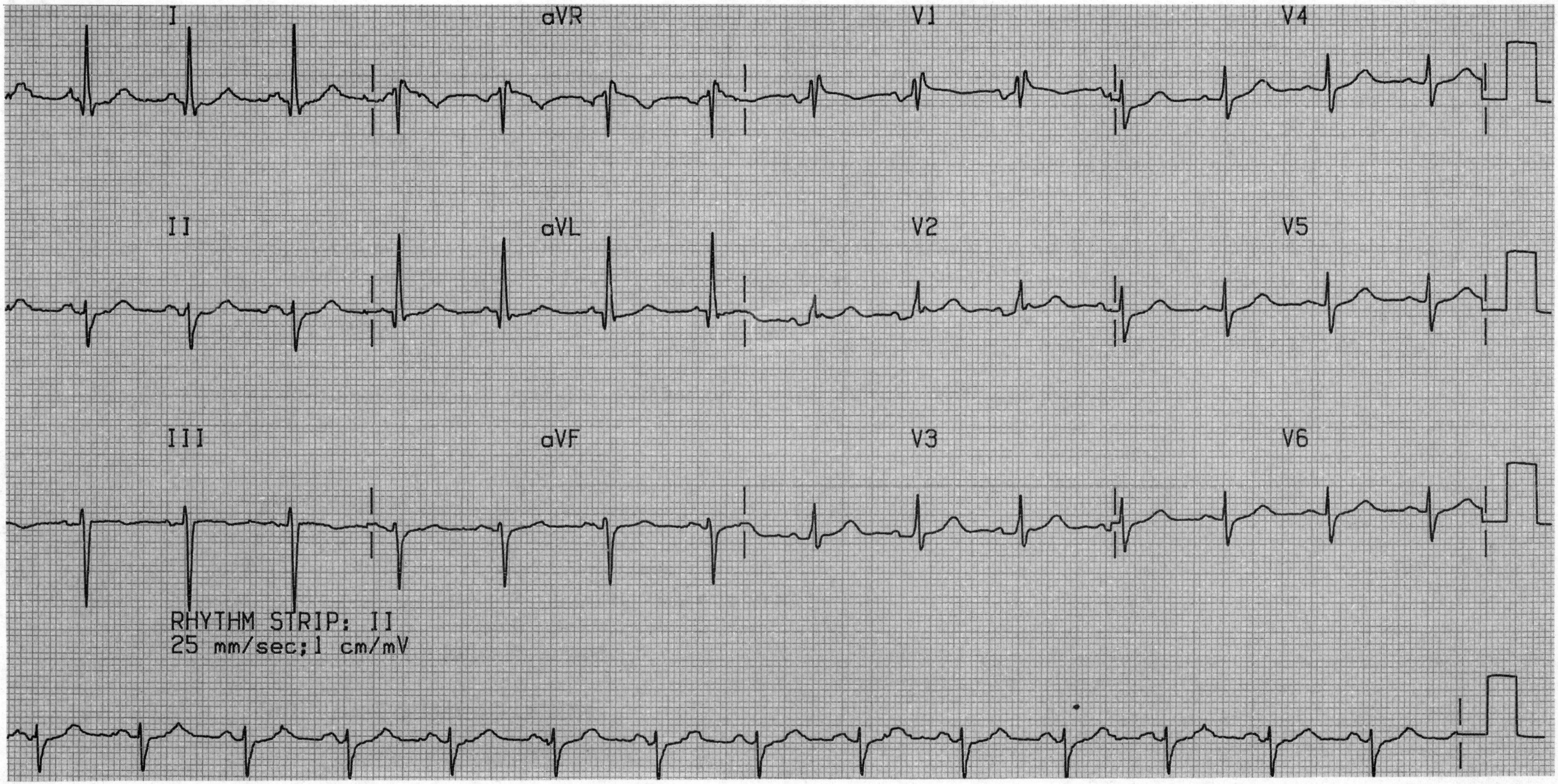

C-17

NARRATIVE INTERPRETATION

Rhythm:	**Sinus**
Rate:	**85**
Intervals:	**PR 0.16, QRS 0.10, QT 0.36**
Axis:	**−45 degrees**

Abnormalities

Axis leftward of −30 degrees. RSR′ pattern lead V1.

Synthesis

Sinus rhythm. Left axis deviation. Left anterior fascicular block. Incomplete RBBB.

TEST ANSWERS: 1, 64, 71, 72.

Comment: Note that the limb-lead voltage criteria for LVH are not present in this example. Isolated left anterior fascicular block (LAFB) can increase the R voltage in I and aVL and the use of standard criteria will often lead to a spurious diagnosis of LVH. A suggested criterion for the diagnosis of LVH in the presence of LAFB is the sum of the S wave in lead III + the maximal precordial R + S voltage in any precordial lead greater than 30. An additional suggested criterion is an R wave in aVL greater than 13. Neither criterion is met in this example.

REFERENCES: Gertsch. Milliken.

C-18

Clinical History

A 78-year-old man with dyspnea.

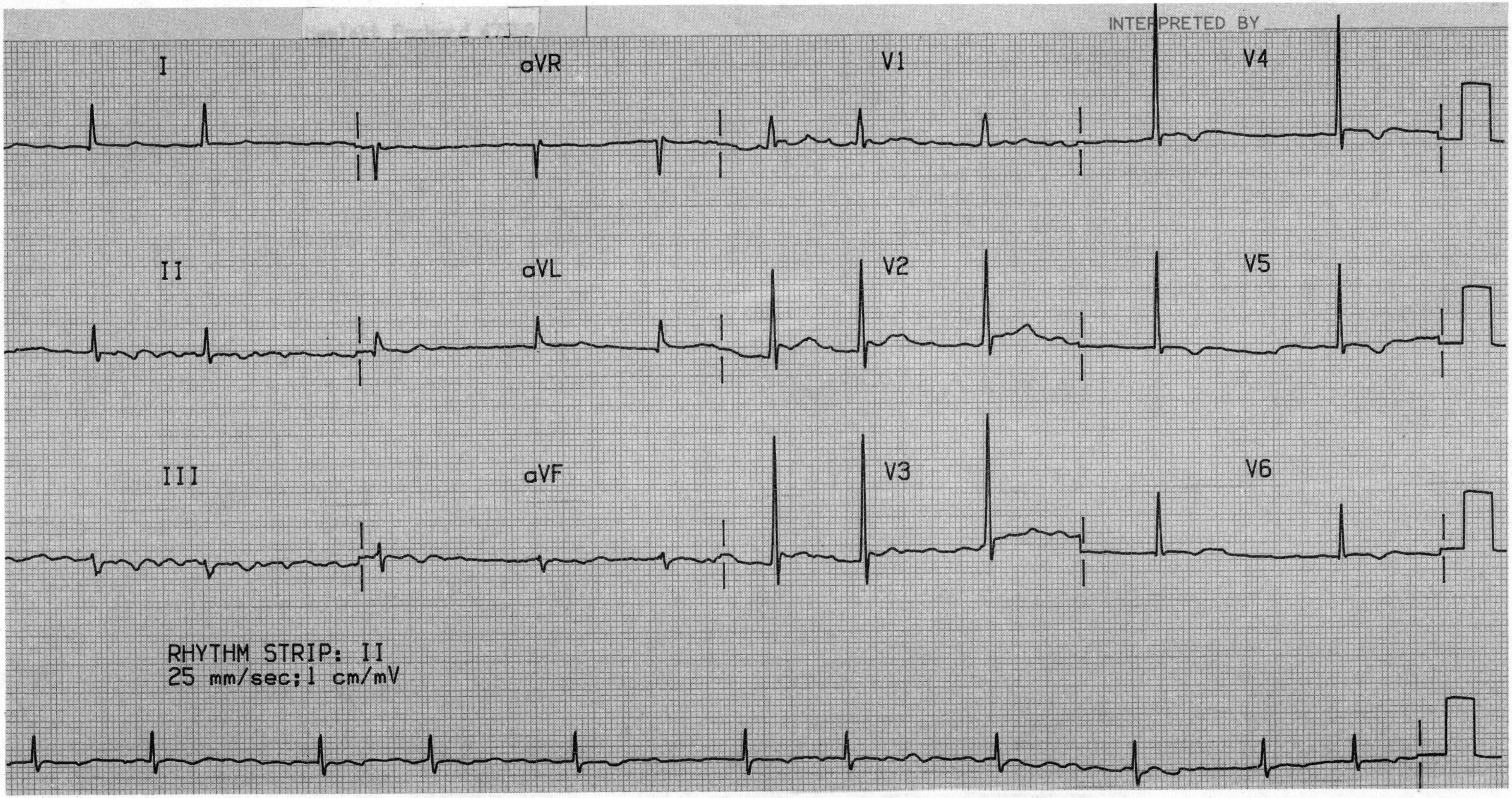

C-18

NARRATIVE INTERPRETATION

Rhythm: **Atrial fibrillation**
Rate: **62 (average)**
Intervals: **PR –, QRS 0.08, QT 0.36**
Axis: **– 15 degrees**

Abnormalities

Tall R waves with R/S greater than 1 leads V1–V3. T wave inverted leads V4–V6.

Synthesis

Atrial fibrillation with controlled ventricular response. Posterior wall MI of indeterminate age. Nonspecific T-wave abnormalities.

TEST ANSWERS: 20, 51, 94, 106.

Comment: This patient had suffered a posterior wall MI a number of years previously. This diagnosis may be made on the basis of tall R waves in leads V1 and V2. The differential diagnosis of tall R waves in the right precordial leads includes RVH, posterior wall MI, normal variant, and misplacement of the chest leads. Other conditions producing tall R waves are AV nodal bypass tract patterns and RBBB. Remember that although the ventricular response is "controlled," it is nonphysiologic secondary to treatment with digoxin.

C-19

Clinical History

A 77-year-old man in the recovery unit after open heart surgery. Previous electrocardiograms are normal.

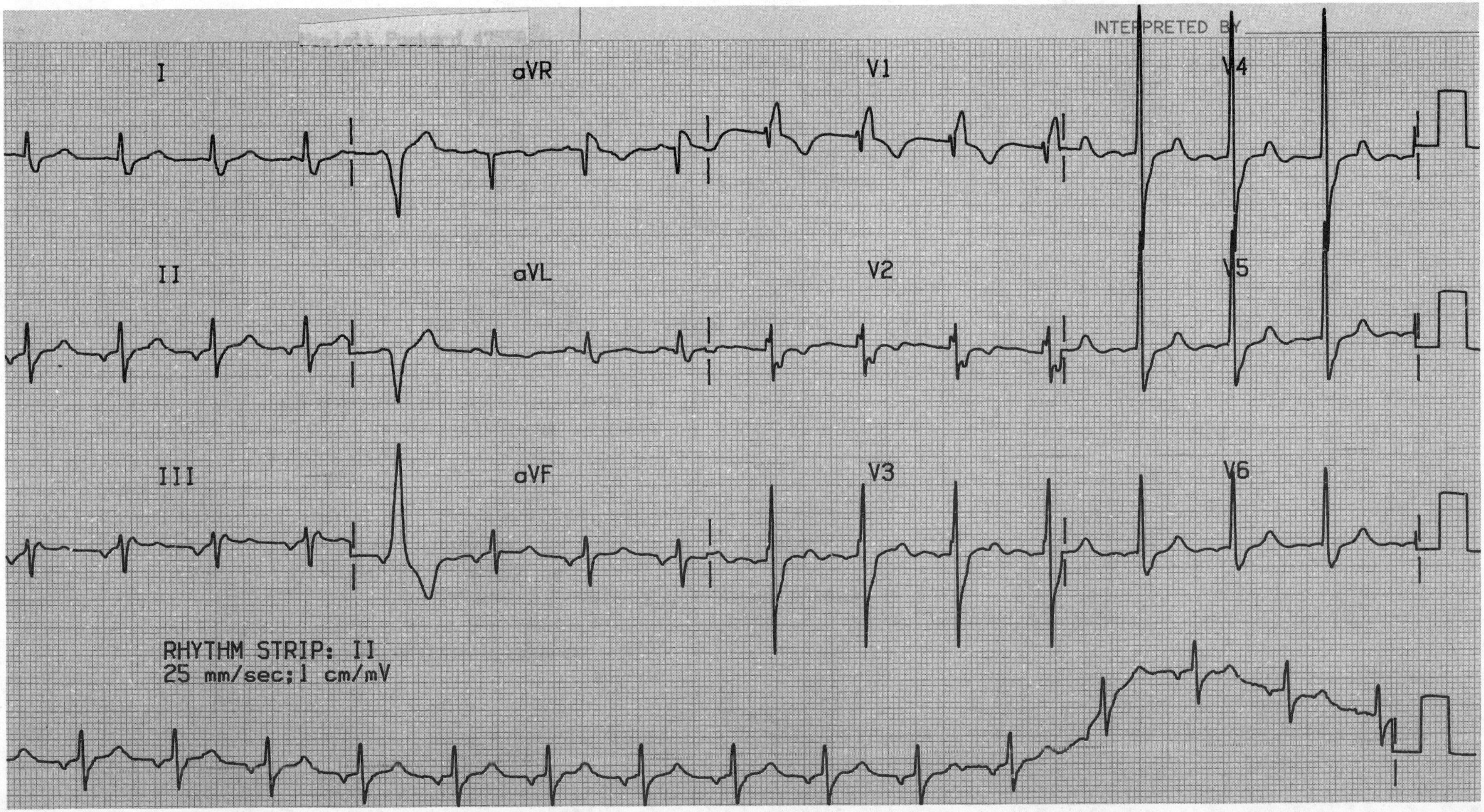

C-19

NARRATIVE INTERPRETATION

Rhythm: **Accelerated AV junctional rhythm**
Rate: **90**
Intervals: **PR 0.12, QRS 0.12, QT 0.36**
Axis: **−30 degrees**

Abnormalities

Inverted P waves leads II, III, aVF with PR interval at lower limit of normal. VPC. Broad, notched QRS with rSR′ and T-wave inversion lead V1.

Synthesis

Accelerated AV junctional rhythm. VPC. RBBB with associated ST-T-wave changes. Normalization of conduction in post VPC complex.

TEST ANSWERS: (9), 23, 26, 70, 104.

Comment: This rhythm is likely to be an accelerated AV junctional rhythm on the basis of the inverted P waves in the inferior leads and a relatively short PR interval. An ectopic atrial rhythm cannot be excluded as the PR interval is borderline. RBBB is evident. An interesting feature of this electrocardiogram can be seen in the sixth beat. Note that after the postextrasystolic pause that the conduction is normalized with loss of the terminal conduction delay from the RBBB. The conduction abnormality returns with the subsequent complex. The development of a new RBBB after coronary bypass surgery does not appear to indicate an adverse prognosis.

REFERENCES: Tuzcu. Thomas. Wexelman.

C-20

Clinical History

A 77-year-old asymptomatic woman.

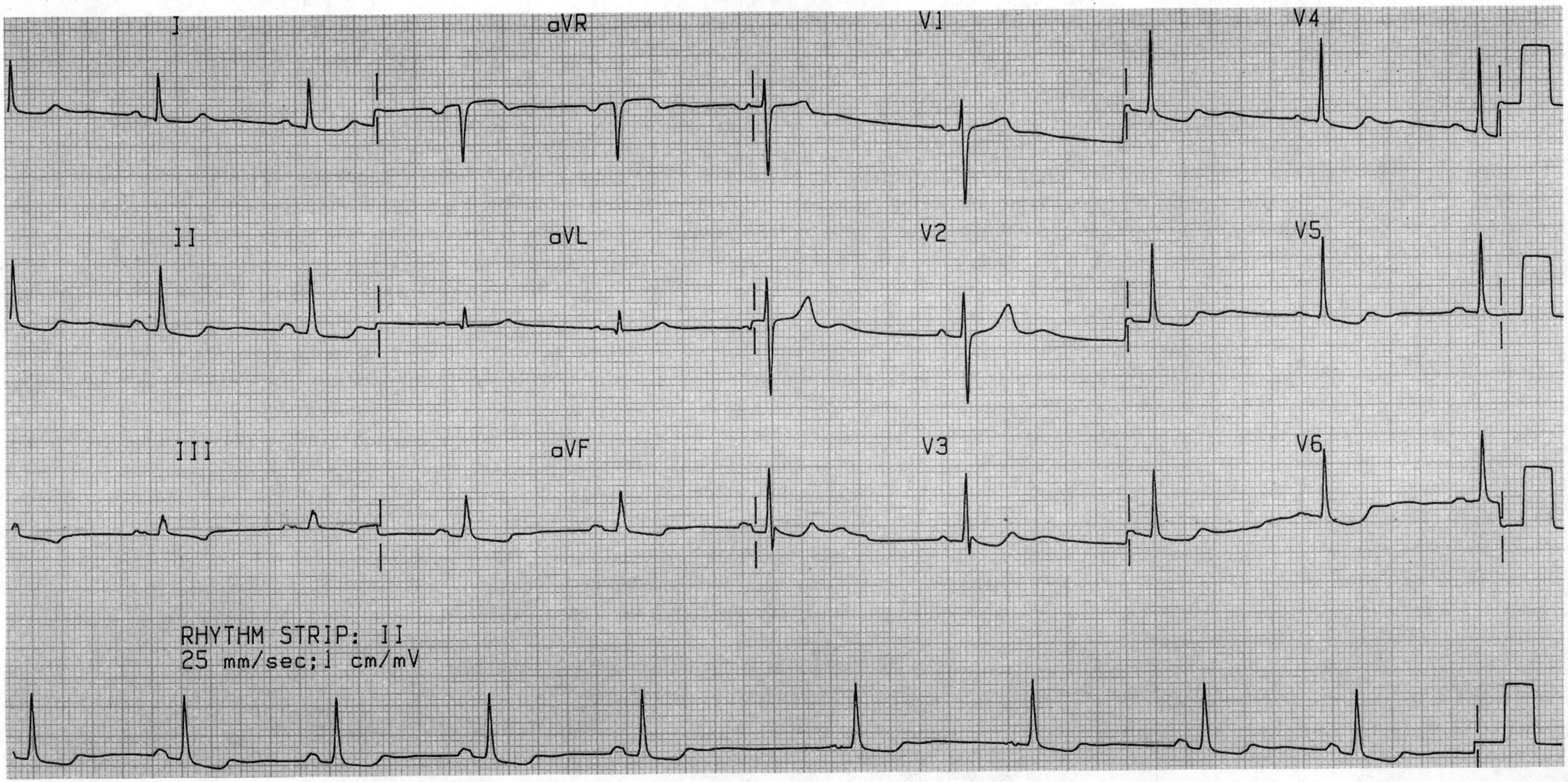

C-20

NARRATIVE INTERPRETATION

Rhythm:	**Sinus bradycardia with sinus pause**
Rate:	**57**
Intervals:	**PR 0.20, QRS 0.08, QT 0.36**
Axis:	**+45 degrees**

Abnormalities

Slow heart rate. Sinus pause. "Low" atrial escape complexes. ST depression leads I, II, aVF, V3–V6. T wave inverted lead III. T wave biphasic lead aVF.

Synthesis

Sinus bradycardia with sinus pause. "Low" atrial escape complexes. Nonspecific ST-T-wave abnormalities.

TEST ANSWERS: 3, 7, 106.

Comment: This patient demonstrates sinus bradycardia with an apparent sinus pause after the fifth complex on the rhythm strip. A subsidiary pacemaker in a "low" atrial site takes over at a slightly slower intrinsic heart rate. The sinus node then again usurps control after two complexes. The escape complexes cannot be called AV junctional as the P wave is not clearly inverted with a short PR interval in the lead II rhythm strip, and there is only one lead to observe with these complexes. This tracing represents a true sinus pause rather than wandering atrial pacemaker and sinus arrhythmia. Sinus arrhythmia should not be diagnosed because the rhythm is regular and abruptly slows, which results in escape complexes. Wandering atrial pacemaker would be characterized only if there were regular R-to-R intervals with a different P-wave configuration and normal PR interval. Criteria for second-degree SA block are also not met in this example.

C-21

Clinical History

A 77-year-old woman in the ICU with respiratory arrest.

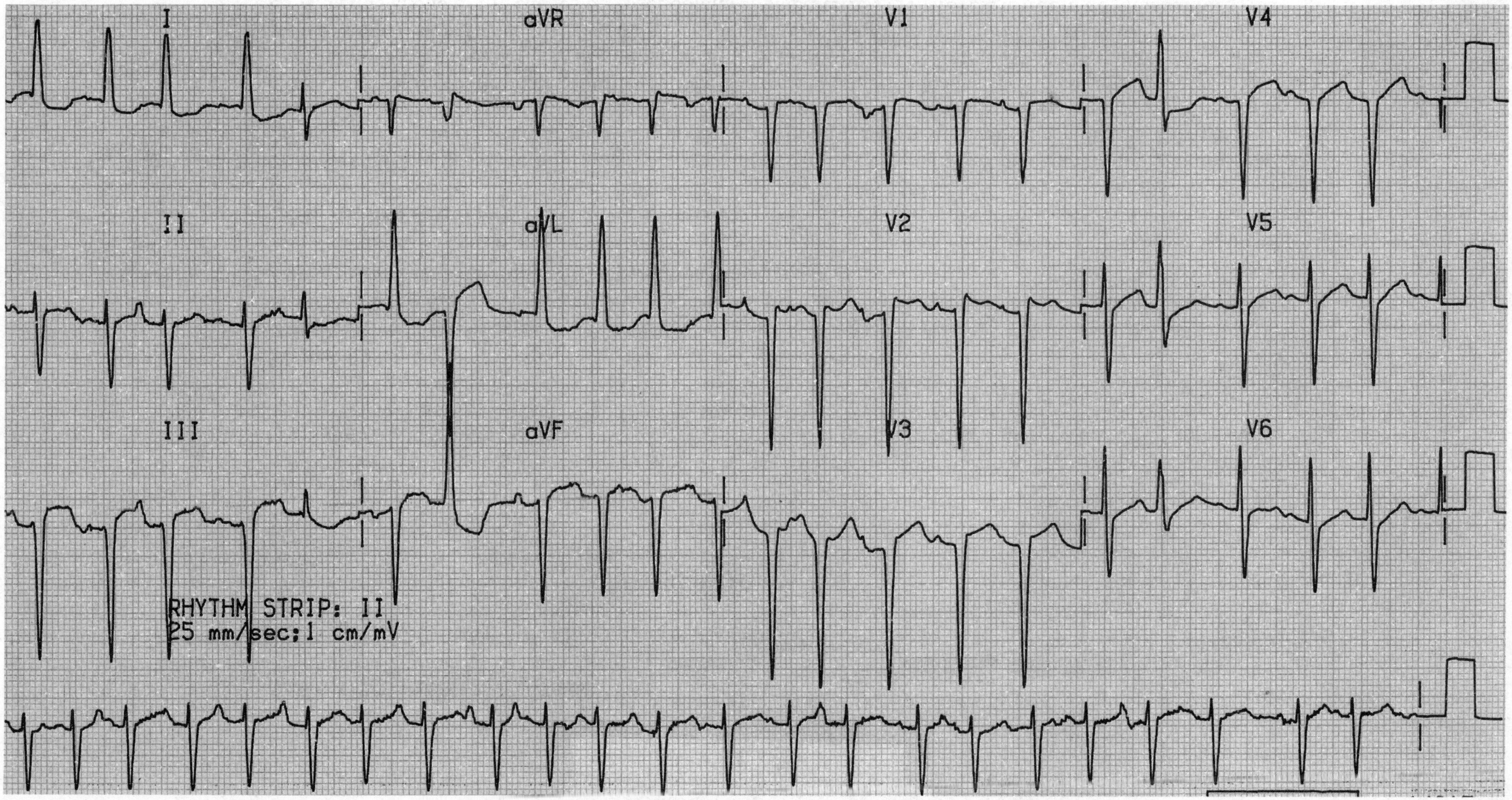

C-21

NARRATIVE INTERPRETATION

Rhythm:	**Multifocal atrial tachycardia**
Rate:	**138**
Intervals:	**PR –, QRS 0.10, QT 0.34**
Axis:	**−45 degrees**

Abnormalities

Rapid heart rate with variable P-wave morphologies. Axis leftward of −30 degrees. Small R wave V2. QS waves leads V3–V4. R wave aVL equals 23. ST elevation leads II, III, aVF, V2–V5. ST depression leads I, aVL. VPCs.

Synthesis

Multifocal atrial tachycardia. VPCs. LVH by voltage criteria limb leads. Associated nonspecific ST abnormalities leads I, aVL. Left axis deviation. Left anterior fascicular block. Anterior wall MI of indeterminate age. Possible acute myocardial injury.

TEST ANSWERS: 14, 26, 64, 72, 78, 84, (100), 103.

Comment: There are quite a number of abnormalities in this tracing. The rhythm is fairly obvious and demonstrates multifocal atrial tachycardia. By definition, there are at least three different P-wave configurations evident in the tachyarrhythmia. Note left axis deviation, likely secondary to a combination of left anterior fascicular block and LVH. The increased voltage in lead aVL is highly specific for LVH. Even allowing for the increase in voltage in aVL in the presence of left anterior fascicular block, there are adequate criteria for LVH. The diagnosis of anterior wall MI may be problematic in the presence of LVH as this is one of the causes of "pseudoinfarction patterns." However, it would be unusual for LVH to produce QS waves in V4. Interestingly, the ST changes present in this example were chronic and probably secondary to LVH, although it would be incorrect to ignore the possibility of acute infarction.

REFERENCES: Milliken. Goldberger I. Goldberger II.

C-22

Clinical History

A 51-year-old man with chest discomfort.

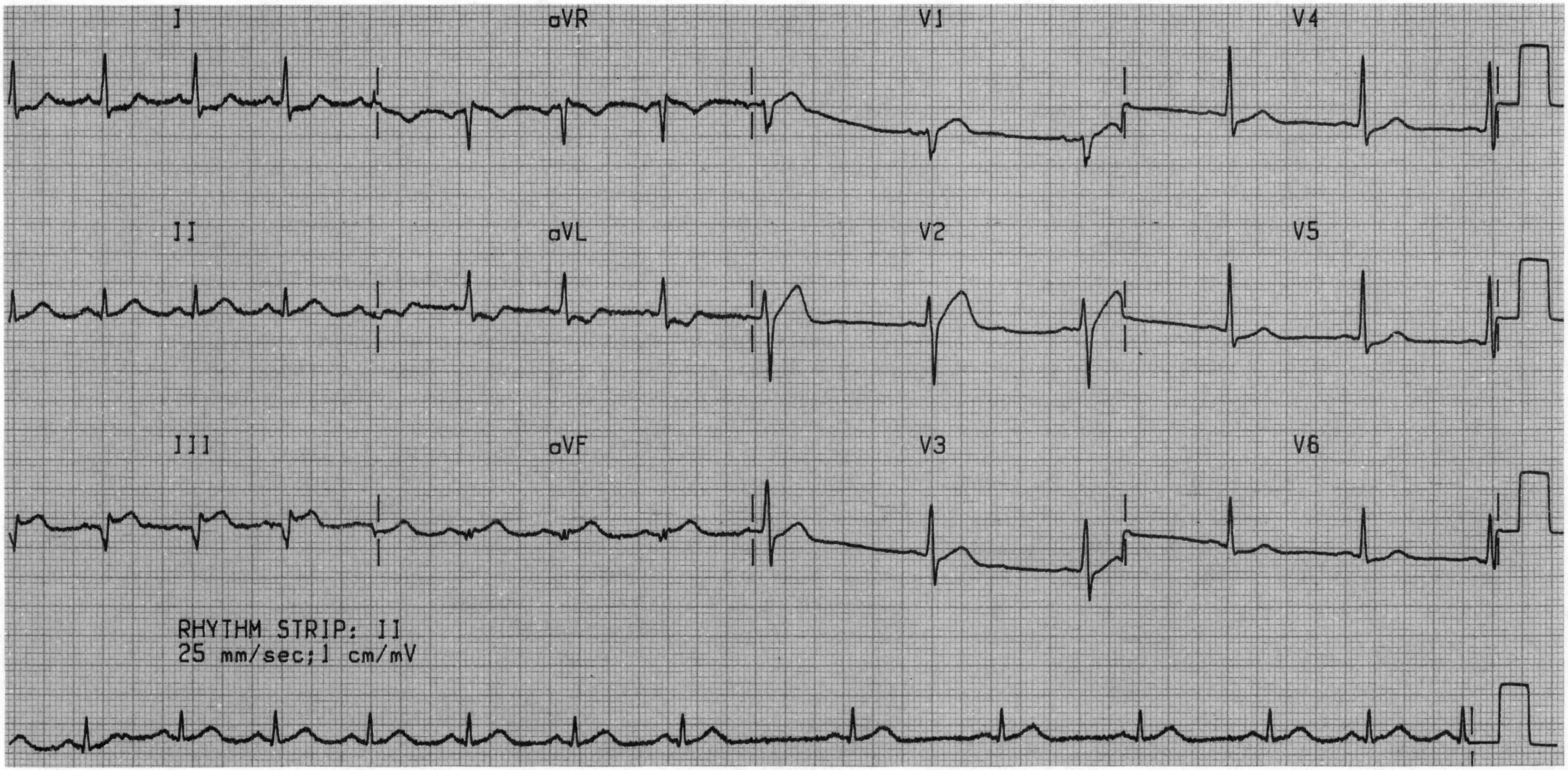

C-22

NARRATIVE INTERPRETATION

Rhythm: **Sinus arrhythmia**
Rate: **90 (average)**
Intervals: **PR 0.16, QRS 0.08, QT 0.36**
Axis: **0 degrees**

Abnormalities

Variation in sinus rate. Small Q wave leads II, aVF. Q wave lead III. ST elevation leads II, III, aVF, V1–V2. ST depression leads I, aVL, V4–V6. T-wave inversion lead aVL.

Synthesis

Sinus arrhythmia. Inferior wall MI with ST abnormalities of acute injury. ST-T-wave abnormalities suggesting either reciprocal change or myocardial ischemia.

TEST ANSWERS: 2, 91, 100, 101.

Comment: Sinus arrhythmia may be divided into two types, respiratory and nonrespiratory. Respiratory sinus arrhythmia is most often seen in the setting of sinus bradycardia and is the result of varying vagal influences within the respiratory cycle. Nonrespiratory sinus arrhythmia is most often seen in patients with organic heart disease or is secondary to medications such as digoxin or morphine. The profound vagal influences often seen in acute inferior wall MI may also produce a marked nonrespiratory sinus arrhythmia, something that is seen in the current example. An additional illustrative point is the ST elevation seen in leads V1–V2 in conjunction with the acute inferior wall MI. A number of investigators have suggested that this represents concomitant right ventricular MI. Right ventricular leads may also be useful in making this diagnosis.

REFERENCES: Robalino. Schweitzer (1990). Lopez-Sendon. Shah.

C-23

Clinical History

A 78-year-old man in the CCU with severe congestive heart failure.

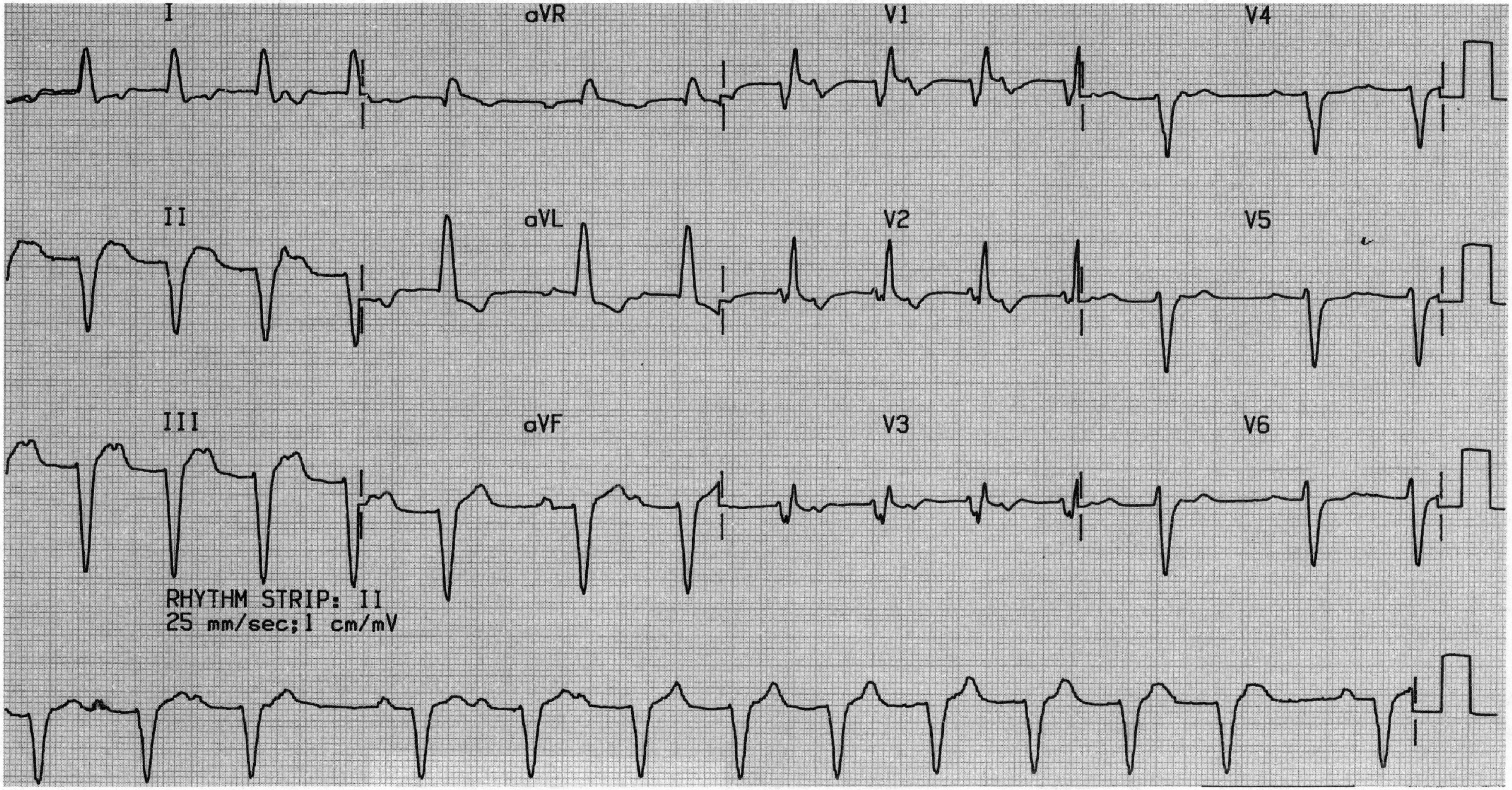

C-23

NARRATIVE INTERPRETATION

Rhythm: **Sinus**
Rate: **84**
Intervals: **PR variable, QRS 0.13, QT 0.40**
Axis: **−75 degrees**

Abnormalities

Gradual prolongation of PR interval with failure to conduct P wave. Axis leftward of −30 degrees. Prolonged QRS duration. rSR′ V1–V3 with associated T-wave inversion leads V1–V3. S wave lead III greater than 15. ST depression leads I, aVL. T-wave inversion leads I, aVL. ST elevation leads II, III, aVF, V1–V2.

Synthesis

Sinus rhythm with second-degree AV block, Mobitz type I (Wenckebach). Left axis deviation. Left anterior fascicular block. RBBB with associated ST-T-wave changes. Probable LVH with associated ST-T-wave abnormalities.

TEST ANSWERS: 1, 43, 64, 70, 72, (78), (103), 104.

Comment: A number of electrocardiographic abnormalities may be seen in this tracing. There is a Wenckebach sequence evident with eventual failure to conduct a P wave. Note that the PR prolongation causes the P waves to be "lost" in the T wave of the preceding QRS complex. This tracing also demonstrates the phenomenon of "masquerading bundle branch block." There is a right bundle branch pattern in the right precordial leads and a QRS pattern in the limb leads that resembles left bundle branch block. A right bundle branch block is indeed present. However, the left axis and left anterior fascicular block, in conjunction with probable LVH, have caused the limb leads to resemble a left bundle branch block pattern. LVH is suggested by the marked voltage in leads III and aVL, even with the left anterior fascicular block.

REFERENCES: Friedman p 208. Rosenbaum.

C-24

Clinical History

A 61-year-old man with palpitations.

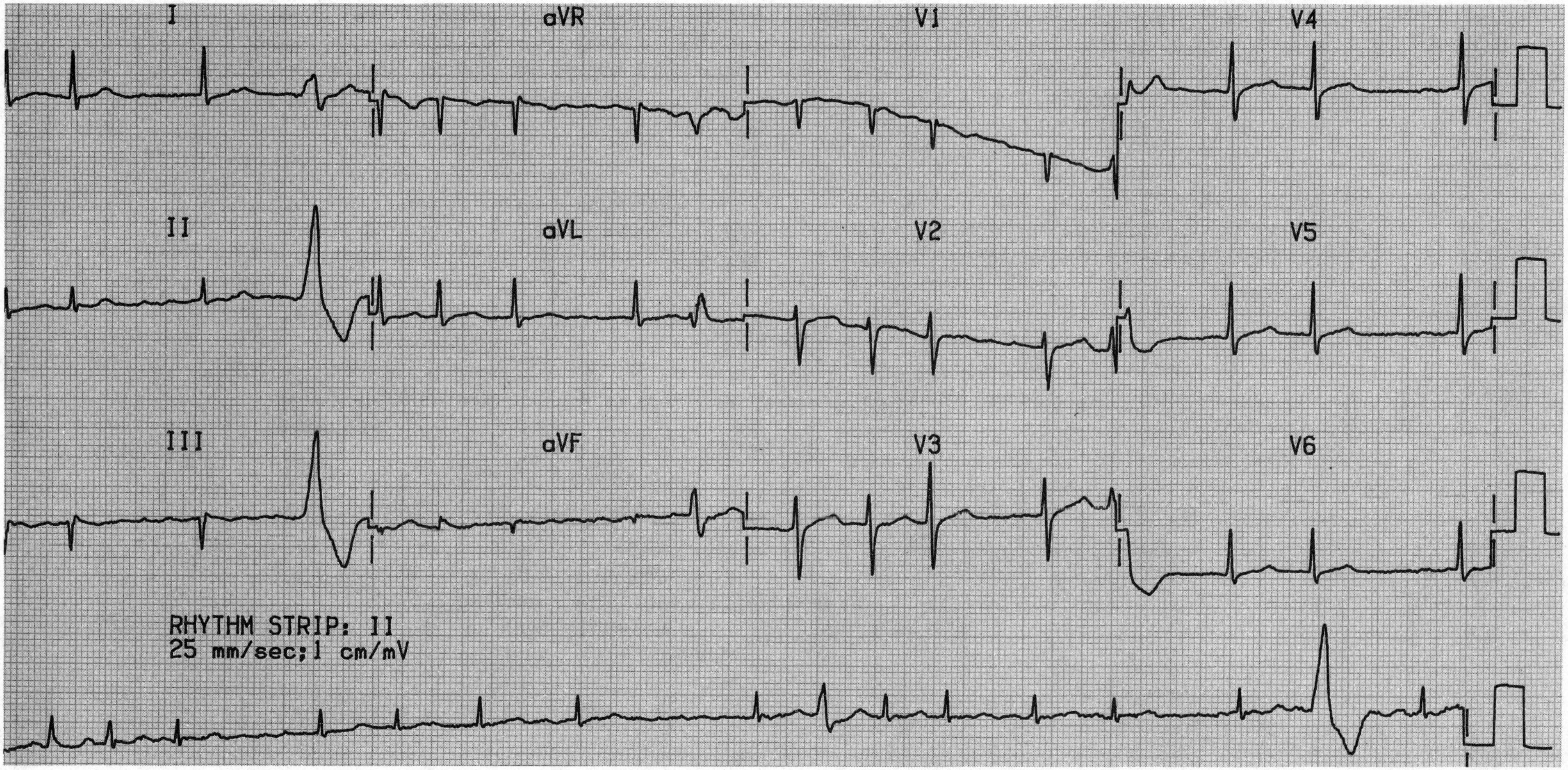

C-24

NARRATIVE INTERPRETATION

Rhythm: **Atrial fibrillation**
Rate: **92 (average)**
Intervals: **PR –, QRS 0.08, QT 0.30**
Axis: **– 15 degrees**

Abnormalities

VPCs. Aberrantly conducted beats.

Synthesis

Atrial fibrillation with a controlled ventricular response. Aberrantly conducted beats. VPCs. Otherwise within normal limits.

TEST ANSWERS: 20, 26, 51, 77.

Comment: This tracing demonstrates that VPCs and aberrantly conducted complexes may resemble each other and coexist. The differentiation of beats of ventricular origin and those conducted aberrantly of supraventricular origin is particularly difficult in patients with atrial fibrillation. Because the cycle lengths are constantly changing in atrial fibrillation, there is a tendency for aberrant conduction by virtue of Ashman's phenomenon. This states that aberrant ventricular conduction is favored by a long-short sequence because the ventricular refractory period is proportional to the preceding cycle length. When the refractory period is longer, the next impulse is more likely to be conducted with aberrancy.

In this example, the next-to-last complex is very wide and is identical to a complex in the limb leads that occurs without a long-short sequence. It is most likely a VPC. The complex six beats earlier in the rhythm strip also occurs after a long-short sequence, but it is less wide and bizarre. This is most likely aberrantly conducted. The sequence in this beat of an extremely long cycle preceding a short cycle should predispose to considerable aberrancy, but it is not as bizarre as the later beat. For this reason aberrancy is suggested by the earlier beat and ventricular ectopy by the later beat. A number of other complexes throughout the tracing also show various degrees of aberrancy.

REFERENCES: Chung pp 494–495. Marriott. Gulamhusein.

C-25

Clinical History

A 61-year-old asymptomatic man.

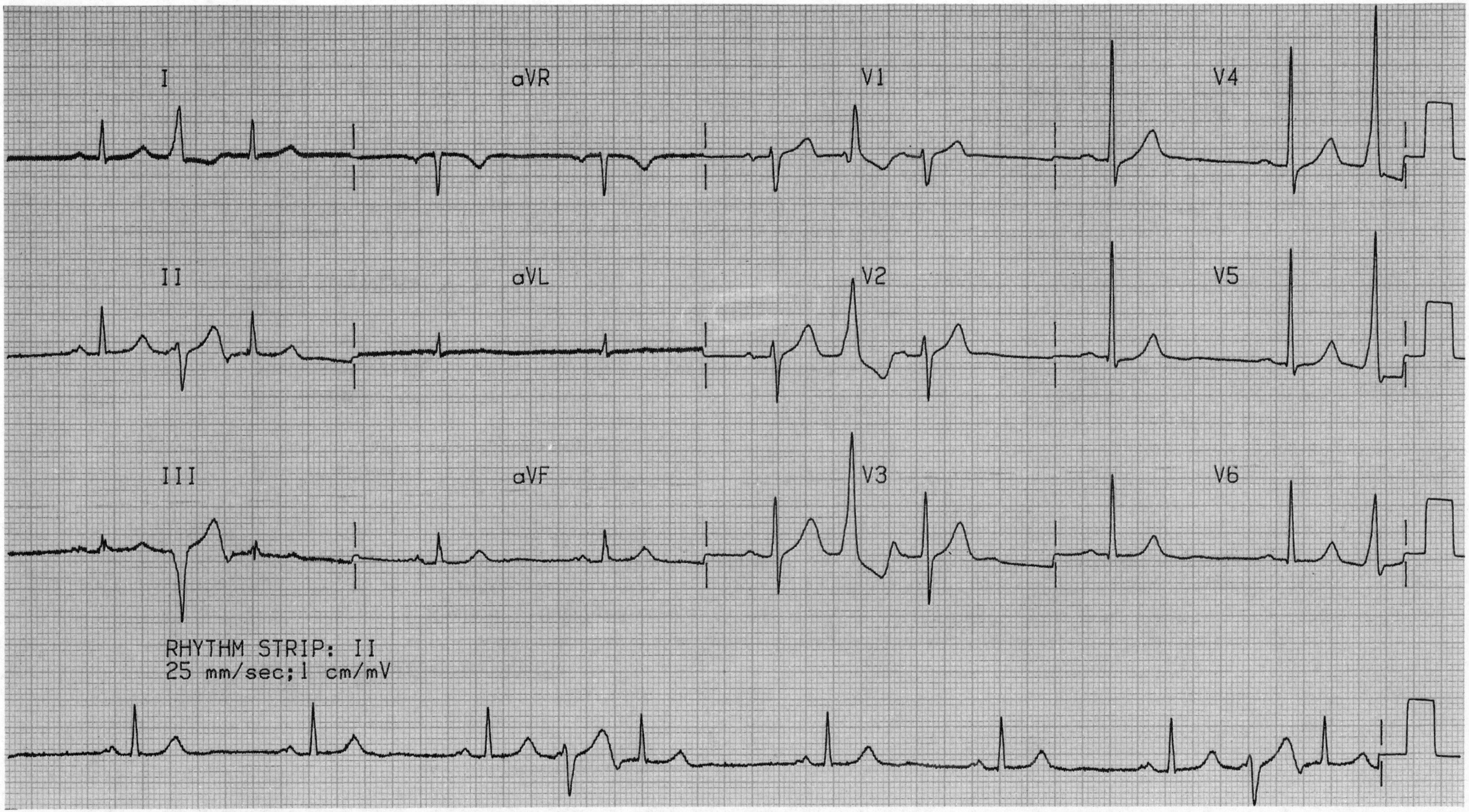

C-25

NARRATIVE INTERPRETATION

Rhythm: **Sinus bradycardia**
Rate: **46**
Intervals: **PR 0.20, QRS 0.08, QT 0.44**
Axis: **+45 degrees**

Abnormalities
Slow heart rate. VPCs. Echo complexes.

Synthesis
Sinus bradycardia. VPCs. Retrograde atrial activation with echo complexes. Otherwise within normal limits.

TEST ANSWERS: 3, 26, 54, 55.

Comment: The basic rhythm of this electrocardiogram is sinus bradycardia. Note that VPCs, which are "sandwiched" between two sinus beats, occur periodically. Usually these beats are interpolated VPCs; however, this is not the case in this example. The narrow complex beat following the VPC is seen to have an inverted P wave preceding it, which indicates retrograde atrial activation. Moreover, the narrow complex beat occurs earlier than would be expected in the sinus mechanism. This indicates that this is an echo, or reciprocal beat. The VPC has depolarized the atria in a retrograde fashion, and the impulse returns to depolarize the ventricles. The remainder of this tracing is within normal limits.

REFERENCE: Chung p 354.

C-26

Clinical History

A 45-year-old woman with atypical chest pain. She has been told she has a history of a "silent" MI.

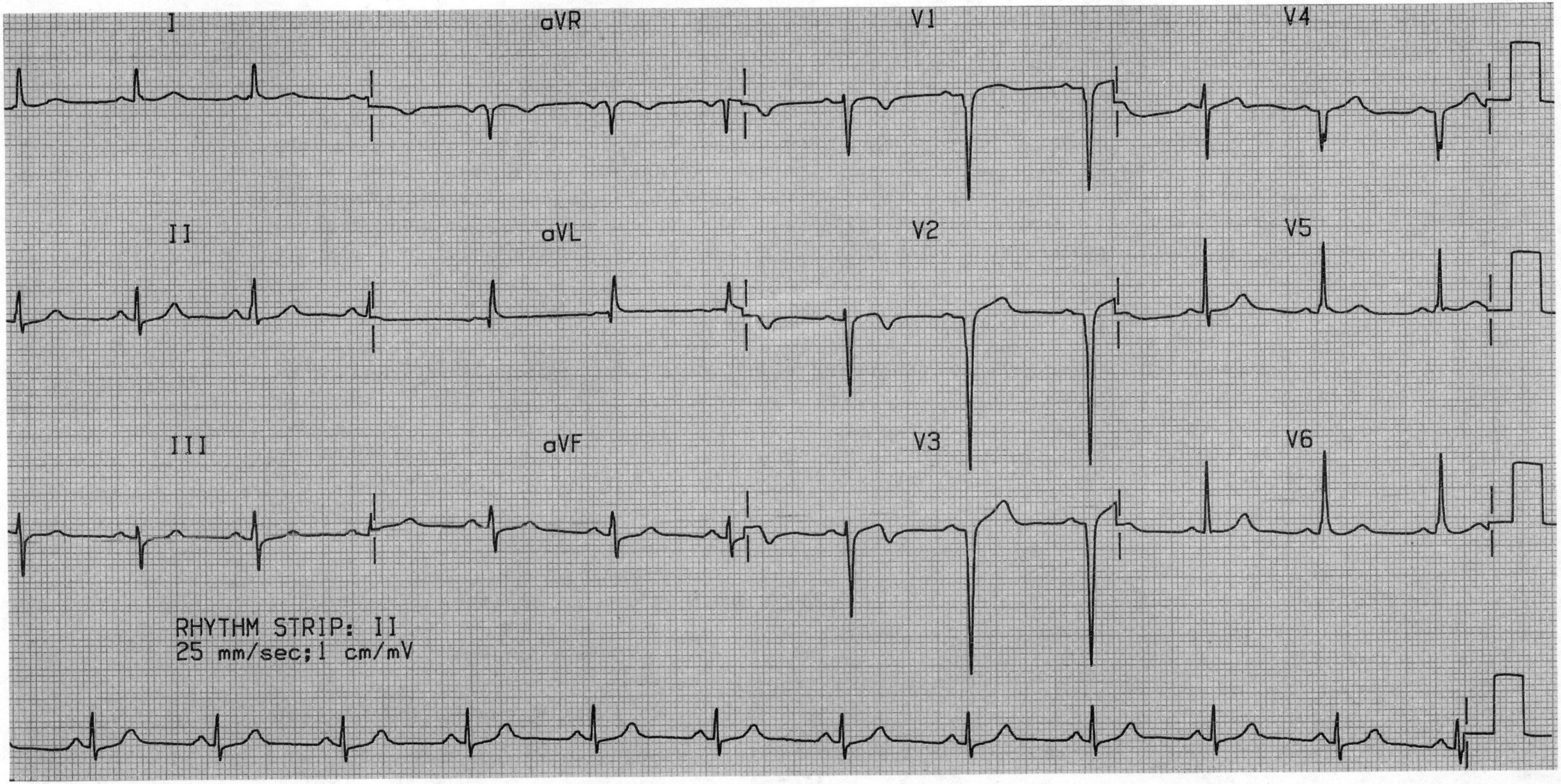

C-26

NARRATIVE INTERPRETATION

Rhythm: **Sinus**
Rate: **70**
Intervals: **PR 0.14, QRS 0.06, QT 0.36**
Axis: **0 degrees**

Abnormalities

Slight ST depression leads III, aVF, V6. ST elevation leads V2–V3. T-wave inversion leads V2–V3. Complexes with shortened PR interval with delta waves and change in QRS axis and configuration.

Synthesis

Sinus rhythm. Nonspecific ST-T-wave abnormalities. Intermittent ventricular preexcitation (WPW).

TEST ANSWERS: 1, 49, 106.

Comment: This tracing demonstrates intermittent ventricular preexcitation (WPW pattern). The second, fifth, eighth, and eleventh complexes of the 12-lead ECG demonstrate normal conduction, whereas the third, ninth, tenth, twelfth, and thirteenth complexes clearly show delta waves, a shortened PR interval, and a change in QRS morphology. Note the "pseudoinfarction" pattern in leads V1–V3 with apparent QS waves that mimic anteroseptal infarction. The WPW pattern is a result of preexcitation of the ventricles via an accessory bypass tract. In classic WPW, there is conduction over an accessory bundle of Kent. Alternative forms include conduction over a paranodal pathway of James or Mahaim fibers. The term *Wolff-Parkinson-White "syndrome"* should be reserved for patients with this pattern who also have tachyarrhythmias. Interestingly, the pattern in the right chest leads is suggestive of underlying coronary heart disease with T-wave inversion. This patient had no clinical evidence of coronary heart disease.

REFERENCES: Klein GJ. Reddy.

C-27

Clinical History

An 88-year-old asymptomatic man.

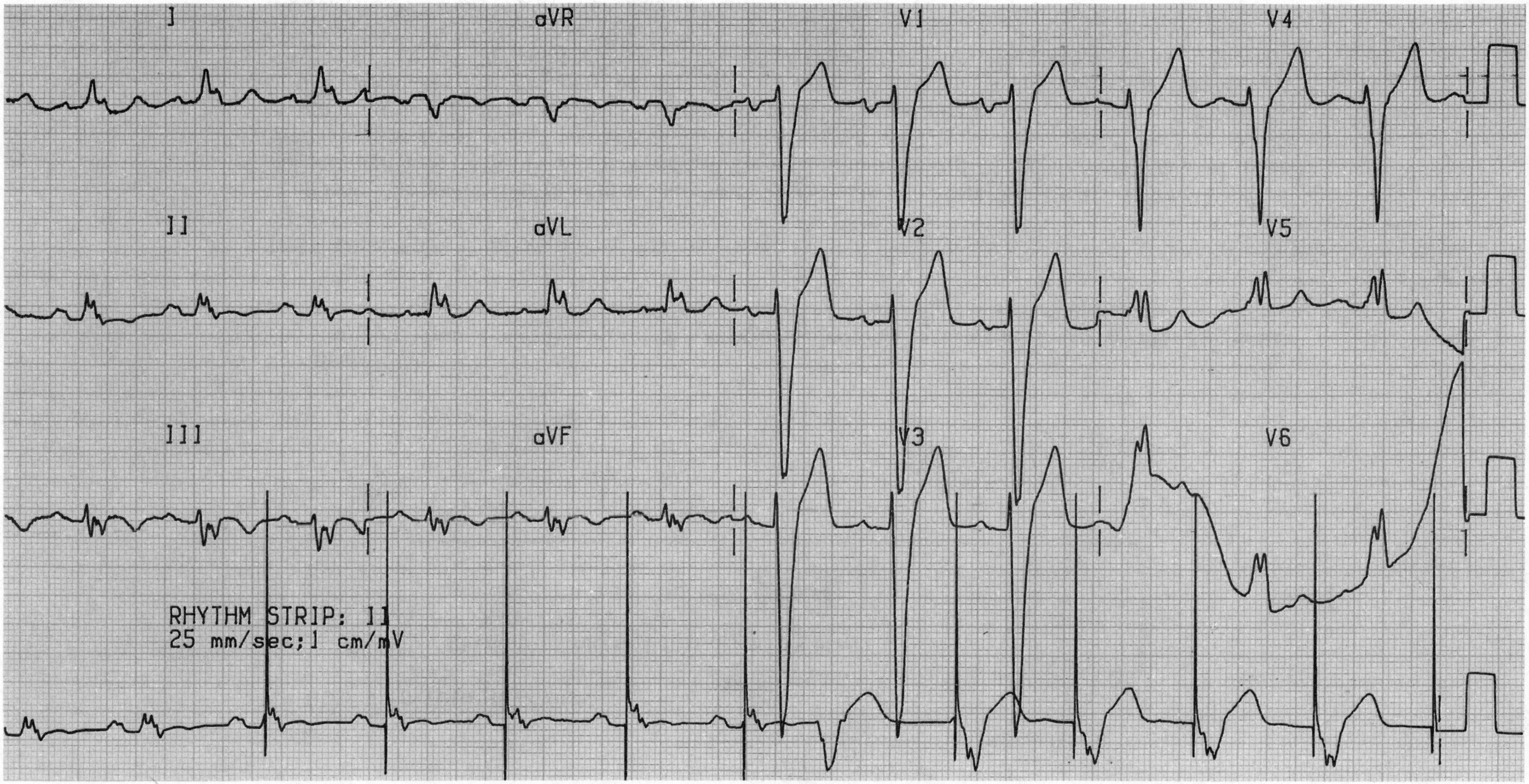

C-27

NARRATIVE INTERPRETATION

Rhythm: **Sinus with first-degree AV block**
Rate: **71**
Intervals: **PR 0.22, QRS 0.16, QT 0.44**
Axis: **0 degrees**

Abnormalities

Prolonged PR interval. Abnormal P terminal force lead V1. Broad, notched QRS leads I, aVL, V5–V6. T waves upright leads I, aVL, V5–V6. VPC. Ventricular pacemaker functioning on demand with appropriate capture, rate 72. Pacemaker pseudofusion complexes.

Synthesis

Sinus rhythm. First-degree AV block. VPC. Ventricular pacemaker on demand with capture. Pacemaker pseudofusion complexes. LBBB. Left atrial abnormality. Nonspecific T-wave abnormalities.

TEST ANSWERS: 1, 26, 35, 42, 60, 74, (104), 106.

Comment: The underlying rhythm is sinus with first-degree AV block and LBBB. Normally, the T waves are inverted with the opposite polarity from the bundle branch block. Thus, T-wave inversion would be expected in leads I and aVL and in the left precordial leads. In this example, the T waves are upright in these leads. This may be a sign of myocardial ischemia, although this is a nonspecific finding. In this patient, the T waves were chronic and were associated only with the conduction abnormality. Also note the pseudofusion pacemaker complexes on the rhythm strip. These are classified as pseudofusion rather than true fusion complexes because the pacemaker does not actually depolarize the ventricles. The QRS morphology is unchanged from baseline. This does not represent pacemaker failure to sense and is simply a manifestation of the intrinsic sinus mechanism's being nearly identical to that of the pacemaker rate. Only after the pause induced by the VPC does the pacemaker truly capture the ventricles.

C-28

Clinical History

An 82-year-old asymptomatic woman with a long history of coronary heart disease who is seen in the office.

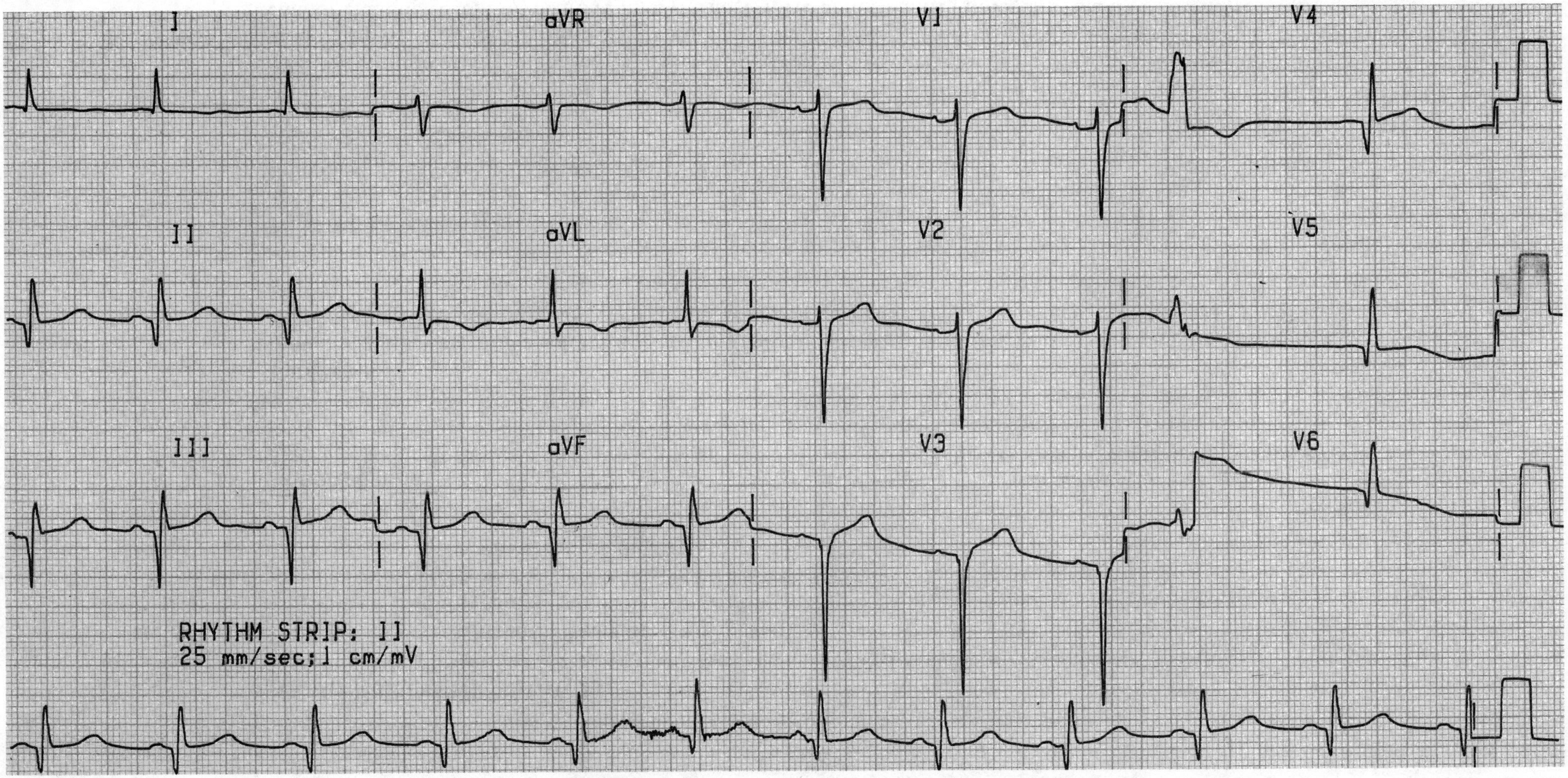

C-28

NARRATIVE INTERPRETATION

Rhythm: **Sinus**
Rate: **68**
Intervals: **PR 0.16, QRS 0.08, QT 0.46**
Axis: **−15 degrees**

Abnormalities

Q waves leads II, III, aVF, V4–V6. QS lead V3. ST elevation leads II, III, aVF, V3–V6. ST depression lead aVL. T wave inverted lead aVL. T wave flat lead I. Prolonged QTc. VPC.

Synthesis

Sinus rhythm. VPC. Inferolateral wall MI of indeterminate age. Anterior wall MI of indeterminate age. ST abnormalities suggestive of ventricular aneurysm. Nonspecific T-wave abnormalities. QTc prolongation.

TEST ANSWERS: 1, 26, 84, (86), 92, 95, 106, 109.

Comment: This tracing illustrates how patients with multiple infarctions may produce complex Q-wave patterns. This patient sustained a prior inferolateral wall infarction with persistent ST elevation in the infarct leads that indicates probable aneurysm formation. There was also a second anterior infarction. A true "lateral" infarction should not be classified owing to the absence of diagnostic Q waves in I and aVL. An anterolateral infarction is also not the best answer because the lateral involvement is most likely an extension of the inferior infarction. In the absence of clinical history or serial tracings, one cannot exclude recent myocardial injury. The T-wave abnormalities in leads I and aVL are most likely related to coronary heart disease but must be categorized as nonspecific findings. The QT interval is slightly prolonged; this also is probably secondary to coronary disease.

C-29

Clinical History

A 38-year-old man with intermittent chest discomfort.

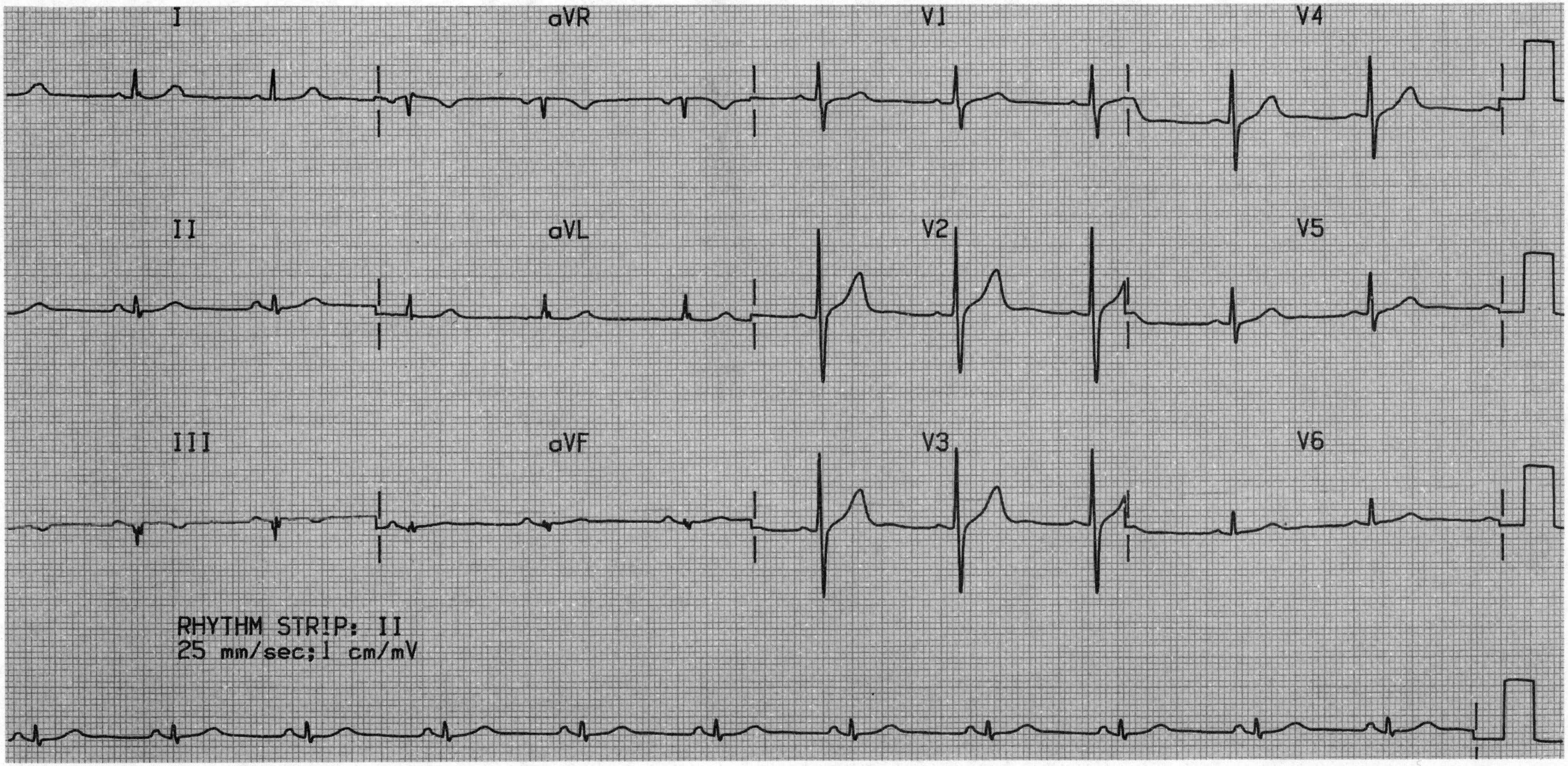

C-29

NARRATIVE INTERPRETATION

Rhythm:	**Sinus**
Rate:	**64**
Intervals:	**PR 0.14, QRS 0.06, QT 0.36**
Axis:	**0 degrees**

Abnormalities

R greater than S wave with upright T wave leads V1–V2. Limb-lead voltage less than 6 mm.

Synthesis

Sinus rhythm. Low voltage limb leads. Posterior MI of indeterminate age.

TEST ANSWERS: 1, 67, 94.

Comment: The tall R waves in the anterior precordial leads should alert the reader to the diagnosis of a posterior wall MI. Note the R/S ratio greater than 1, with an upright T wave in lead V1. Patients with a posterior wall MI often have a coexistent inferior wall MI, although this is not evident in this tracing. An R/S ratio greater than 1 may be seen in lead V2 in up to 10 percent of normal persons, but this would be highly unusual in lead V1 in the absence of pathology. At the time of clinical evaluation, this electrocardiogram was interpreted as suggestive but not diagnostic of posterior wall MI. Nevertheless, the patient was admitted to the hospital for clinical evaluation. The wisdom of this decision and the definitive diagnosis became apparent a number of hours later (see following ECG).

C-30

Clinical History

A 38-year-old man with recurrent chest discomfort. Tracing taken 6 h after previous electrocardiogram.

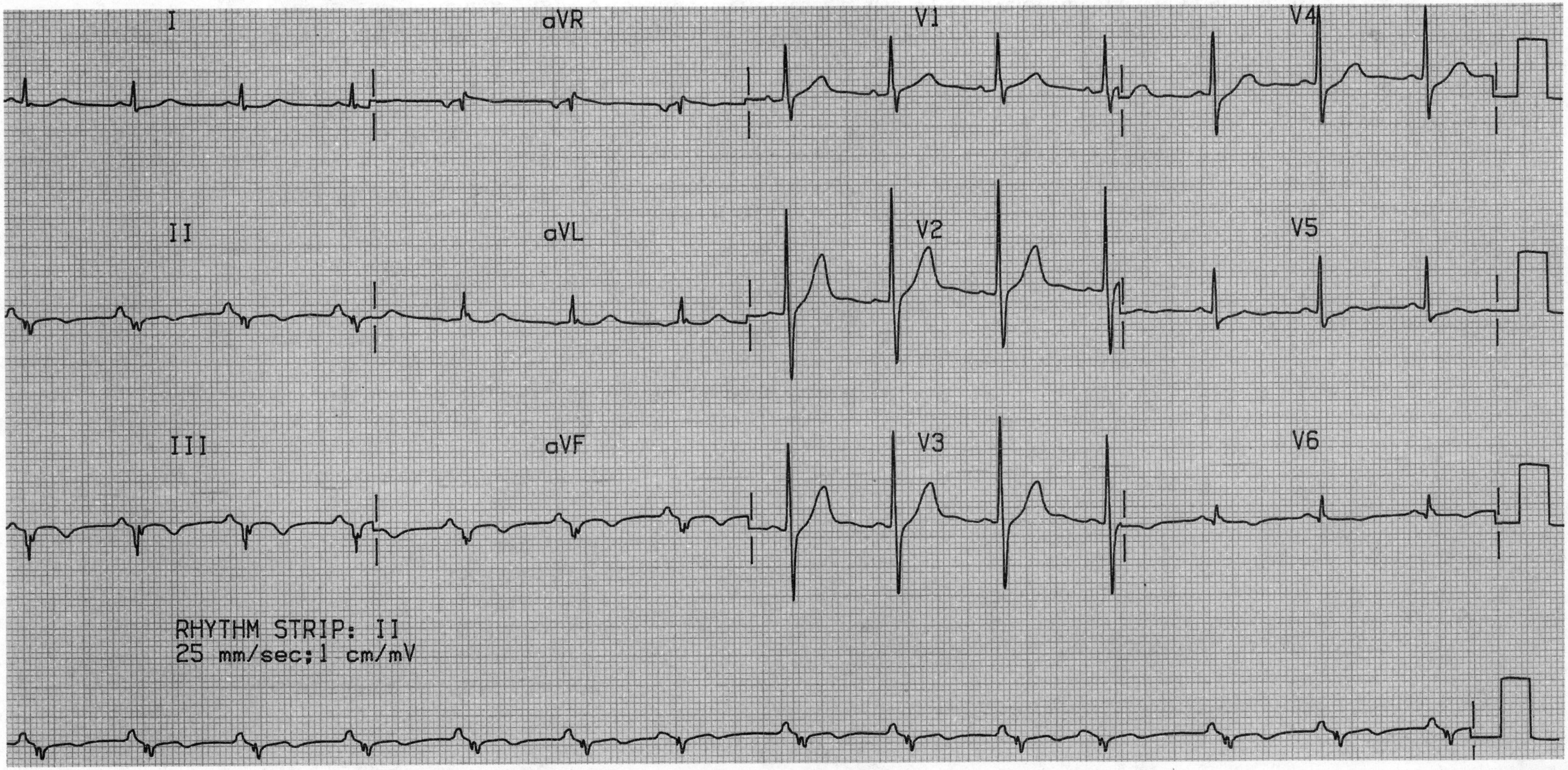

C-30

NARRATIVE INTERPRETATION

Rhythm: **Sinus**
Rate: **80**
Intervals: **PR 0.14, QRS 0.08, QT 0.36**
Axis: **−45 degrees**

Abnormalities

APCs. Limb-lead voltage less than 6 mm. Axis leftward of −30 degrees. Q waves leads II, III, aVF, V6. R greater than S wave with upright T wave leads V1–V2. ST depression leads I, aVL, V4, V5. ST elevation leads II, III, aVF, V6. T-wave inversion leads II, III, aVF, V6.

Synthesis

Sinus rhythm. APCs. Low-voltage limb leads. Inferior wall MI with ST-T-wave abnormalities suggesting acute myocardial injury. Acute posterior wall MI. Left axis deviation. Left anterior fascicular block (LAFB). ST-T-wave abnormalities suggesting myocardial ischemia.

TEST ANSWERS: 1, 10, 64, 67, 72, 91, 93, 100, 101, (106).

Comment: This patient demonstrates an acute inferior wall MI. When this tracing is compared with the previous tracing, extension of the prior posterior wall MI is also seen. Note the "growth" in the R waves in leads V1 and V2. The tracing is characterized as demonstrating an acute posterior MI only in comparison with the previous electrocardiogram. Criteria are also now present for combined inferior wall MI and LAFB as a terminal R wave is now seen in lead aVR and occurs after the terminal R wave in aVL. The "notching" of the QRS in the inferior leads is also supportive of combined inferior wall MI and LAFB.

REFERENCES: Warner (*Am Heart J*). Fisher. Louridas.

C-31

Clinical History

A 68-year-old man with cardiomegaly and dyspnea. Medications include digoxin.

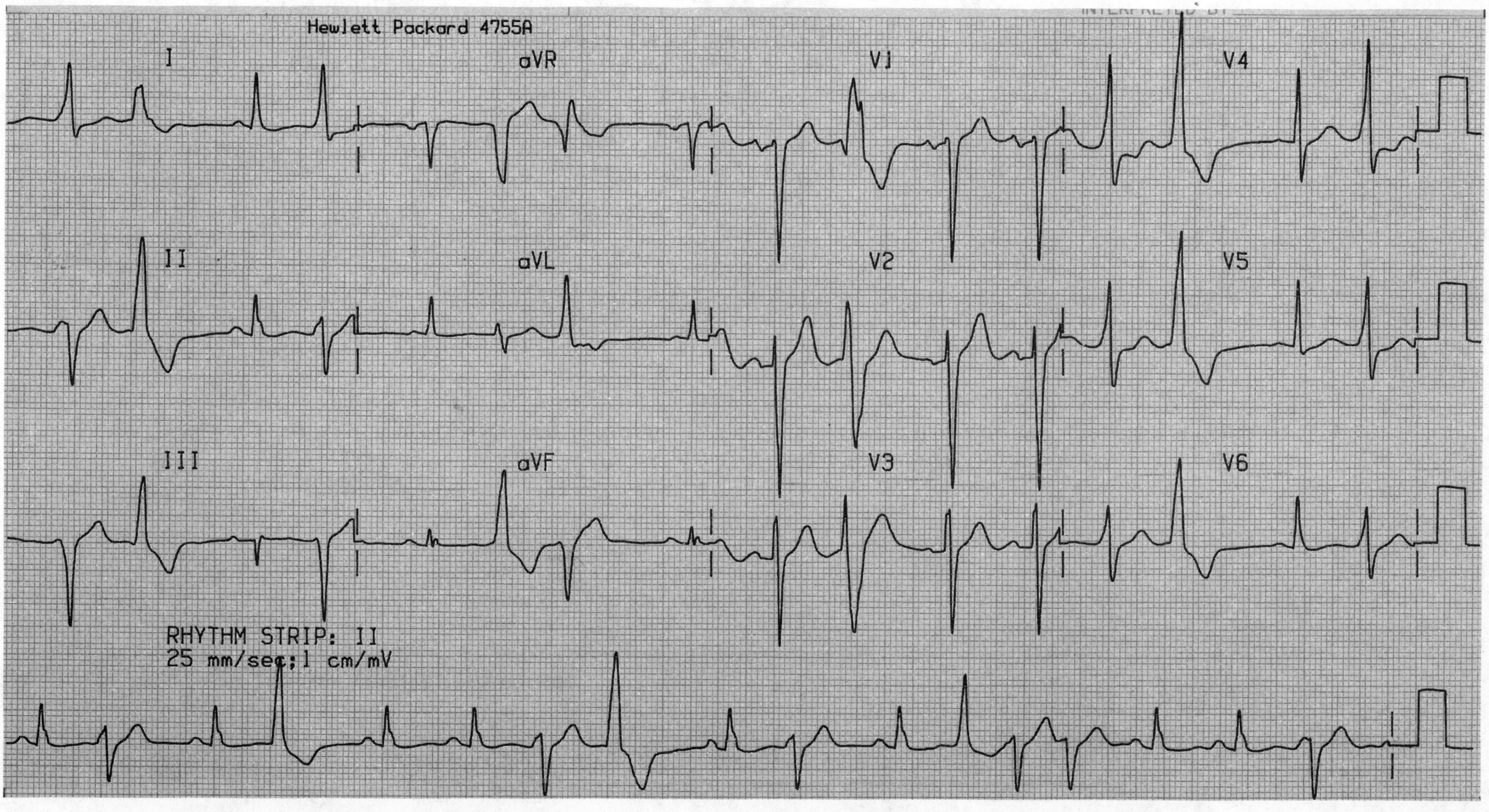

C-31

NARRATIVE INTERPRETATION

Rhythm: **Sinus**
Rate: **96**
Intervals: **PR 0.16, QRS 0.08, QT 0.40**
Axis: **+15 degrees**

Abnormalities

VPCs. Paired VPCs, multiform VPCs. Ventricular tachycardia on rhythm strip. Abnormal P terminal force V1. Slight ST depression leads I, II, V5–V6. Diffuse T-wave flattening limb leads. SV2 + RV5 greater than 35.

Synthesis

Sinus rhythm. Frequent VPCs with paired, multiform VPCs. Ventricular tachycardia (multiform triplet) on rhythm strip. Left atrial abnormality. LVH. Associated ST-segment abnormalities. Non-specific T-wave abnormalities.

TEST ANSWERS: 1, 27, 28, 30, 60, 78, 103, (106).

Comment: This patient had congestive heart failure and massive cardiomegaly on the basis of an idiopathic dilated cardiomyopathy. Interestingly, voltage criteria for LVH are borderline. Chronic ventricular ectopy, which is often multiform, is commonly seen in these patients. A minor illustrative point regarding this tracing is low T voltage in the limb leads. T-wave flattening is a bit subjective but should be noted. The T wave should be upright in leads I and II and at least 0.5 mm in amplitude. There is virtually no T-wave voltage in the limb leads. This is a nonspecific finding that, in addition to mild ST depression, may be associated with digitalis.

REFERENCE: Friedman pp 75, 329.

C-32

Clinical History

A 72-year-old man with aortic stenosis.

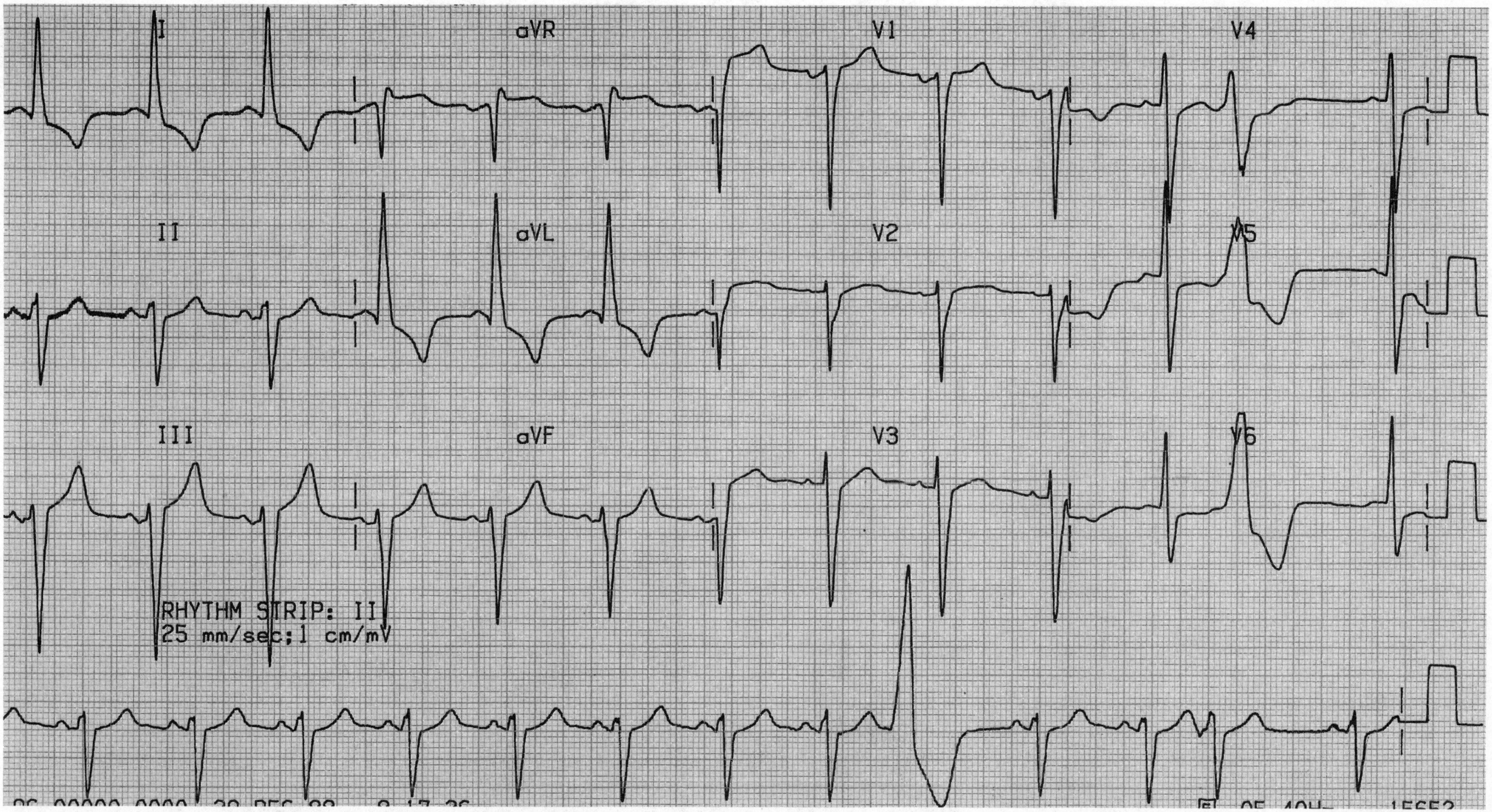

C-32

NARRATIVE INTERPRETATION

Rhythm: **Sinus**
Rate: **78**
Intervals: **PR 0.14, QRS 0.12, QT 0.40**
Axis: **−45 degrees**

Abnormalities

Axis leftward of −30 degrees. Abnormal P terminal force lead V1. R wave aVL greater than 13. Prolonged QRS interval. ST depression leads I, aVL, V5–V6. T-wave inversion leads I, aVL. Flat T wave leads V5–V6. VPC. JPC.

Synthesis

Sinus rhythm. VPC. JPC. Left axis deviation. LVH by voltage criteria with associated ST-T-wave abnormalities. Intraventricular conduction delay. Left atrial abnormality.

TEST ANSWERS: 1, 25, 26, 60, 64, 76, 78, 103.

Comment: This tracing demonstrates a number of interesting findings. The patient had significant cardiomegaly and echocardiographic LVH secondary to aortic stenosis, yet precordial voltage criteria are absent for LVH. The probable explanation is that the marked left axis deviation resulted in superior displacement of the QRS forces in the lateral precordial leads, which produced relatively small R waves and deep S waves in leads V5 and V6. In contrast, there is a marked increase in limb-lead voltage, which is diagnostic for LVH. Despite the shift in axis, one should generally not make the diagnosis of left anterior fascicular block in the presence of an intraventricular conduction delay. Note also that despite a prolonged QRS, there are insufficient criteria for LBBB. Septal Q waves remain in leads I and aVL, and a relatively narrow R wave is present in leads V5 and V6.

REFERENCES: Chou p 101. Gertsch. Milliken.

C-33

Clinical History

A 43-year-old man with palpitations.

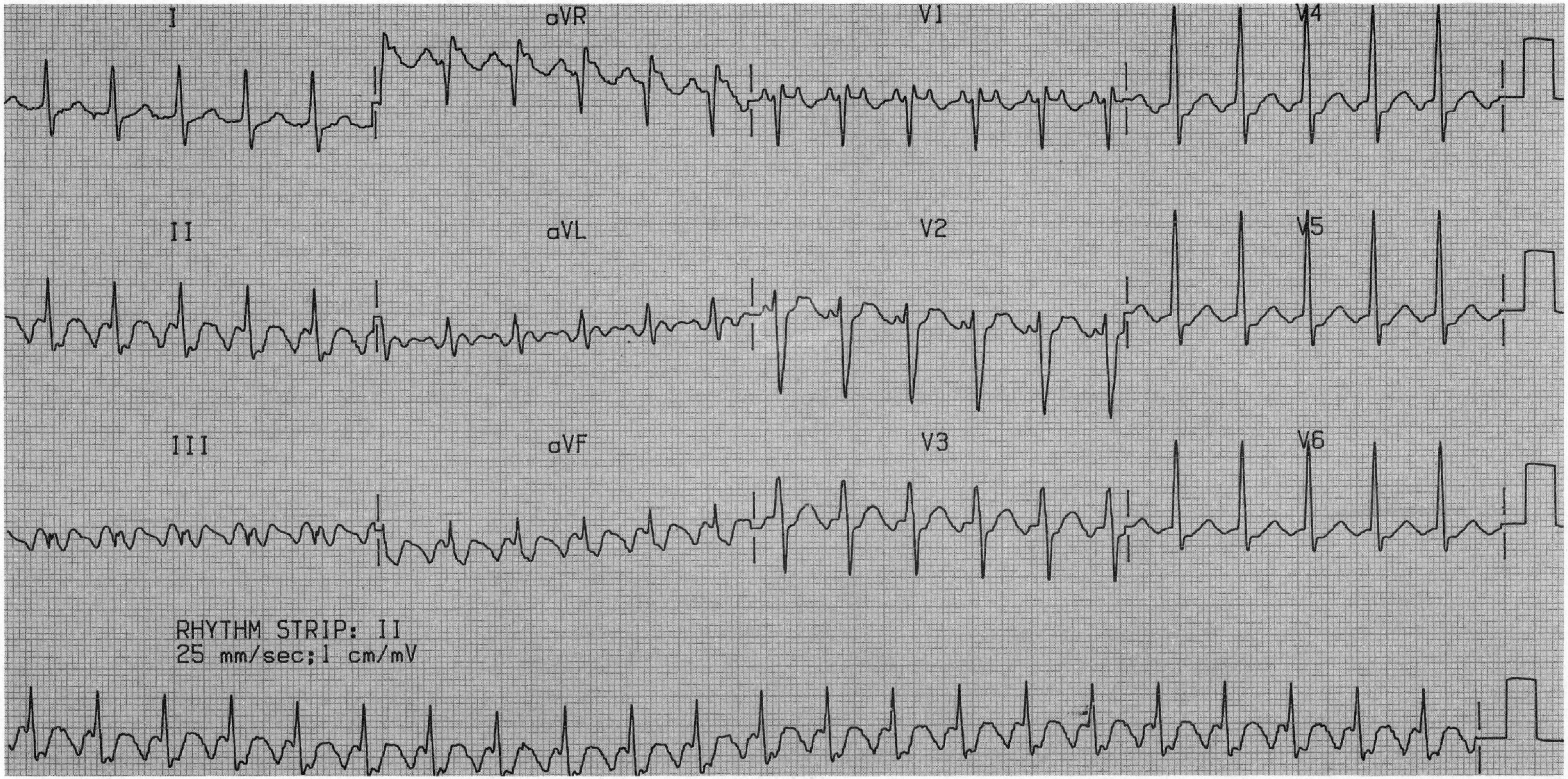

C-33

NARRATIVE INTERPRETATION

Rhythm: **Atrial flutter with 2:1 AV conduction**
Rate: **Atrial 270, ventricular 135**
Intervals: **PR –, QRS 0.08, QT 0.32**
Axis: **Indeterminate**

Abnormalities
Generalized ST depression.

Synthesis
Atrial flutter with 2:1 AV conduction. Generalized ST-segment depression, possibly artifactual from superimposition of inverted flutter (P) wave.

TEST ANSWERS: 19, 50, (106).

Comment: The rhythm disturbance is fairly obvious with characteristic "sawtooth" inverted flutter waves evident in leads II, III, and aVF. A more difficult determination is whether or not there are additional ST or T-wave abnormalities. There is an inverted flutter wave superimposed on the ST segment immediately following the QRS, and the author has concluded that these findings may be artifactual. The determination of abnormal ST-T-wave findings often requires comparison with additional tracings after conversion to sinus rhythm (see next tracing).

C-34

Clinical History

A 43-year-old asymptomatic man. Medications include quinidine and digoxin.

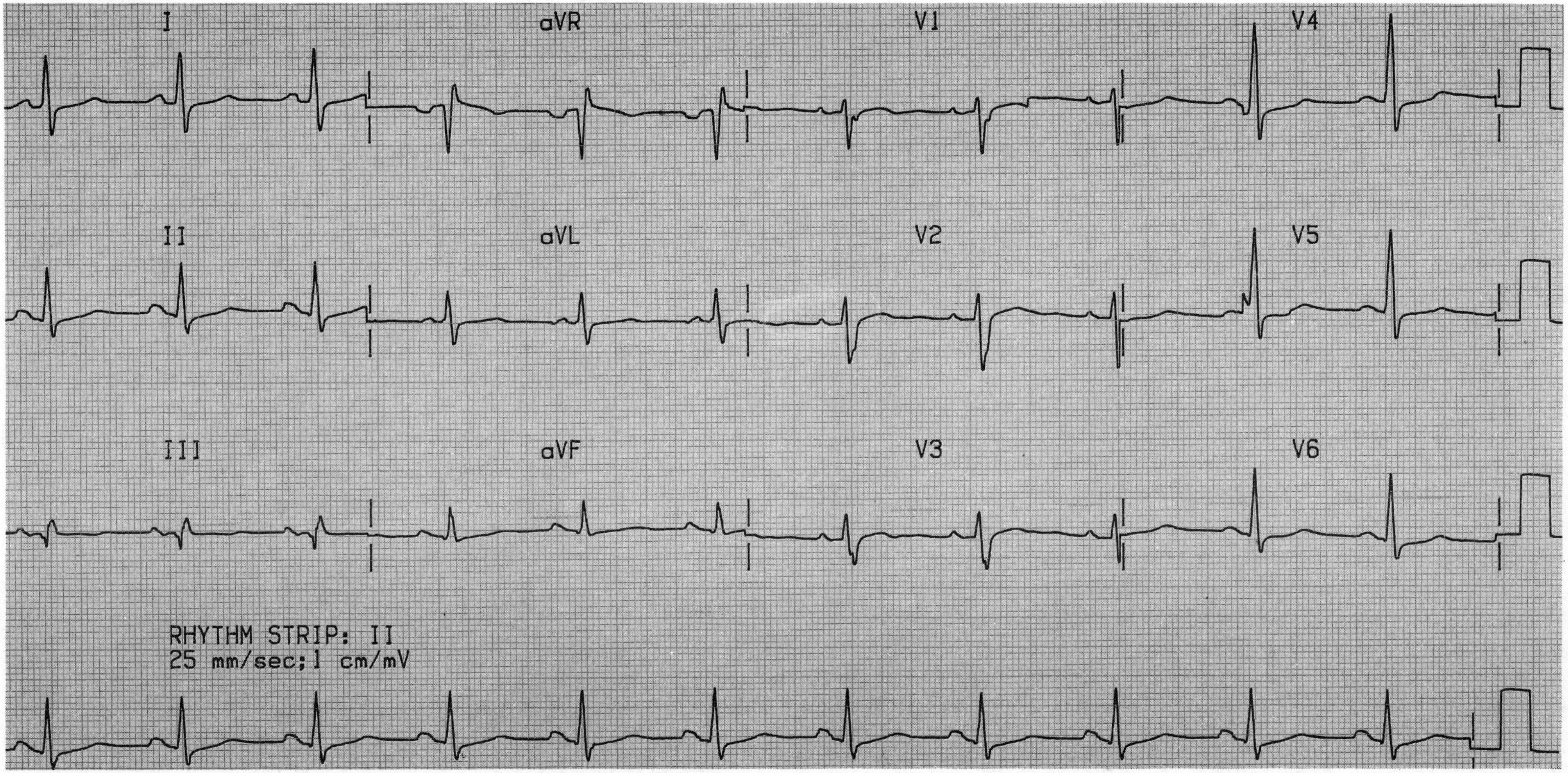

C-34

NARRATIVE INTERPRETATION

Rhythm:	**Sinus**
Rate:	**68**
Intervals:	**PR 0.18, QRS 0.08, QT 0.42**
Axis:	**+60 degrees**

Abnormalities
ST depression leads I, II, aVF, V4–V6. Prolonged QTc interval.

Synthesis
Sinus rhythm. Nonspecific ST abnormalities. Prolonged QTc.

TEST ANSWERS: 1, 106, 109.

Comment: This tracing represents the postcardioversion electrocardiogram from the previous tracing. The slight ST abnormalities are much less marked than on the previous tracing, which demonstrated artifactual ST abnormalities from the superimposed flutter waves. The QT prolongation is likely secondary to treatment with quinidine.

C-35

Clinical History

A 34-year-old female nurse with chest pain on inspiration.

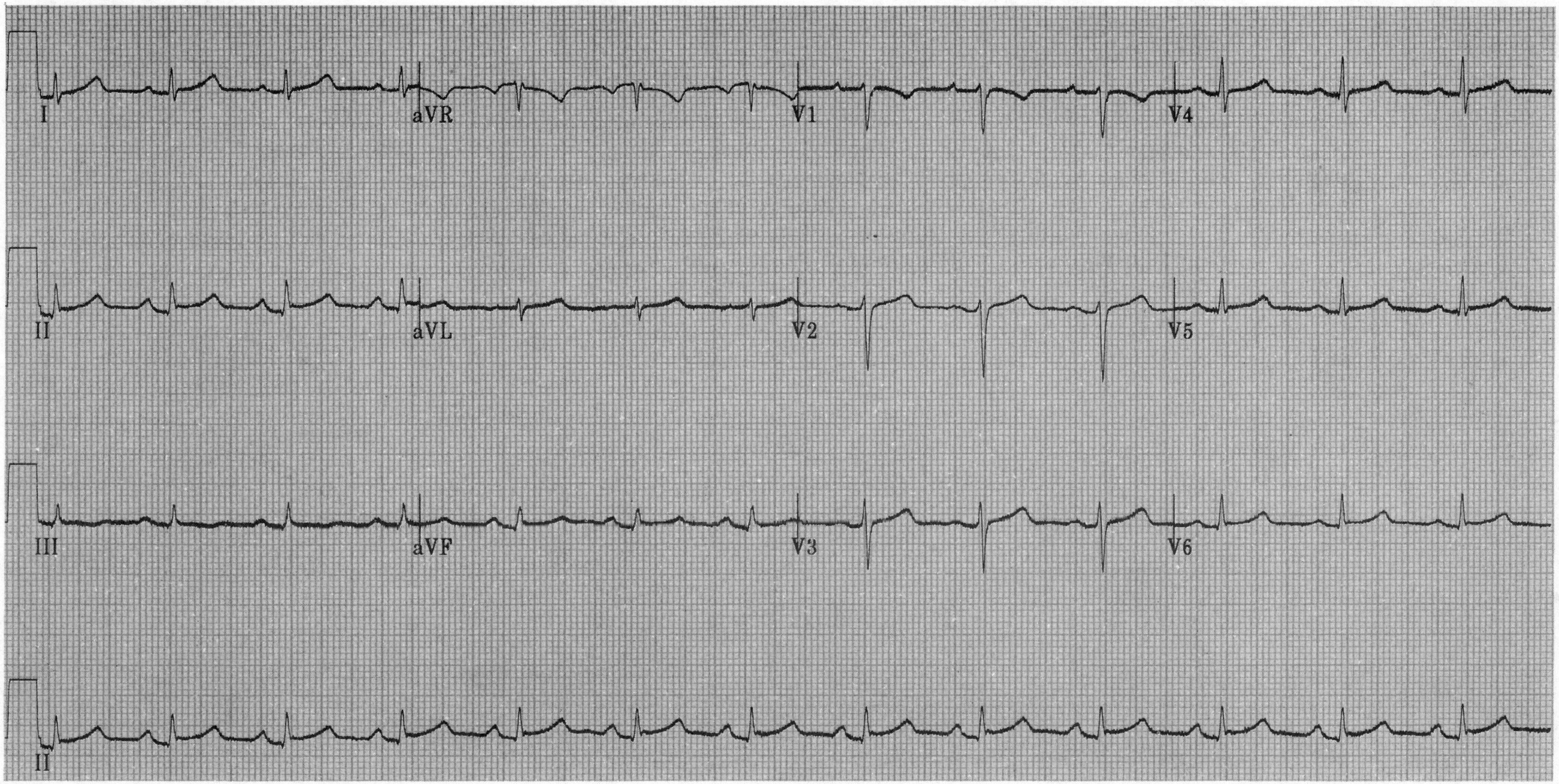

C-35

NARRATIVE INTERPRETATION

Rhythm: Sinus
Rate: 77
Intervals: PR 0.18, QRS 0.08, QT 0.38
Axis: +60 degrees

Abnormalities

PR depression leads II, aVF. ST elevation with upward concavity leads I, II, aVF, V3–V6.

Synthesis

Sinus rhythm. PR depression and generalized ST elevation suggestive of early acute pericarditis.

TEST ANSWERS: 1, 63, 105.

Comment: PR depression, often most prominent in the inferior leads, is an early finding in acute pericarditis. Diffuse ST elevation with upward concavity is characteristic but is often difficult to differentiate from a normal variant. ST elevation in pericarditis is most often diffuse, although it may also be localized to a few leads. In such circumstances, it may be difficult to differentiate these findings from those found in acute myocardial injury. ST elevation with MI, however, characteristically demonstrates downward concavity.

REFERENCES: Spodick (1976). Gintzon.

C-36

Clinical History

A 74-year-old man with recurrent chest discomfort on his third day in the CCU.

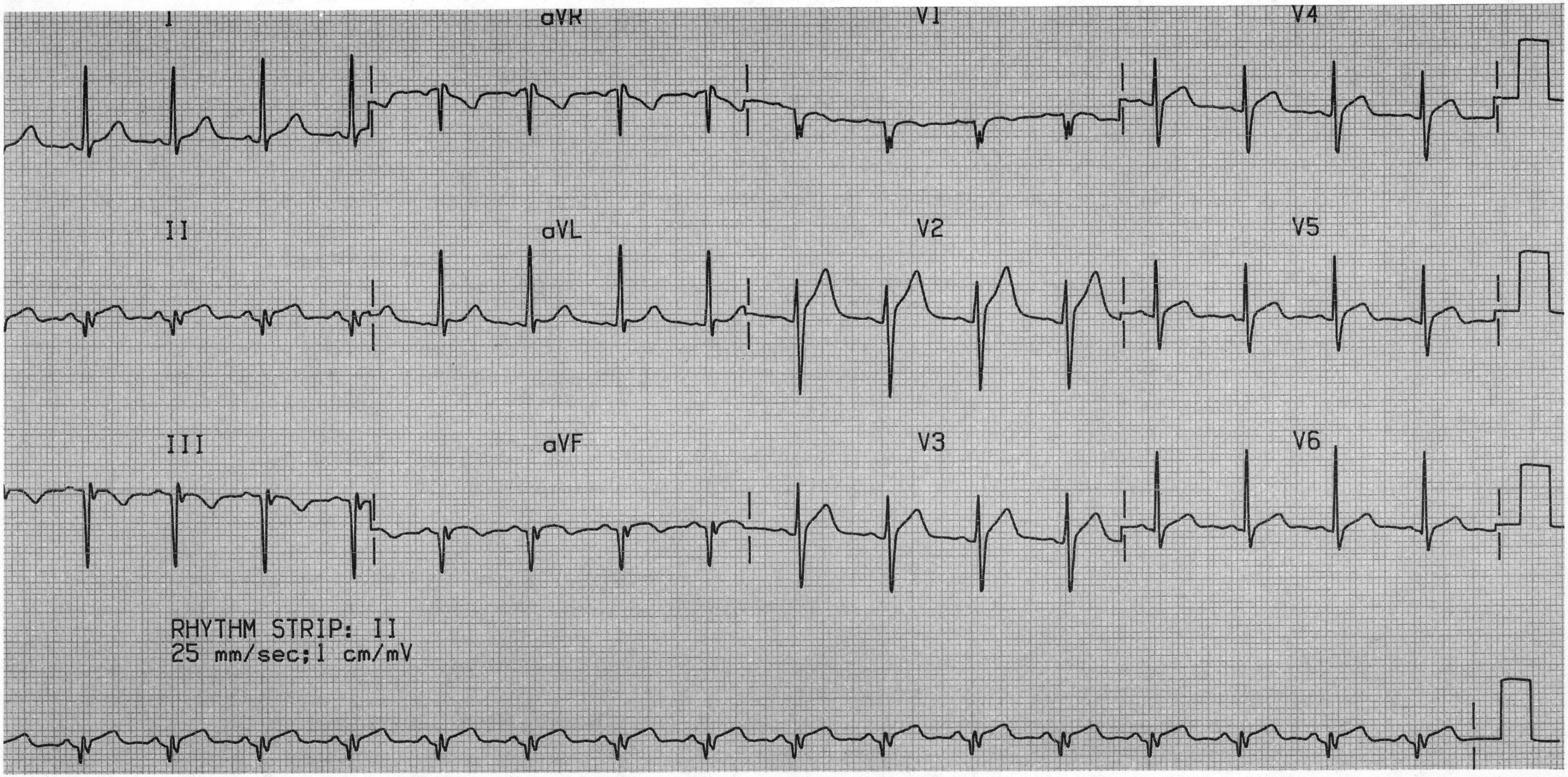

C-36

NARRATIVE INTERPRETATION

Rhythm: **Sinus**
Rate: **99**
Intervals: **PR 0.14, QRS 0.08, QT 0.36**
Axis: **−35 degrees**

Abnormalities

Axis leftward of −30 degrees. Q waves leads II, III, aVF. ST elevation leads II, III, aVF, V2–V6. Slight ST elevation leads I, aVL. T-wave inversion leads III, aVF. R wave lead aVL greater than 11 mm.

Synthesis

Sinus rhythm. Inferior wall MI with ST-T-wave abnormalities in leads II, III, aVF suggestive of recent myocardial injury. Additional ST abnormalities leads I, aVL, V2–V6 suggestive of anterolateral myocardial injury. Borderline left axis deviation. LVH by voltage criteria.

TEST ANSWERS: 1, 64, 78, 91, 100.

Comment: This tracing illustrates a patient who demonstrates anterolateral myocardial injury shortly after an inferior wall MI. A Q-wave infarction pattern is present in the inferior limb leads but is not yet present in the precordial leads. Note that a left anterior fascicular block (LAFB) is not present because of the R waves in the inferior leads. In LAFB, S waves should be present in these leads. Remember that not all patients with left axis deviation have an LAFB.

REFERENCES: Friedman p 280. Spodick (1987).

C-37

Clinical History

A 63-year-old woman with severe dyspnea and chest discomfort.

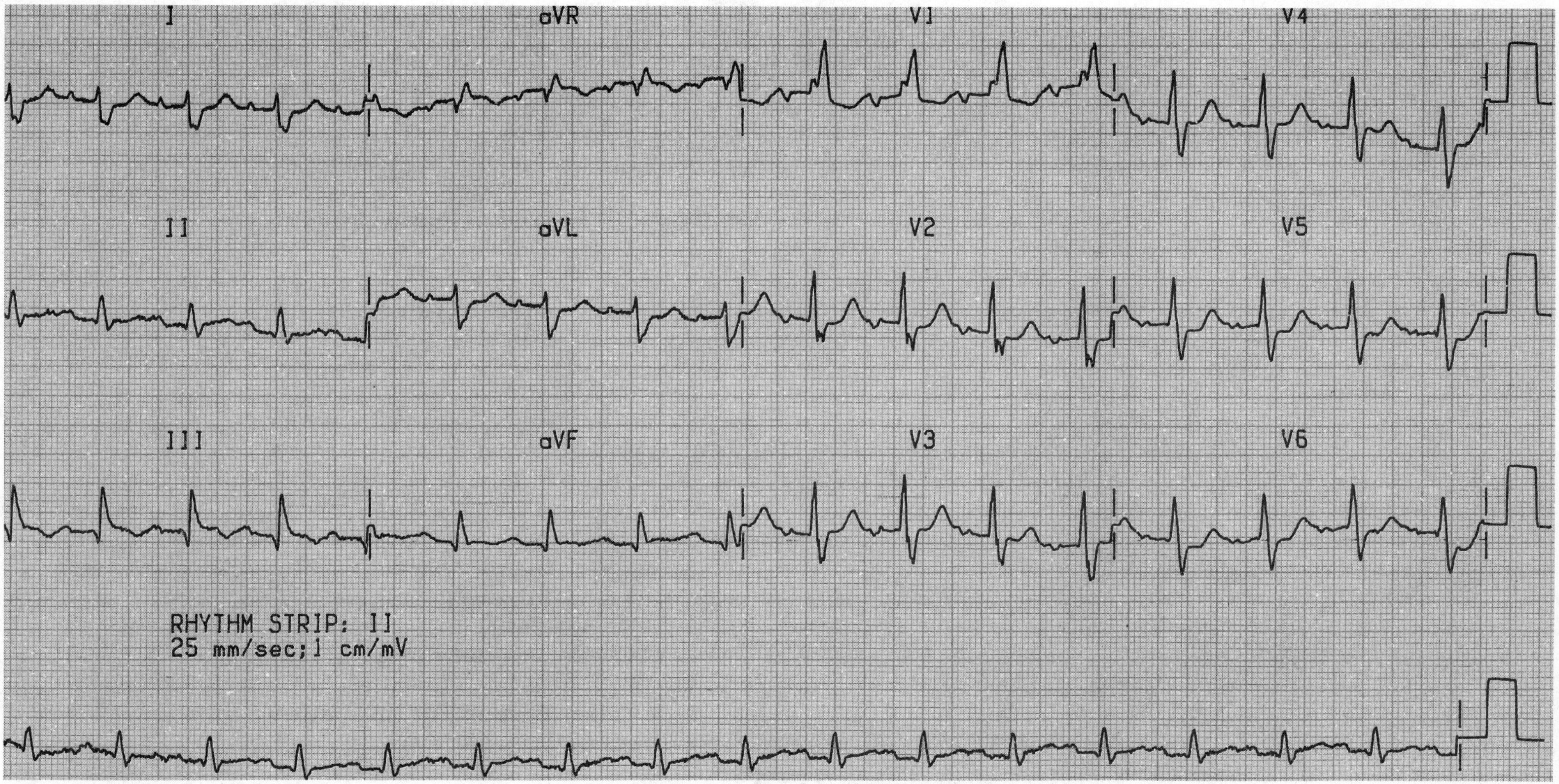

C-37

NARRATIVE INTERPRETATION

Rhythm: **Sinus with first-degree AV block**
Rate: **96**
Intervals: **PR 0.21, QRS 0.12, QT 0.36**
Axis: **+120 degrees**

Abnormalities

Axis rightward of +90 degrees. Prolonged PR interval. Abnormal P terminal force lead V1. Q waves leads II, III, aVF. ST elevation leads II, III, aVF. Broad, notched R wave with rR′ pattern and T-wave inversion lead V1.

Synthesis

Sinus rhythm. First-degree AV block. Right axis deviation. Left atrial abnormality. RBBB with associated ST-T-wave abnormalities. Left posterior fascicular block. Inferior wall MI with ST-T-wave abnormalities suggestive of acute myocardial injury.

TEST ANSWERS: 1, 42, 60, 65, 70, 73, 91, 100, 104.

Comment: This patient has a number of conduction abnormalities in the presence of an acute MI. Diagnostic Q waves are not yet present, but there are early Q waves and ST-segment abnormalities indicative of acute inferior wall MI. The combination of a myocardial infarction with multiple conduction abnormalities is particularly ominous. The posterior fascicle derives its blood supply from both the left anterior descending and posterior descending coronary arteries. One series found a 20 percent incidence of progression to complete heart block in patients with acute MI and concomitant bilateral bundle branch block and first-degree AV block.

REFERENCES: Hindman I. Hindman II. Alpert JS. Haft.

C-38

Clinical History

A 61-year-old man with a systolic murmur.

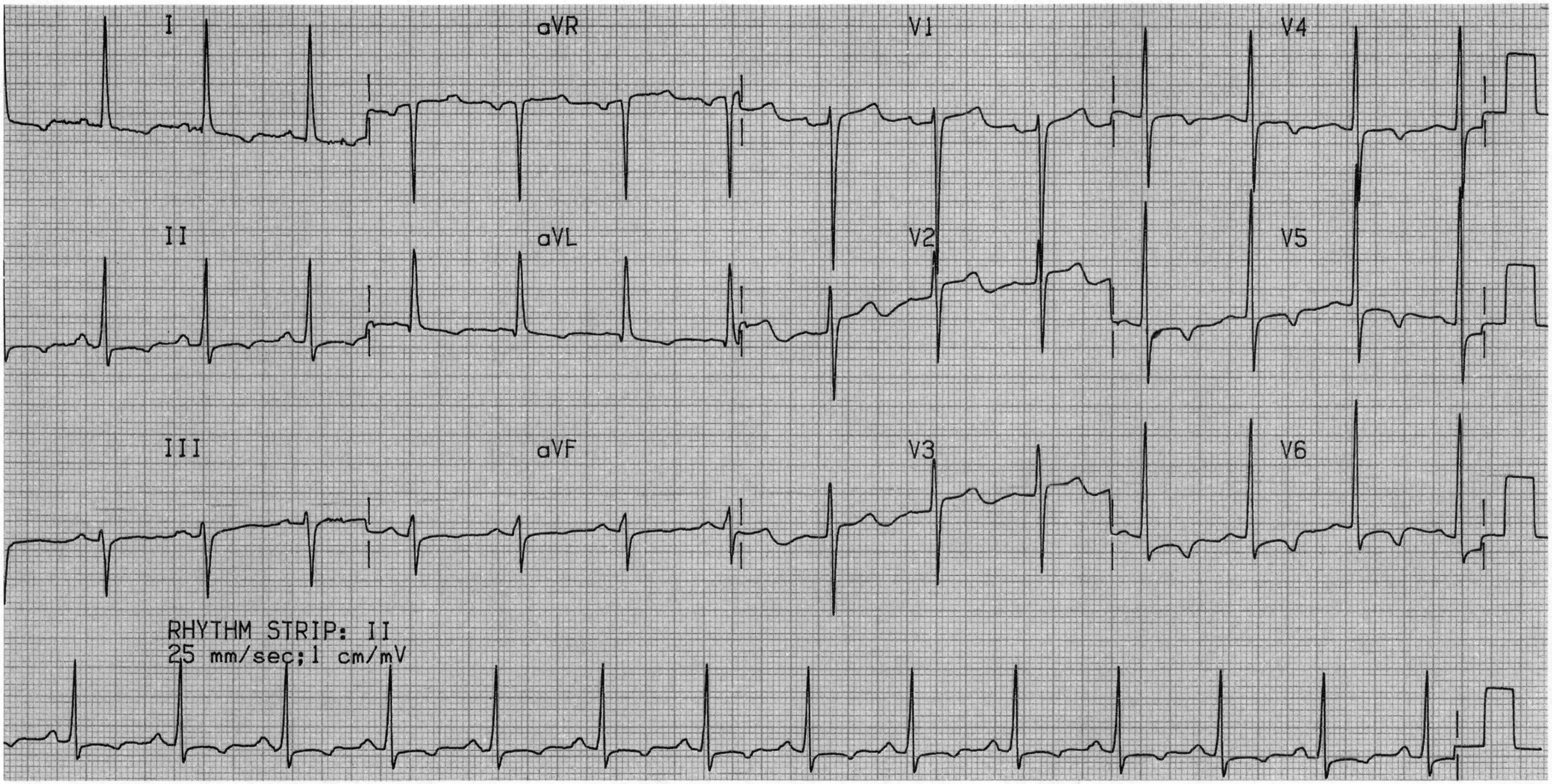

C-38

NARRATIVE INTERPRETATION

Rhythm: **Sinus**
Rate: **84**
Intervals: **PR 0.18, QRS 0.08, QT 0.36**
Axis: **−15 degrees**

Abnormalities

R wave in aVL greater than 11. R1 + S3 greater than 25. ST depression lead V6. T-wave inversion leads I, II, aVL, V4–V6.

Synthesis

Sinus rhythm. LVH. Associated ST-T-wave abnormalities.

TEST ANSWERS: 1, 78, 103.

Comment: Note that the more familiar precordial voltage criteria for LVH are absent in this tracing. However, two different limb-lead voltage criteria are present. These have proved to be less sensitive than precordial voltage standards but are highly specific for LVH when they are present. This patient had marked cardiomegaly secondary to chronic mitral insufficiency.

REFERENCE: Romhilt (1968 and 1969).

C-39

Clinical History

A 41-year-old asymptomatic man seen preoperatively for minor surgery.

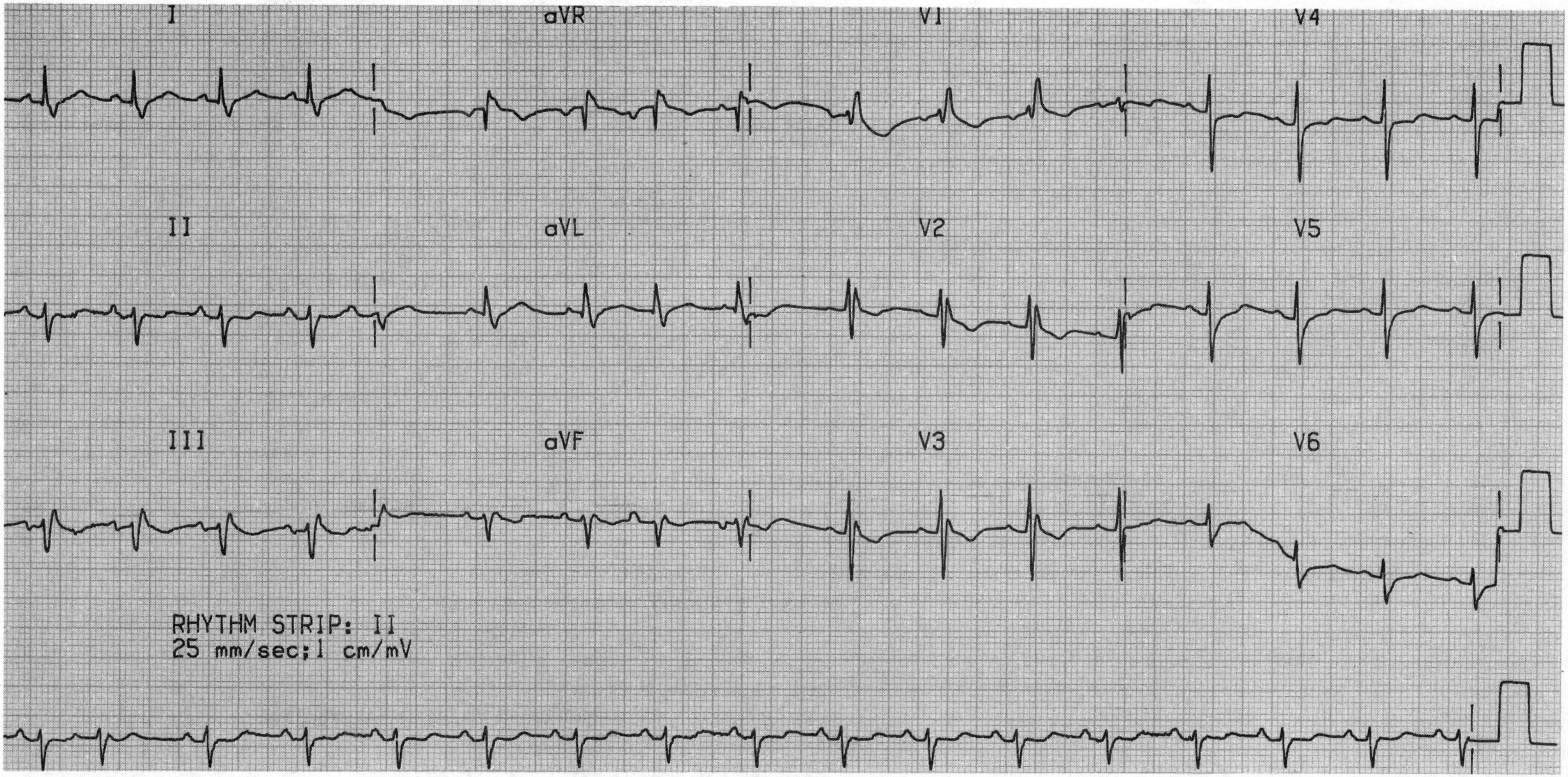

C-39

NARRATIVE INTERPRETATION

Rhythm: Sinus
Rate: 99
Intervals: PR 0.16, QRS 0.11, QT 0.30
Axis: −45 degrees

Abnormalities

Broad QRS with rsR′ leads V1–V3 and T-wave inversions leads V1–V3. Axis leftward of −30 degrees. APCs.

Synthesis

Sinus rhythm. APCs. Left axis deviation. Left anterior fascicular block. Incomplete RBBB with associated ST-T-wave changes.

TEST ANSWERS: 1, 10, 64, 71, 72, 104.

Comment: This patient had no evidence of clinical cardiac disease despite the conduction abnormalities. The tracing shows an incomplete RBBB as the QRS duration does not quite reach 0.12 s. A left anterior fascicular block (LAFB) is also present. RBBB and LAFB may rarely be seen in young, normal persons. In one study of 23,700 healthy airmen, this electrocardiographic diagnosis was found in 0.1 percent. In patients with underlying cardiac disease, bifascicular block may indicate an adverse prognosis. It is important to note, however, that the excess mortality is not a result of progression to complete AV block.

REFERENCES: Barrett. McAnulty. Liao.

C-40

Clinical History

A 45-year-old asymptomatic woman in the recovery room after minor surgery.

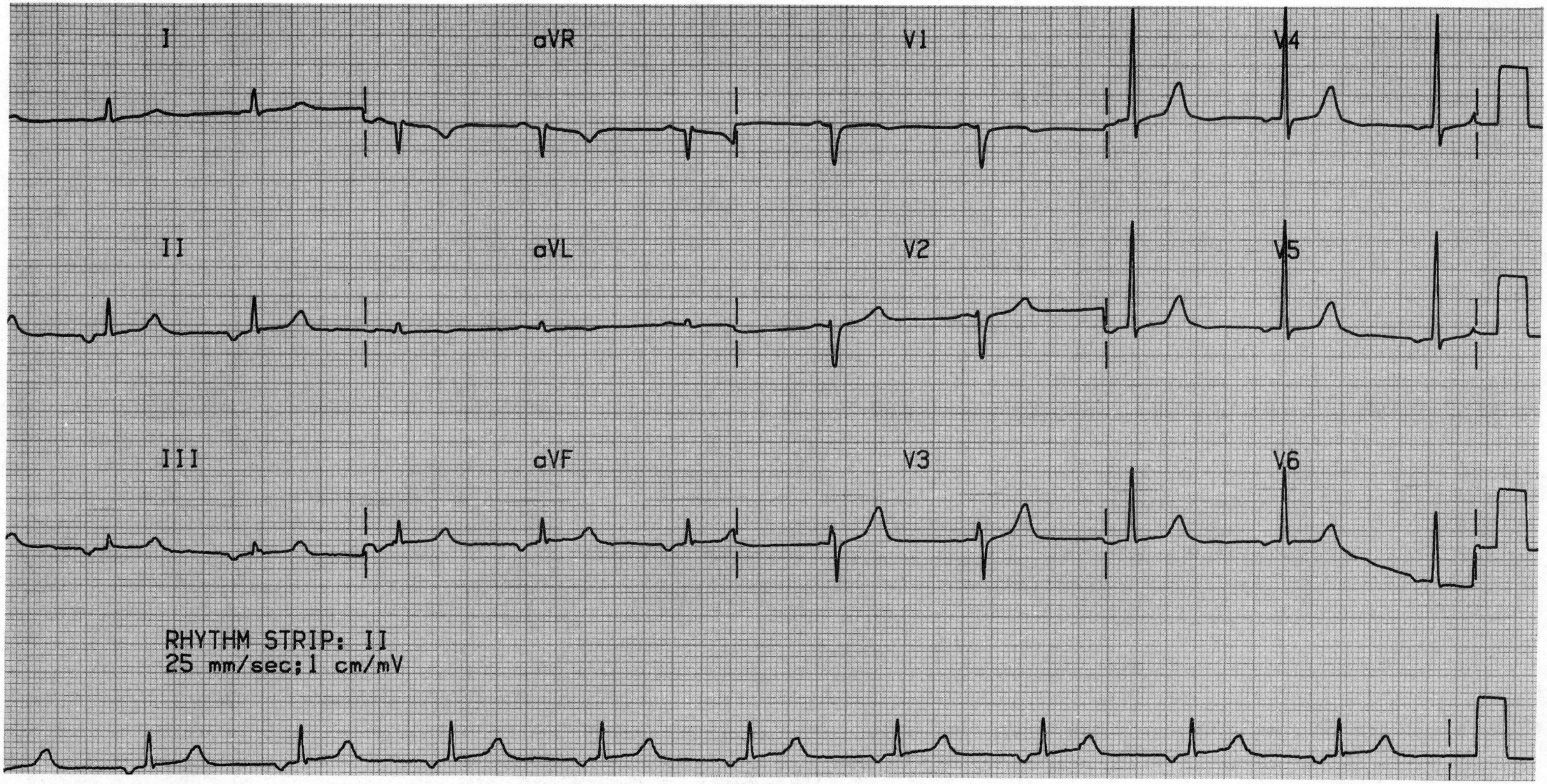

C-40

NARRATIVE INTERPRETATION

Rhythm:	**Ectopic atrial rhythm**
Rate:	**58**
Intervals:	**PR 0.14, QRS 0.08, QT 0.42**
Axis:	**+60 degrees**

Abnormalities
Retrograde P waves with slow heart rate.

Synthesis
Ectopic atrial rhythm. Otherwise within normal limits.

TEST ANSWER: 9.

Comment: Inverted P waves are easily seen in leads II, III, and aVF. This finding rules out a sinus mechanism. This rhythm may originate in either a low atrial site or the AV junction. Whereas an inverted P wave with a short PR interval suggests an AV junctional site, a normal PR interval can occur with either an ectopic atrial rhythm or AV junctional rhythm with antegrade AV conduction delay. Older textbooks of electrocardiography have referred to the rhythm displayed in the present example as "coronary sinus rhythm," a term no longer in use.

TEST D

D-1

Clinical History

An 89-year-old asymptomatic woman.

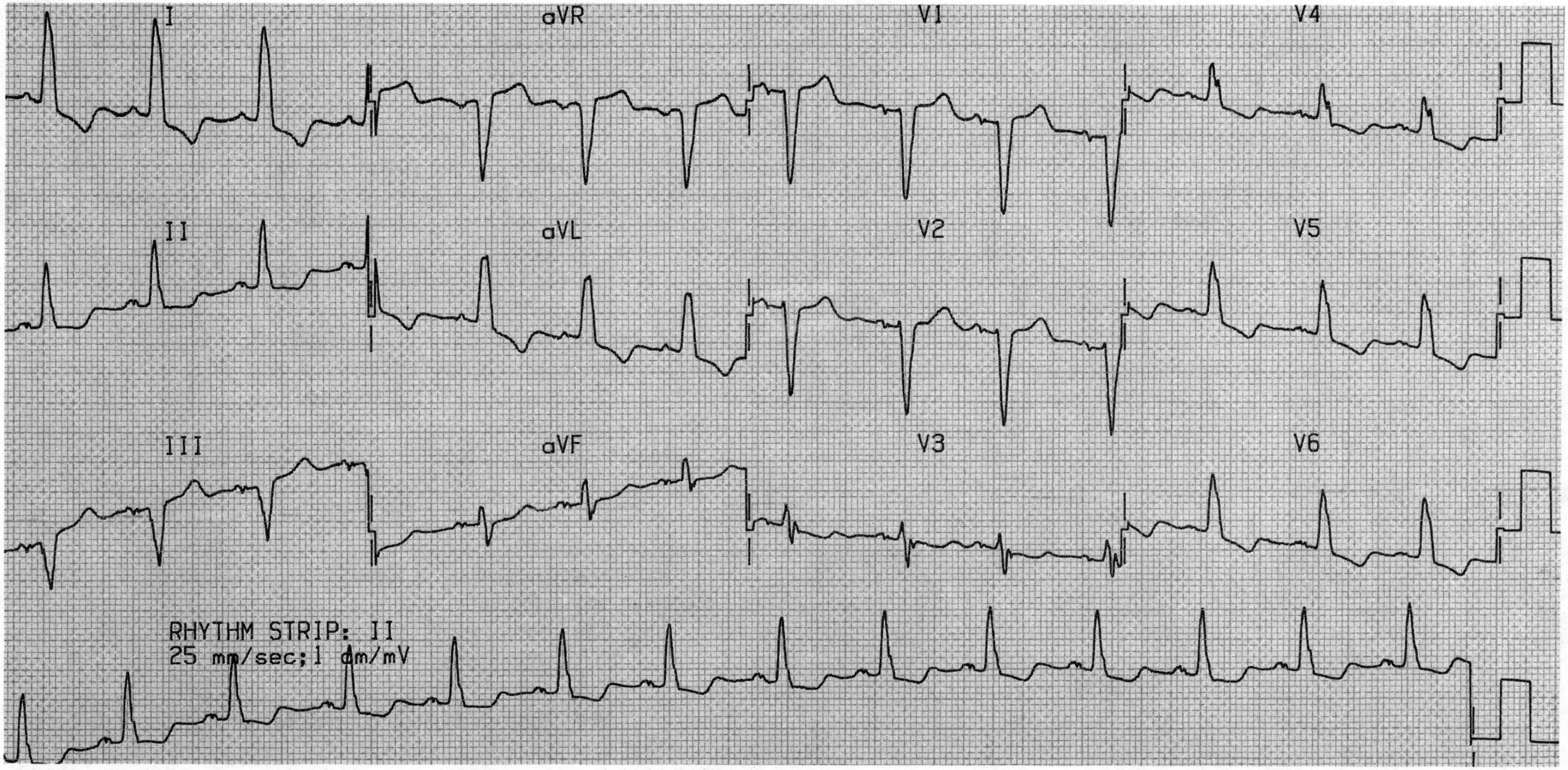

D-1

NARRATIVE INTERPRETATION

Rhythm:	**Sinus**
Rate:	**80**
Intervals:	**PR 0.16, QRS 0.11, QT 0.40**
Axis:	**0 degrees**

Abnormalities

Prolonged QRS interval. Abnormal Lewis index (see below). ST depression leads I, II, aVL, V4–V6. T-wave inversion leads I, aVL, V4–V6.

Synthesis

Sinus rhythm. Intraventricular conduction delay. LVH by voltage criteria. ST-T-wave abnormalities associated with ventricular hypertrophy.

TEST ANSWERS: 1, 76, 78, 103.

Comment: This tracing is actually a bit more difficult to interpret than it appears on first glance. Criteria for LBBB are not present as the QRS duration is not quite 0.12 s. Incomplete LBBB is suggested by the prolonged QRS interval and absent septal Q waves in the lateral leads. However, additional supporting criteria for incomplete LBBB are absent, such as a delay in the intrinsicoid deflection or notching of the upstroke of the R wave in the lateral leads. LVH is most likely present on the basis of the intraventricular conduction delay and associated ST-T-wave abnormalities, as well as the presence of an abnormal Lewis index. The Lewis index is the sum of the R wave in lead I and S wave in lead III, minus the R wave in III and S wave in I. A Lewis index of 17 or more is a highly specific criterion for LVH.

D-2

Clinical History

A 68-year-old asymptomatic man.

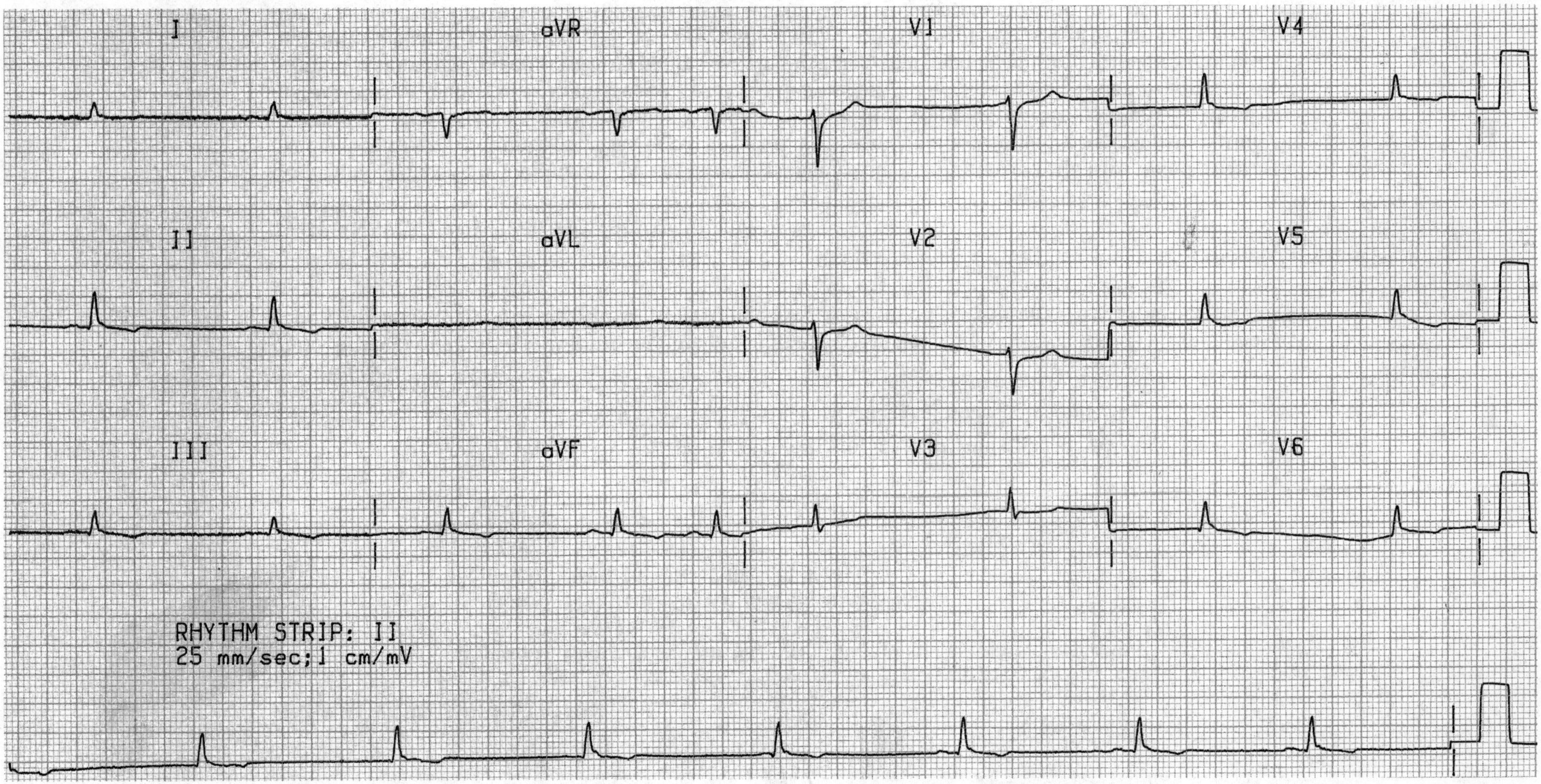

D-2

NARRATIVE INTERPRETATION

Rhythm:	**Sinus bradycardia, AV junctional escape complexes (rhythm)**
Rate:	**Sinus rate 50, AV junctional rate 45**
Intervals:	**PR 0.16, QRS 0.08, QT 0.36**
Axis:	**+60 degrees**

Abnormalities

Slow heart rate. APC followed by second premature complex and sinus pause. AV junctional escape complexes (rhythm). ST depression leads V4–V5. T-wave inversion leads II, III, aVF, V4–V6.

Synthesis

Sinus bradycardia. APC with probable reciprocal (echo) complex. Sinus pause with AV junctional escape complexes (rhythm). Period of isorhythmic AV dissociation on rhythm strip. Nonspecific ST-T-wave abnormalities.

TEST ANSWERS: 3, 7, 10, (22), 24, 53, 54, 106.

Comment: When first looking at the rhythm strip, one could easily mistake this for wandering atrial pacemaker to the AV junction. This is not the case in this example. The likely mechanism is that the intrinsic rhythm is sinus bradycardia at a rate of 50. The fifth complex of the tracing is an atrial premature beat, which results in an "echo" beat (sixth complex). The sinus node is depolarized in a retrograde fashion and is temporarily suppressed. A subsidiary pacemaker in the AV junction then takes over until the sinus pacemaker recovers and again usurps control. A period of isorhythmic AV dissociation is evident on the rhythm strip where the P waves and QRS complexes occur in close proximity but are unrelated.

D-3

Clinical History

A 69-year-old woman with dyspnea and a history of cardiac surgery for congenital heart disease.

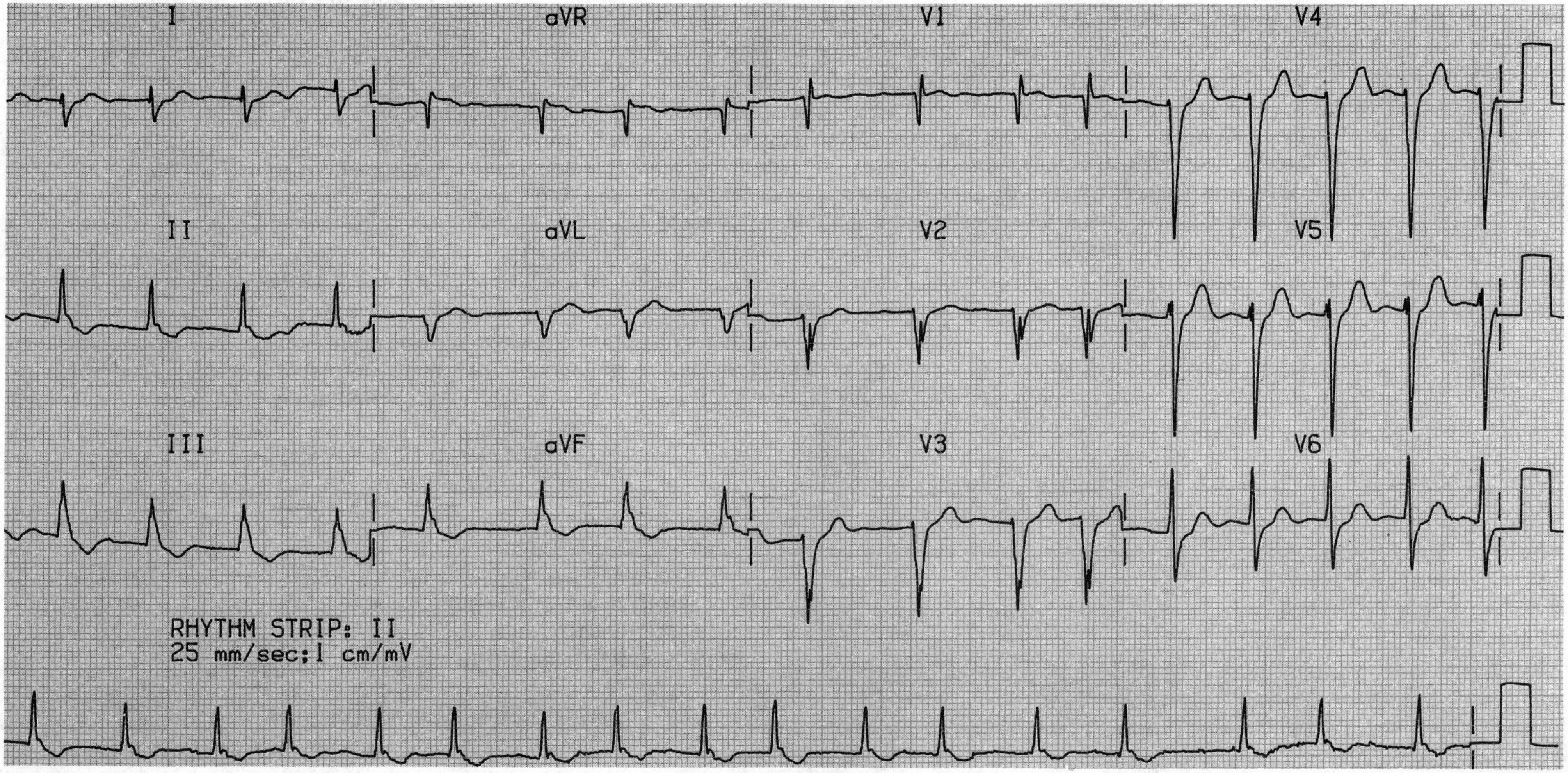

D-3

NARRATIVE INTERPRETATION

Rhythm: **Atrial fibrillation**
Rate: **100 (average)**
Intervals: **PR –, QRS 0.10, QT 0.30**
Axis: **+105 degrees**

Abnormalities

Axis rightward of +90 degrees. qR pattern V1. R-wave voltage less than 3 mm leads V1–V3. T-wave inversion leads II, III, aVF.

Synthesis

Atrial fibrillation with a moderate ventricular response. Right axis deviation. RVH. Nonspecific ST-wave abnormalities. Poor R-wave progression.

TEST ANSWERS: 20, 50, 65, 66, 79, 106.

Comment: This patient had a history of repair of an atrial septal defect with moderate pulmonary hypertension. The right axis deviation is characteristic of an ostium secundum type of atrial septal defect. In contrast, left axis deviation is usually seen in persons with an ostium primum defect. Left posterior fascicular block is also a cause of right axis deviation; however, in this tracing, there are additional signs of RVH to explain the rightward axis. The qR pattern in lead V1 is a very specific sign of RVH, although an rSR′ pattern is more typical of an ostium secundum atrial septal defect. The poor R-wave progression is also likely to be secondary to RVH as are the deep S waves in the left precordial leads.

REFERENCE: Chou p 276.

D-4

Clinical History

A 67-year-old woman following mitral valve replacement. The patient is prescribed digoxin.

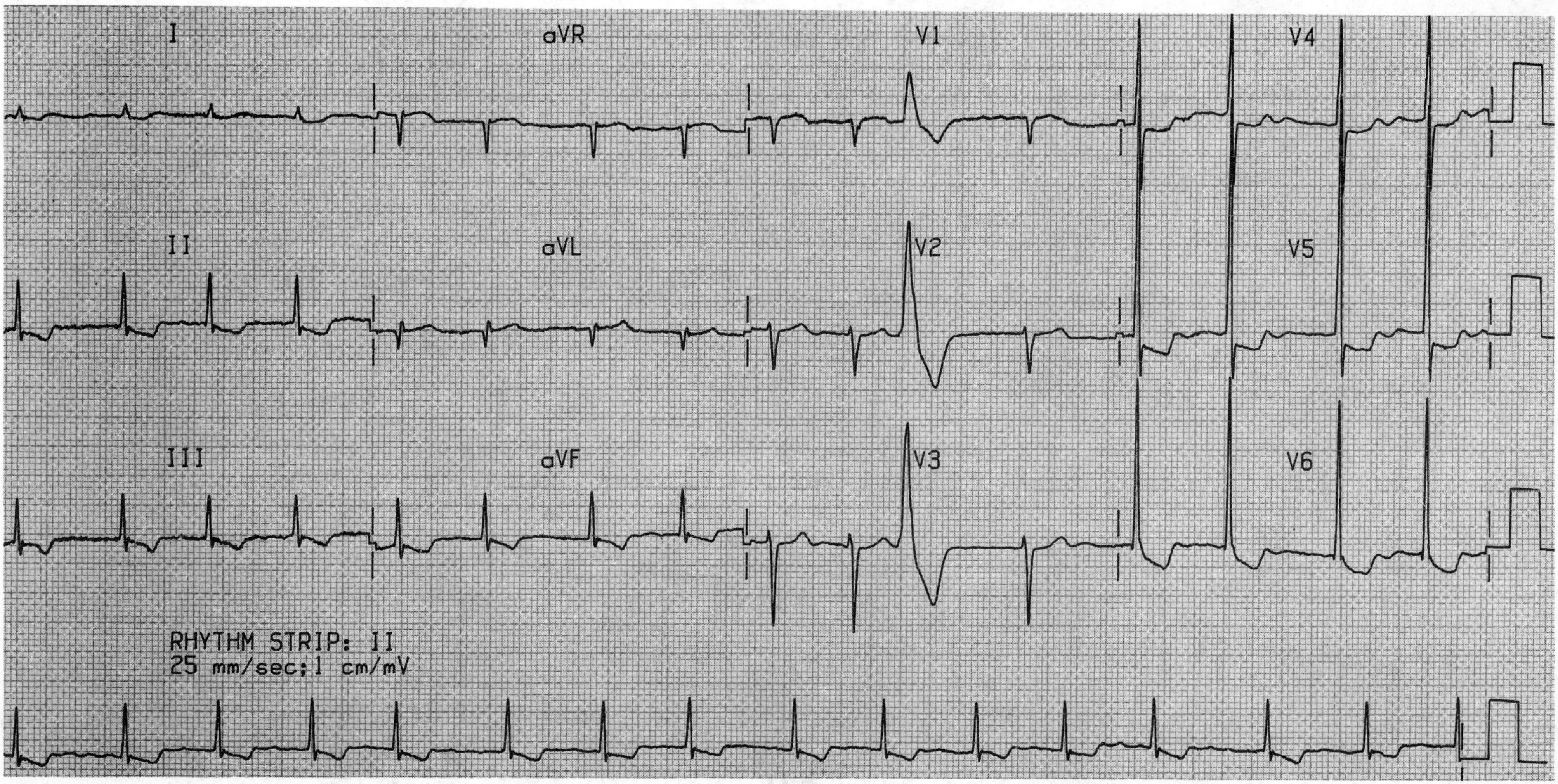

D-4

NARRATIVE INTERPRETATION

Rhythm: **Atrial fibrillation**
Rate: **90 (average)**
Intervals: **PR –, QRS 0.08, QT 0.26**
Axis: **+75 degrees**

Abnormalities

ST depression leads I, II, III, aVF, V4–V6. T-wave inversion leads II, III, aVF, V4–V6. SV2 + RV5 greater than 35. R wave leads V1–V3 less than 3 mm. VPC. Prominent U waves in leads V4–V6.

Synthesis

Atrial fibrillation with a controlled ventricular response. VPC. LVH with associated ST-T-wave abnormalities. Poor R-wave progression. Prominent U waves.

TEST ANSWERS: 20, 26, 51, 66, 78, 103, 110.

Comment: This patient had LVH secondary to chronic mitral regurgitation. Characteristic findings of increased voltage in the precordial leads, generalized ST-T-wave abnormalities, and poor R-wave progression are evident. Some of the ST depression is also likely to be secondary to the effects of digoxin. Note also the relatively short QT interval, likely secondary to digoxin. The wide complex beat is ventricular in origin based on its configuration and should not be misinterpreted as aberrant conduction. A monophasic QRS in lead V1 is unlikely to be supraventricular with aberrancy. Note also that the Q wave in aVL is a normal finding and is not reflective of a high lateral wall MI in the absence of a significant Q wave in lead I. The prominent U waves are most likely associated with LVH.

D-5

Clinical History

A 46-year-old man in the CCU.

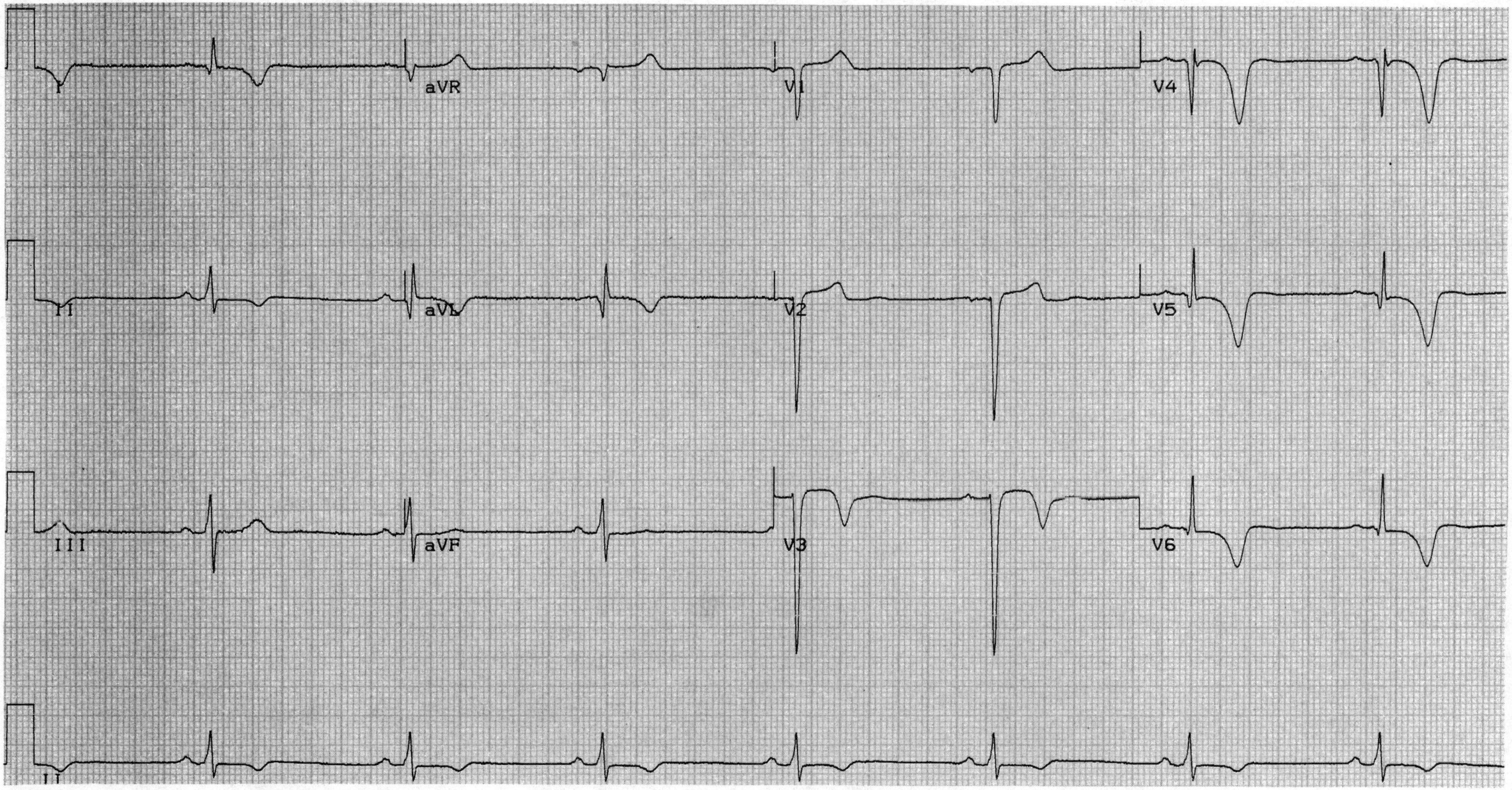

D-5

NARRATIVE INTERPRETATION

Rhythm:	**Sinus bradycardia**
Rate:	**45**
Intervals:	**PR 0.18, QRS 0.08, QT 0.44**
Axis:	**+15 degrees**

Abnormalities

Slow heart rate. Q waves leads I, aVL, V4–V5. "Micro" R waves leads V1–V3. ST "coved" with slight elevation leads I, aVL, V1–V5. T-wave inversion leads I, II, aVL, V3–V6.

Synthesis

Sinus bradycardia. Extensive anterior and lateral wall MI with ST-T-wave changes suggestive of recent myocardial injury.

TEST ANSWERS: 3, (66), (85), 87, 89, 100, (101).

Comment: This patient sustained an extensive anterior and lateral wall MI 36 h earlier. Q waves developed in the lateral limb leads, as well as in V4 and V5. A "micro" R wave remained in the anterior precordial leads. The small Q wave in lead V6 cannot be truly categorized as pathologic despite the clinical picture and is therefore not mentioned as an abnormality.

D-6

Clinical History

An 80-year-old man with a history of aortic valve replacement. He is treated with digoxin.

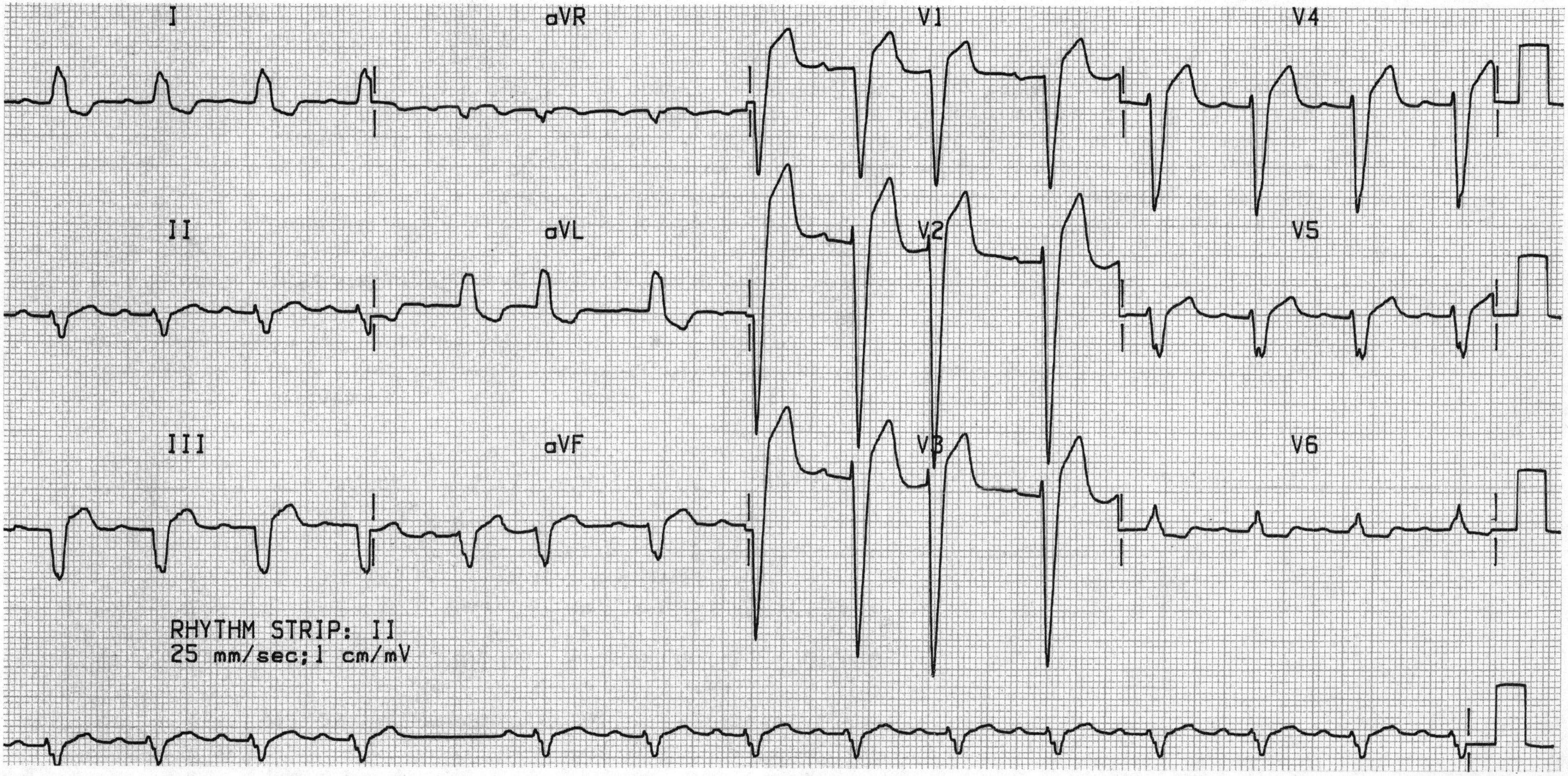

D-6

NARRATIVE INTERPRETATION

Rhythm: **Sinus with first-degree AV block**
Rate: **84**
Intervals: **PR 0.24, QRS 0.13, QT 0.34**
Axis: **−45 degrees**

Abnormalities
Prolonged PR interval. APCs. Blocked APCs. Left axis deviation. Broad, slurred R wave leads I, aVL, V6 with ST depression and T-wave inversion.

Synthesis
Sinus rhythm. First-degree AV block. APCs. Blocked APC on rhythm strip. LBBB. Associated ST-T-wave abnormalities. Left axis deviation.

TEST ANSWERS: 1, 10, 12, 42, 64, 74, 104.

Comment: At first glance, the rhythm strip appears to indicate a Wenckebach sequence with a short PR interval following a pause. On closer observation, there is no shortening of the preceding RR intervals or prolongation of the PR intervals prior to the pause. APCs are clearly noted in the tracing, and a search for a nonconducted APC should be made to explain the pause. Note that the T wave prior to the pause is slightly more prominent than other complexes owing to a nonconducted APC. The PR interval of the next beat is shorter than the others and is probably due to transient improvement of AV conduction following the pause. Left axis deviation is present in this example, although LBBB may occur with a normal, left, or right frontal plane axis.

REFERENCE: Howard.

D-7

Clinical History

A 55-year-old man with palpitations.

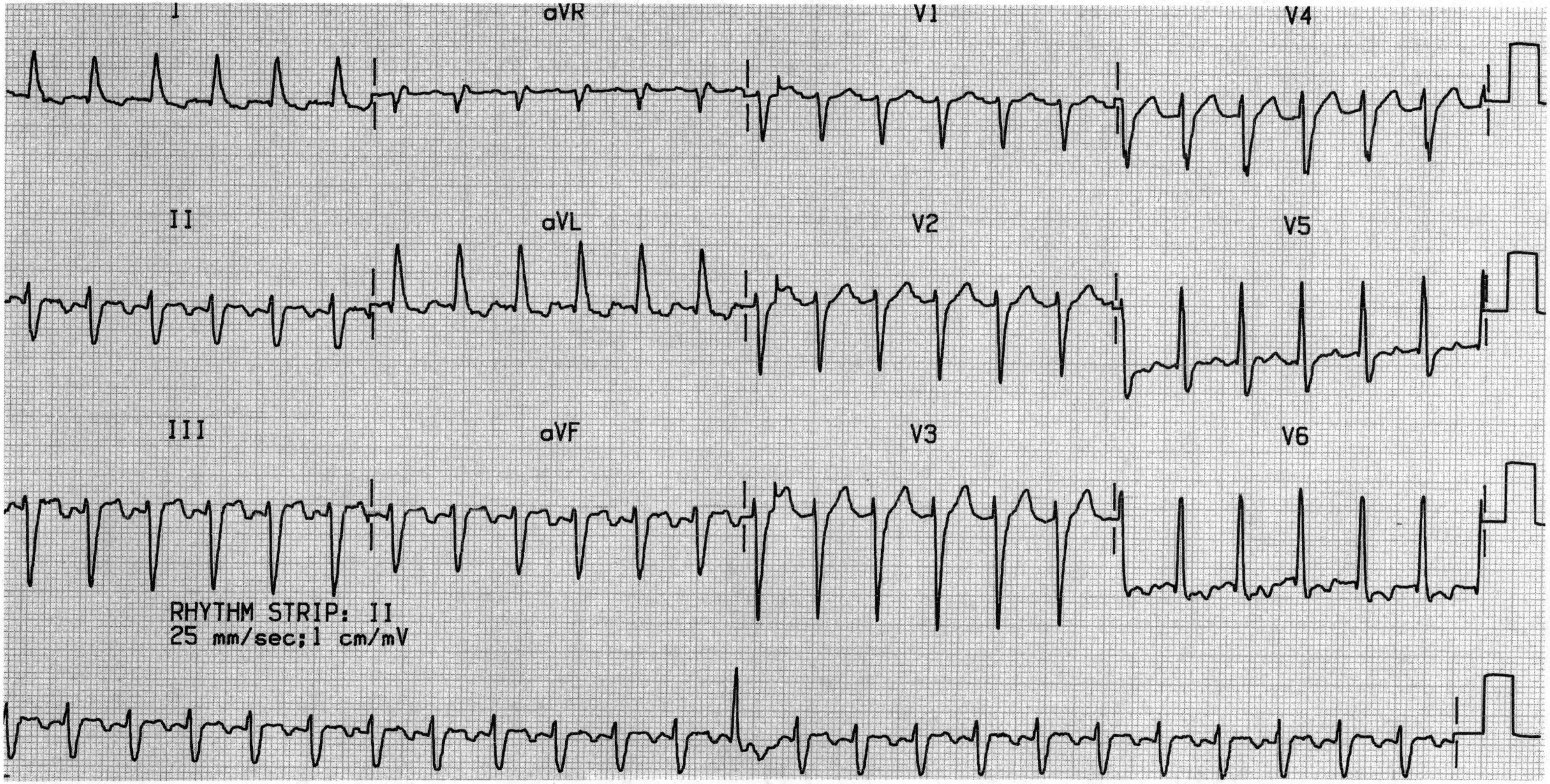

D-7

NARRATIVE INTERPRETATION

Rhythm:	**Atrial flutter with 2:1 AV conduction**
Rate:	**Atrial rate 144, ventricular rate 72**
Intervals:	**PR –, QRS 0.12, QT 0.28**
Axis:	**−45 degrees**

Abnormalities

Axis leftward of −30 degrees. QRS prolongation. ST depression leads I, aVL, V6. T-wave inversion leads I, aVL, V6. VPC.

Synthesis

Atrial flutter with 2:1 AV conduction. VPC. Left axis deviation. Intraventricular conduction delay with associated nonspecific ST-T-wave abnormalities.

TEST ANSWERS: 19, 26, 50, 64, 76, 104, (106).

Comment: At first examination, it would be difficult for the reader to differentiate the atrial flutter seen in this example from supraventricular tachycardia. The inverted P waves in leads II, III, and aVF could easily be mistaken for T waves related to the preceding QRS complex. The ventricular rate of about 150 should always make one suspect atrial flutter with 2:1 AV conduction. In clinical practice, it is often impossible to differentiate these two entities without "uncovering" the underlying flutter waves. Methods to accomplish this include performing carotid sinus pressure or using medications that increase the block at the AV node (see next tracing). Left axis deviation is present in this example, but the diagnosis of left anterior fascicular block (LAFB) is deferred because of the prolonged QRS duration. In most circumstances, LAFB requires a QRS duration of 0.11 s or less. Nonspecific intraventricular conduction delay is interpreted here because of the prolonged QRS duration without criteria for LBBB. Note the preservation of septal Q waves in leads I and aVL, which precludes the diagnosis of LBBB. Limb lead criteria for LVH are borderline.

D-8

Clinical History

A 55-year-old man with palpitations administered 5 mg of verapamil HCl intravenously in the emergency department.

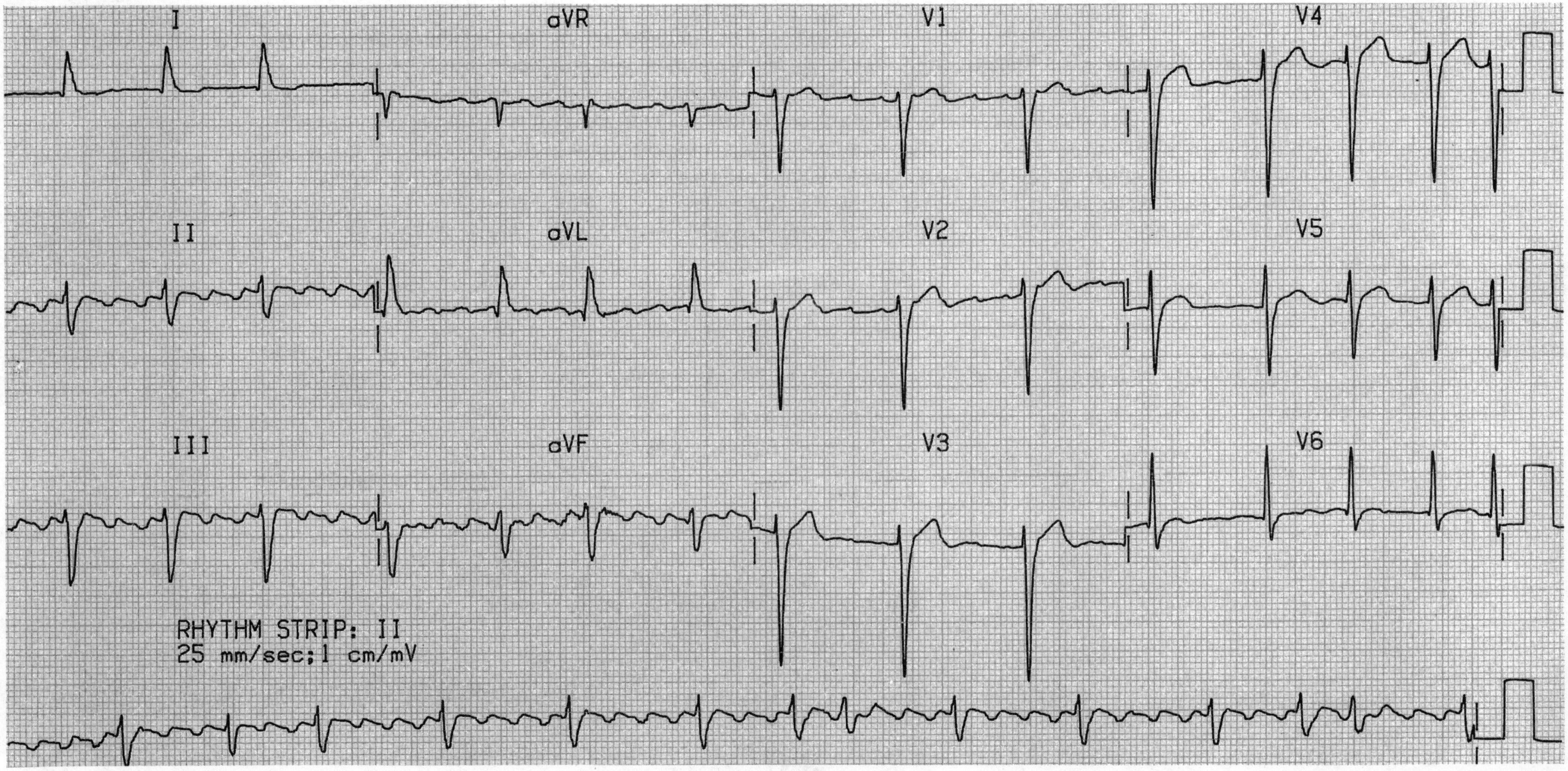

D-8

NARRATIVE INTERPRETATION

Rhythm:	**Atrial flutter with variable AV conduction**
Rate:	**Atrial 144, ventricular 85 (variable)**
Intervals:	**PR –, QRS 0.12, QT 0.30**
Axis:	**−45 degrees**

Abnormalities
Axis leftward of −30 degrees. Prolonged QRS duration.

Synthesis
Atrial flutter with variable AV conduction. Left axis deviation. Nonspecific intraventricular conduction delay.

TEST ANSWERS: 19, 51, 64, 76.

Comment: As noted in the previous tracing, it is often necessary to perform maneuvers to allow the flutter waves to become evident. The diagnosis of atrial flutter is now easily made. Useful bedside tools to differentiate atrial flutter from supraventricular tachycardia (SVT) include carotid sinus pressure or the Valsalva maneuver. Both may convert SVT but will only slow the ventricular rate of atrial flutter. Intravenous administration of AV blocking agents such as adenosine, verapamil, or short-acting beta blockers such as esmolol is also helpful in making a rapid diagnosis. In the previous example, the 2:1 conduction ratio was a physiologic response of the AV node. In this tracing, the conduction response is now nonphysiologic secondary to treatment with verapamil.

D-9

Clinical History

A 75-year-old woman with a history of heart failure. She is prescribed digoxin.

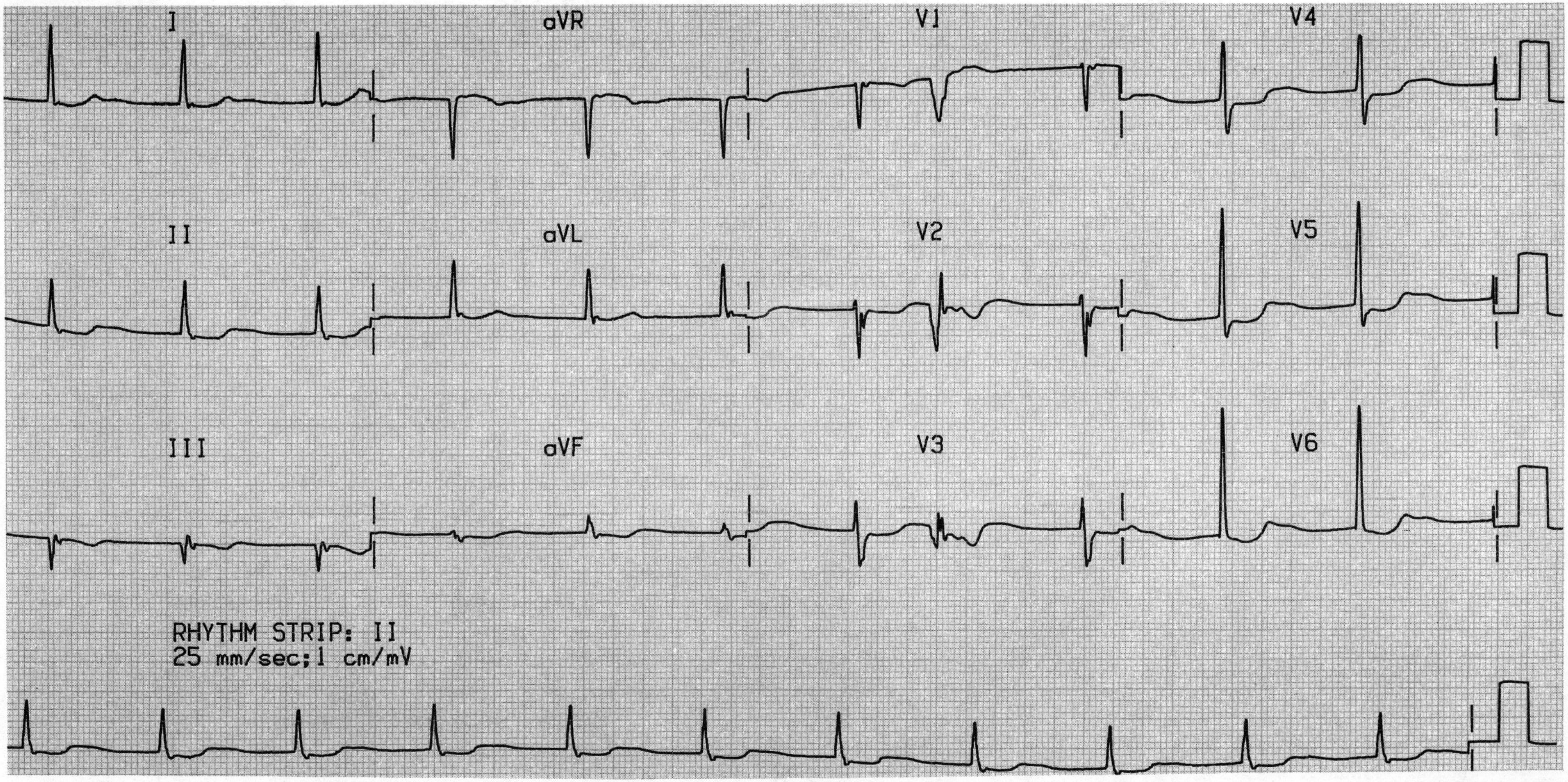

D-9

NARRATIVE INTERPRETATION

Rhythm: **Accelerated AV junctional rhythm**
Rate: **65**
Intervals: **PR –, QRS 0.08, QT 0.36**
Axis: **+15 degrees**

Abnormalities

P waves not evident. ST depression leads I, II, aVL, aVF, V2–V6. VPC.

Synthesis

Accelerated AV junctional rhythm. VPC. Diffuse nonspecific ST abnormalities.

TEST ANSWERS: 23, 26, 106.

Comment: This tracing demonstrates a characteristic rhythm of digitalis toxicity. Digitalis toxicity may manifest as depression of spontaneous pacemakers or depression of conduction or with ectopic rhythms. Nonparoxysmal junctional tachycardia, otherwise known as *accelerated AV junctional rhythm,* is diagnosed in this example on the basis of absent P waves and a relatively fast rate for an AV junctional rhythm. The retrograde P waves may actually be present just after the QRS complex but are not clearly seen. Diffuse ST depression is also noted secondary to administration of digoxin. Ventricular ectopy is also present, and it is important to remember that this is the most frequent cardiac arrhythmia associated with digoxin toxicity.

REFERENCES: Fisch. Smith.

D-10

Clinical History

A 59-year-old woman admitted to the ICU after a cerebral vascular accident.

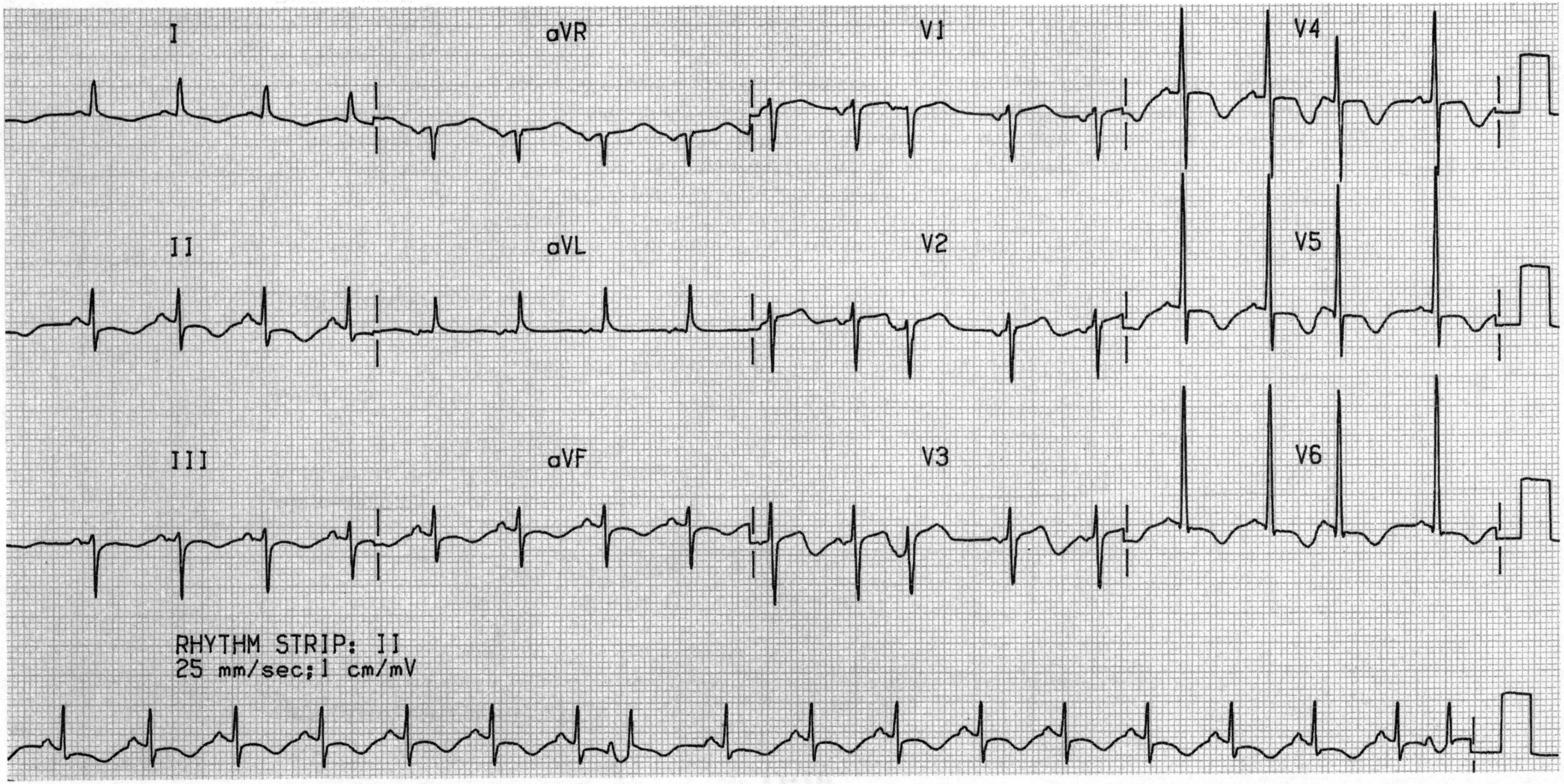

D-10

NARRATIVE INTERPRETATION

Rhythm: **Sinus tachycardia**
Rate: **102**
Intervals: **PR 0.14, QRS 0.08, QT 0.40**
Axis: **−15 degrees**

Abnormalities

Rapid heart rate. ST depression leads I, II, aVF, V5–V6. T-wave inversion leads I, II, III, aVF, V2–V6. QT prolonged for heart rate. APCs.

Synthesis

Sinus tachycardia. APCs. Diffuse, nonspecific ST-T-wave abnormalities. QTc prolongation.

TEST ANSWERS: 4, 10, (11), (102), 106, 109.

Comment: Electrocardiographic abnormalities are frequently seen in patients with cerebral vascular accidents. These include disorders of conduction and repolarization as well as a variety of cardiac arrhythmias. Two studies of a total of 250 patients with acute stroke found QT prolongation in 33 percent, ST-T-wave abnormalities in 45 percent, and abnormal U waves in 18 percent. Supraventricular ectopy, seen in the present tracing, has been reported in 5 to 13 percent of patients with acute stroke. The ST-T-wave abnormalities in patients with central nervous system events often cannot be distinguished from those seen in myocardial ischemia. Moreover, coronary and cerebral ischemic events may occur simultaneously.

REFERENCE: Fass.

D-11

Clinical History

A 72-year-old man seen in routine follow-up. He has a history of hypertension and coronary heart disease.

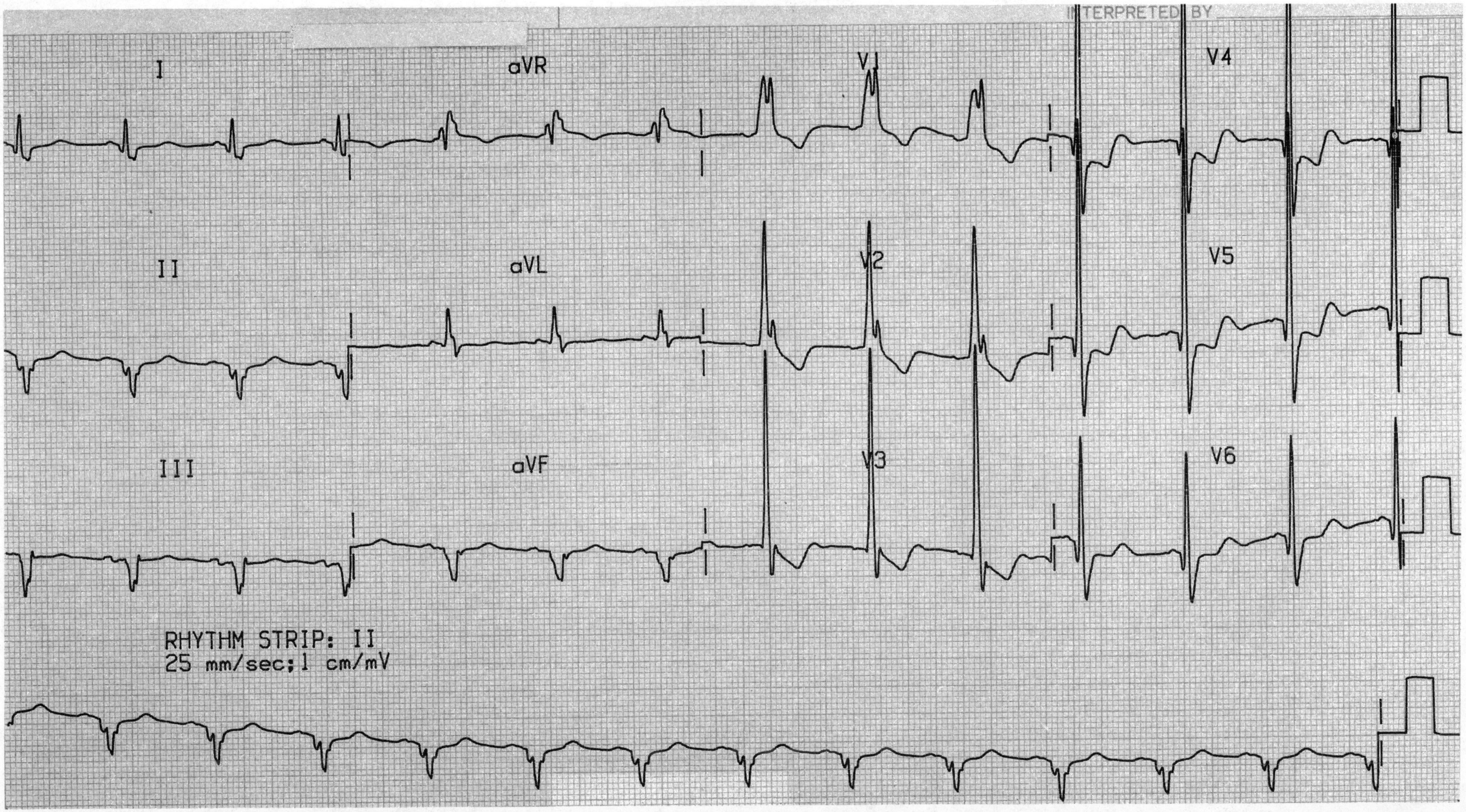

D-11

NARRATIVE INTERPRETATION

Rhythm: **Sinus**
Rate: **79**
Intervals: **PR 0.14, QRS 0.14, QT 0.40**
Axis: **−60 degrees**

Abnormalities

Axis leftward of −30 degrees. Broad, notched QRS with RsR′ with T-wave inversion leads V1–V2. Q waves leads II, III, aVF. R wave lead V5 greater than 35.

Synthesis

Sinus rhythm. RBBB with associated ST-T-wave changes. Left axis deviation. Left anterior fascicular block. Inferior wall MI of indeterminate duration. Probable LVH.

TEST ANSWERS: 1, 64, 70, 72, (78), 92, 104.

Comment: Remember that in RBBB, the initial forces (0.06 s) are unaffected by the conduction abnormality, and standard diagnostic criteria for MI still apply. The Q waves in the inferior leads are diagnostic of this patient's prior inferior wall MI. The tall, broad, initial R wave in lead V1 might also suggest a coexisting posterior wall MI. However, this diagnosis is very difficult in the presence of RBBB alone, and particularly so with coexisting left anterior fascicular block. LVH is also suggested by unusually pronounced R waves in the left precordial leads.

REFERENCES: Benchimol. Cooksey p 431. Friedman p 289.

D-12

Clinical History

An 82-year-old woman presenting in pulmonary edema.

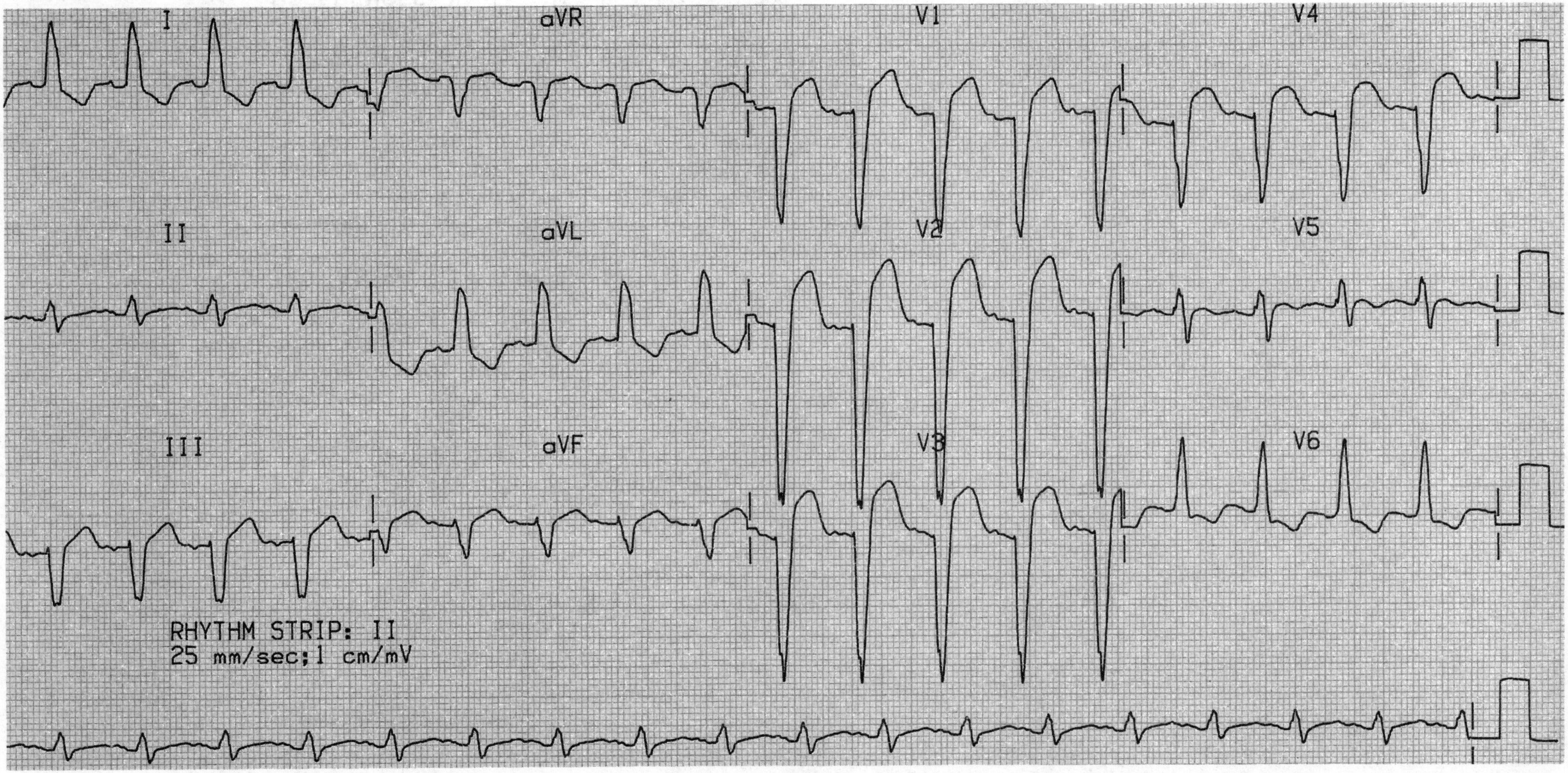

D-12

NARRATIVE HISTORY

Rhythm: **Sinus**
Rate: **110**
Intervals: **PR 0.16, QRS 0.12, QT 0.36**
Axis: **−15 degrees**

Abnormalities

Rapid heart rate. Broad QRS with slurred R waves and T-wave inversion leads I, aVL, V6. Prominent ST-segment elevation leads V1–V4.

Synthesis

Sinus tachycardia. LBBB with associated ST-T-wave changes. Clinical correlation required to exclude myocardial injury.

TEST ANSWERS: 4, 74, (100), 104.

Comment: The electrocardiographic diagnosis of acute MI is often impossible in patients with LBBB. The ST elevation seen primarily in the right precordial leads in this example is not diagnostic of myocardial injury and may be found in uncomplicated LBBB. Some authors have noted that ST elevation more than 7 mm in a direction opposite the main QRS complex is suggestive of acute infarction. In this example, the ST elevation seen in leads V1–V5 is somewhat suspicious for myocardial injury and warrants some comment. In reality, it was due to the conduction delay alone. In the absence of serial tracings, clinical correlation, or other supporting evidence, this diagnosis cannot be definitive.

REFERENCES: Wackers. Hands. Friedman p 290.

D-13

Clinical History

An 80-year-old woman admitted for elective hip surgery.

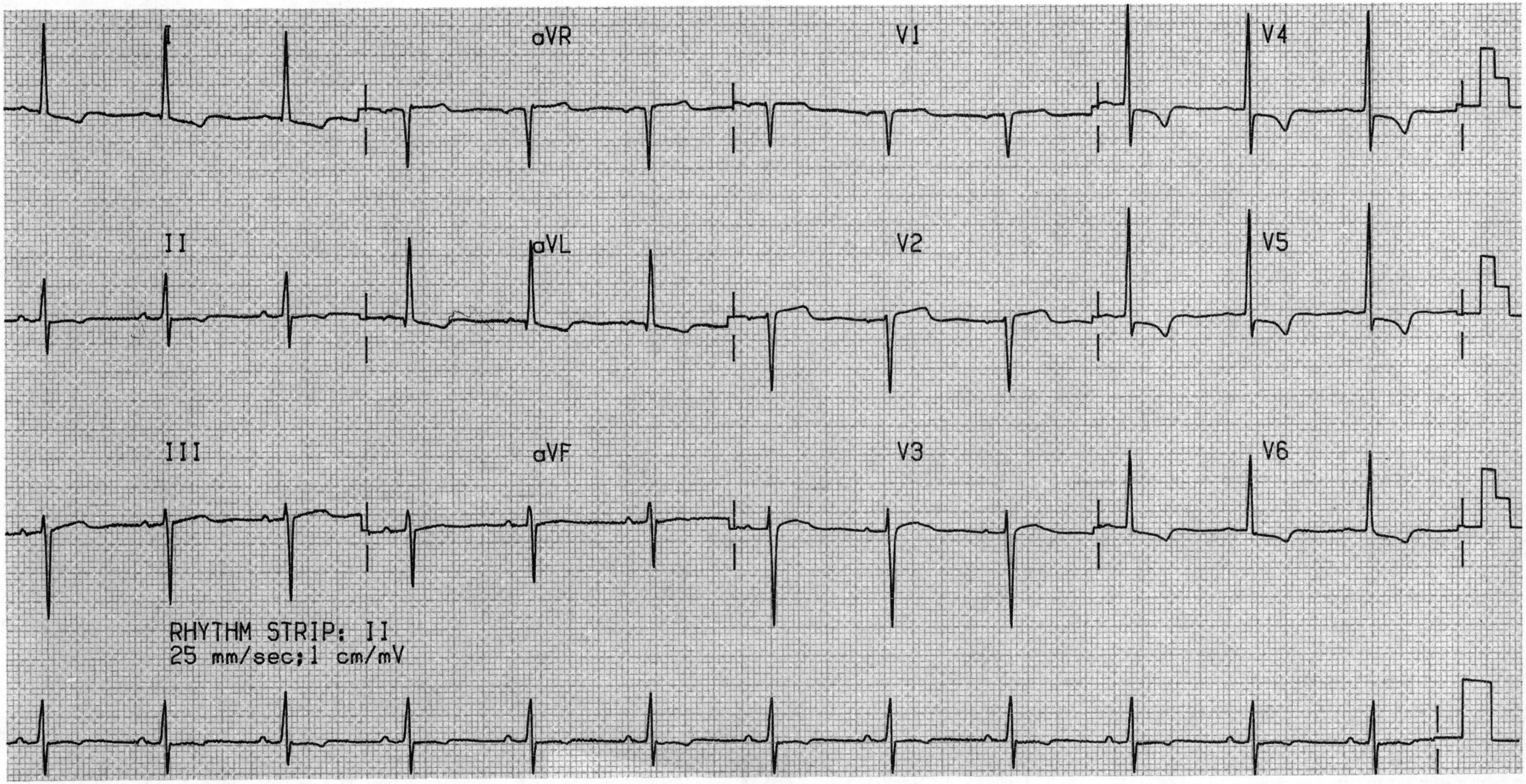

D-13

NARRATIVE INTERPRETATION

Rhythm: **Sinus**
Rate: **70**
Intervals: **PR 0.16, QRS 0.08, QT 0.34**
Axis: **−15 degrees**

Abnormalities

SV2 + RV5 greater than 35. R wave lead aVL greater than 11. ST depression leads I, aVL, V4–V6. T-wave inversion leads I, II, aVL, V4–V6.

Synthesis

Sinus rhythm. LVH with associated ST-T-wave abnormalities.

TEST ANSWERS: 1, 78, 103.

Comment: On first glance, classic precordial voltage criteria for LVH are not present in this tracing. Remember, however, to check the standardization. The precordial leads are recorded at one-half standard. Additional limb lead criteria may also be cited, such as R lead I + S lead III greater than 25. Relatively new criteria that have also been proposed are met by this tracing as well (R in lead aVL + S in lead V3 > 28 mm in men, or > 20 mm in women).

REFERENCE: Casale.

D-14

Clinical History

A 42-year-old woman with dyspnea.

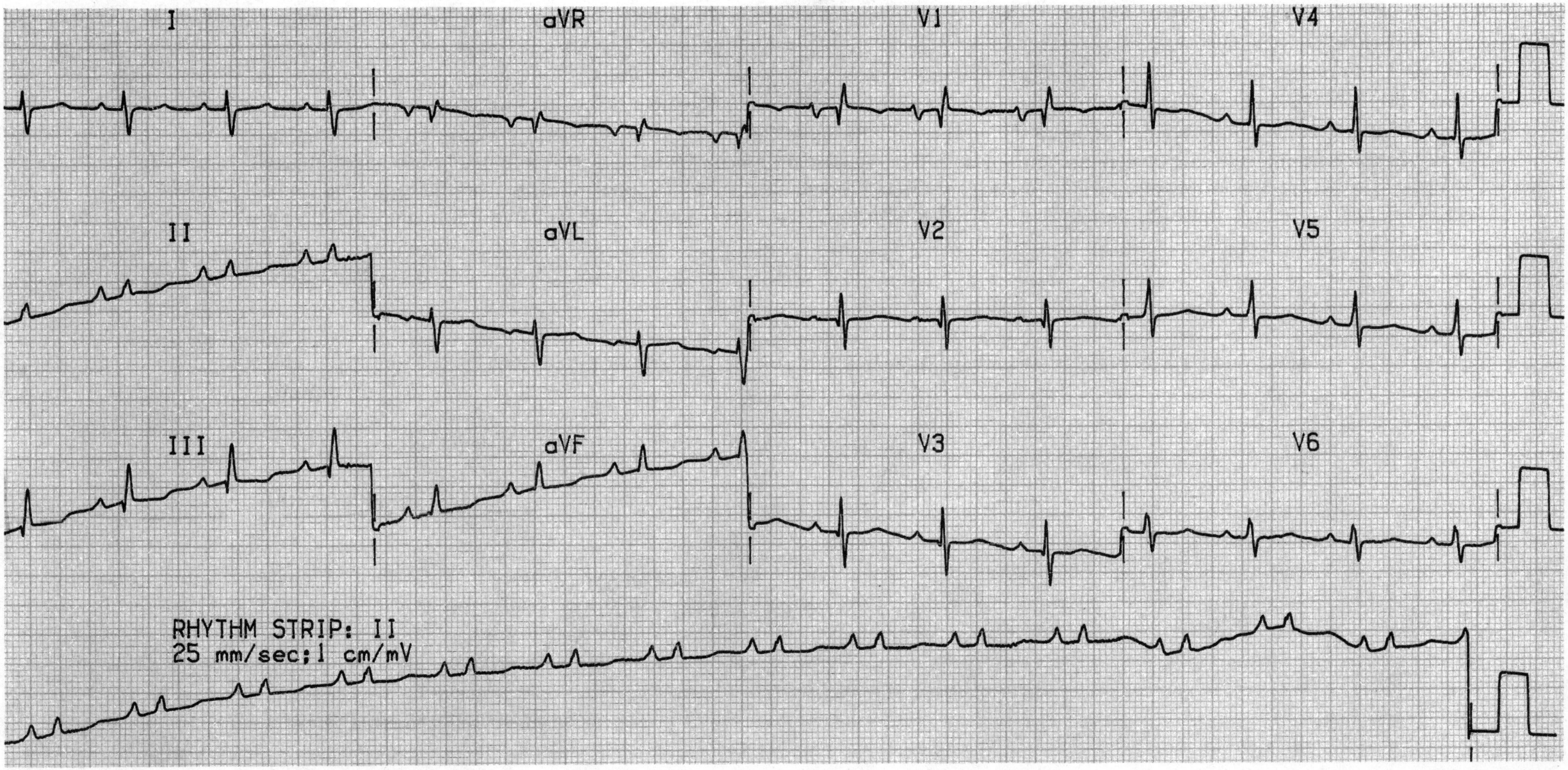

D-14

NARRATIVE INTERPRETATION

Rhythm: **Sinus**
Rate: **86**
Intervals: **PR 0.20, QRS 0.08, QT 0.34**
Axis: **+120 degrees**

Abnormalities
Axis rightward of +90 degrees. QR lead V1. R wave less than S lead V6. Abnormal P terminal force lead V1. T-wave inversion lead III. Biphasic T wave lead II, aVF.

Synthesis
Sinus rhythm. Right axis deviation. RVH. Left atrial abnormality. Nonspecific ST-T-wave abnormalities.

TEST ANSWERS: 1, 60, 65, 79, 106.

Comment: This tracing demonstrates many diagnostic features of RVH. There is marked right axis deviation. A QR pattern, seen in lead V1, is a very specific criterion for RVH. The S wave is slightly greater than the R wave in lead V6. Right atrial hypertrophy is suggested in lead II but does not quite meet definitive criteria. Causes of RVH commonly seen in clinical practice include primary pulmonary hypertension, cor pulmonale, right ventricular volume overload from left-to-right cardiac communications, and mitral stenosis.

D-15

Clinical History

A 55-year-old woman with sudden onset of lightheadedness.

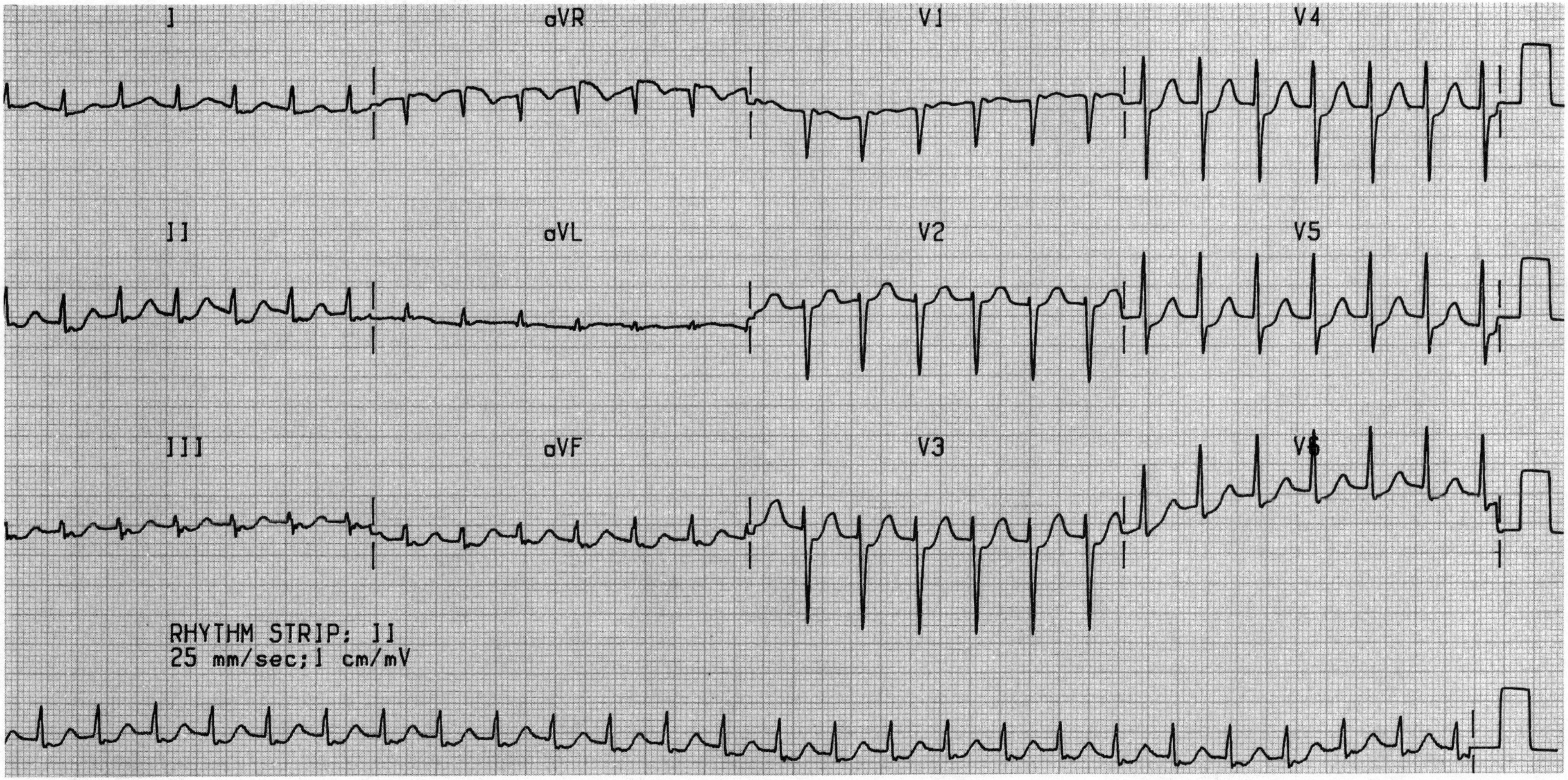

D-15

NARRATIVE INTERPRETATION

Rhythm: **Supraventricular tachycardia**
Rate: **155**
Intervals: **PR –, QRS 0.06, QT 0.28**
Axis: **+30 degrees**

Abnormalities

Rapid heart rate. ST depression leads II, III, aVF, V3–V6.

Synthesis

Supraventricular tachycardia. Nonspecific ST-segment abnormalities.

TEST ANSWERS: 18, 106.

Comment: This example demonstrates a supraventricular tachycardia (SVT). The most common mechanism for SVT in adults is AV nodal reentrant tachycardia. In this form of SVT, the P wave is characteristically hidden in or, as in this example, occurs slightly after the QRS complex. The reentry circuit is located in the AV node and has two separate pathways with different conduction properties. As in all reentrant mechanisms, a premature stimulus is blocked in the pathway with the longer refractory period and is conducted in the pathway with the shorter refractory period. The impulse is then conducted retrograde via the recovered limb and a new cycle is begun. Nonspecific ST-segment abnormalities are present in this electrocardiogram. These are often seen in normal persons at these high heart rates and may not reflect myocardial ischemia.

REFERENCES: Manolis. Kalbfleisch. Bar (*Am J Cardiol*).

D-16

Clinical History

A 44-year-old man with palpitations after drinking heavily.

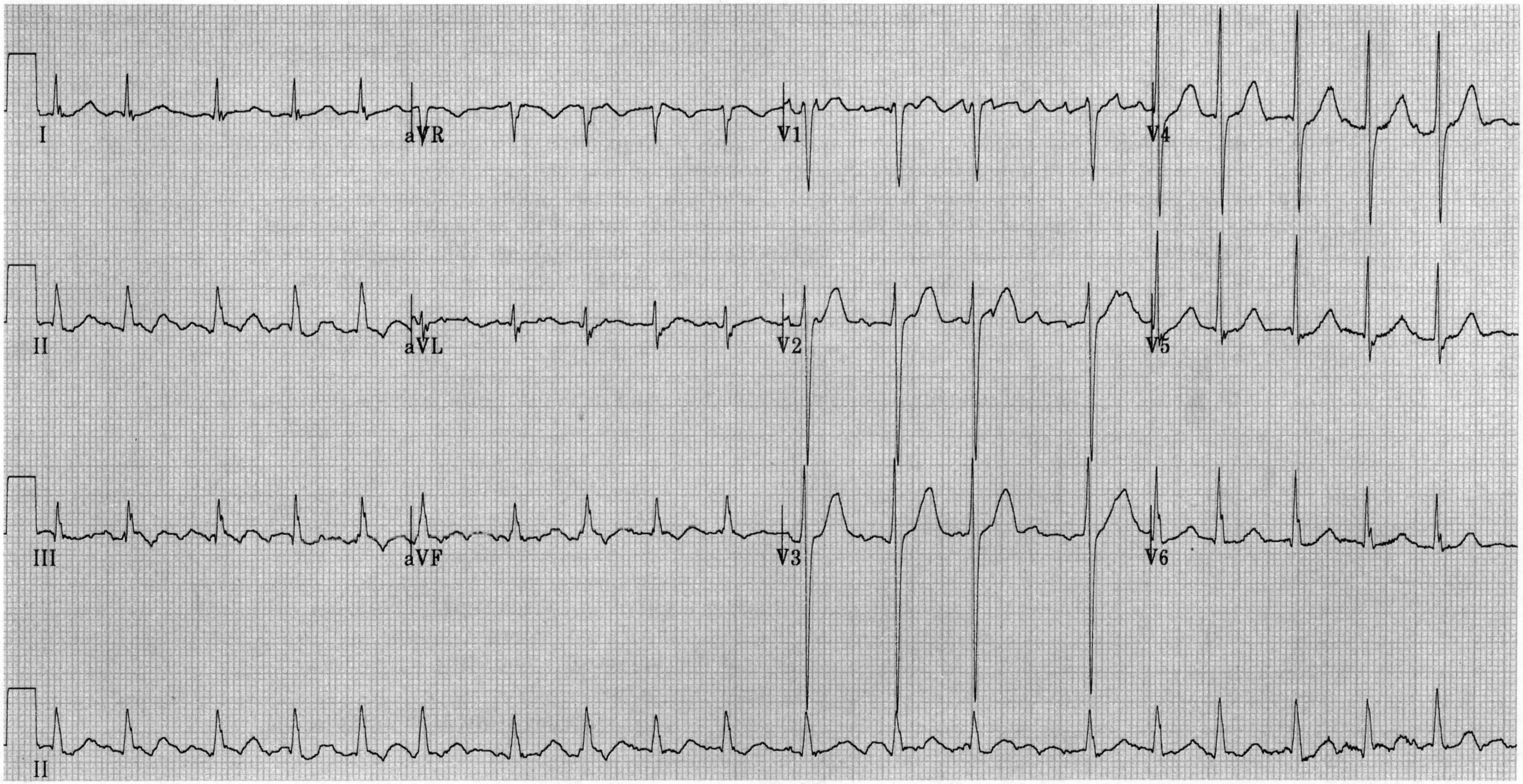

D-16

NARRATIVE INTERPRETATION

Rhythm:	**Atrial fibrillation**
Rate:	**116 (average)**
Intervals:	**PR –, QRS 0.08, QT 0.36**
Axis:	**+60 degrees**

Abnormalities
Rapid heart rate.

Synthesis
Atrial fibrillation with rapid ventricular response. Otherwise within normal limits.

TEST ANSWERS: 20, 50.

Comment: The relationship of heavy alcohol consumption and atrial fibrillation of new onset has been coined the "holiday heart syndrome." Whereas this relationship has not been corroborated in all studies, there is little doubt that alcohol may play a role in the genesis of atrial arrhythmias in patients without other demonstrable cardiac disease. Note that the fibrillatory waves appear somewhat organized or "coarse," particularly in lead V1. Some authors have noted a correlation between coarse fibrillatory waves and an abnormal P terminal force with resumption of sinus rhythm, indicative of left atrial enlargement (see next tracing).

REFERENCES: Chou p 337. Koskinen.

D-17

Clinical History

A 44-year-old man treated with an antiarrhythmic agent for new-onset atrial fibrillation.

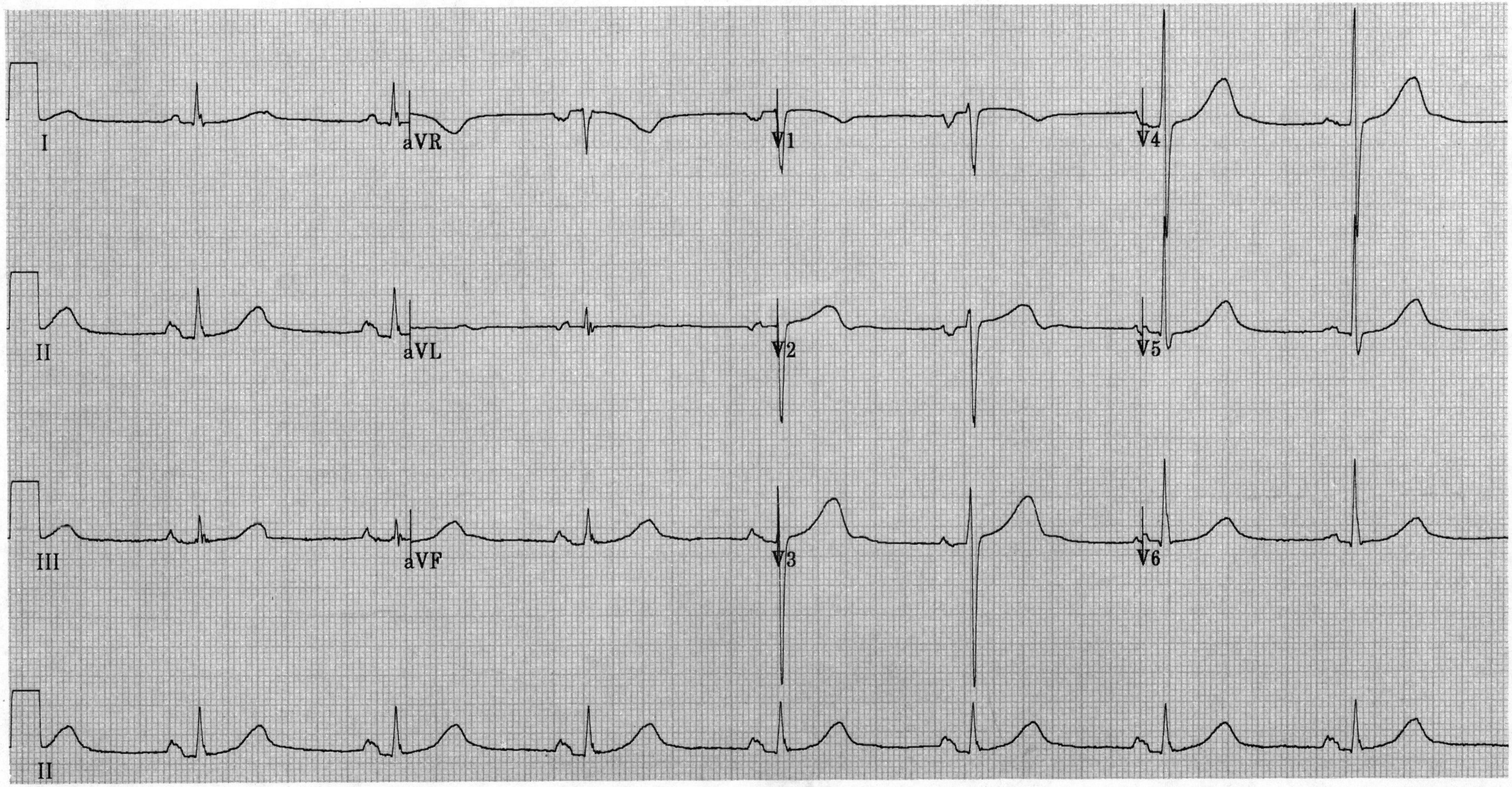

D-17

NARRATIVE INTERPRETATION

Rhythm: Sinus
Rate: 60
Intervals: PR 0.20, QRS 0.08, QT 0.54
Axis: +45 degrees

Abnormalities

Abnormal P terminal force lead V1. Prolonged QT interval for heart rate.

Synthesis

Sinus rhythm. Left atrial abnormality. Prolonged QTc interval.

TEST ANSWERS: 1, 60, 109.

Comment: The patient described in the previous tracing was treated with intravenous digoxin and procainamide and converted from atrial fibrillation to sinus rhythm. Although the rhythm has normalized, there is now a marked prolongation of the QT interval. This is perhaps a more dangerous phenomenon as it may predispose to malignant ventricular arrhythmias. Torsades de pointes, a potentially lethal arrhythmia, may be seen in patients with a prolonged QTc interval from type I antiarrhythmic agents such as procainamide. This arrhythmia is defined by ventricular tachycardia with cycles of differing polarity, such that it appears to be "turning around the point" of the baseline of the electrocardiogram.

REFERENCE: Stratmann.

D-18

Clinical History

A 41-year-old man seen for evaluation of a forearm rash. He has a history of a tick bite 3 weeks earlier.

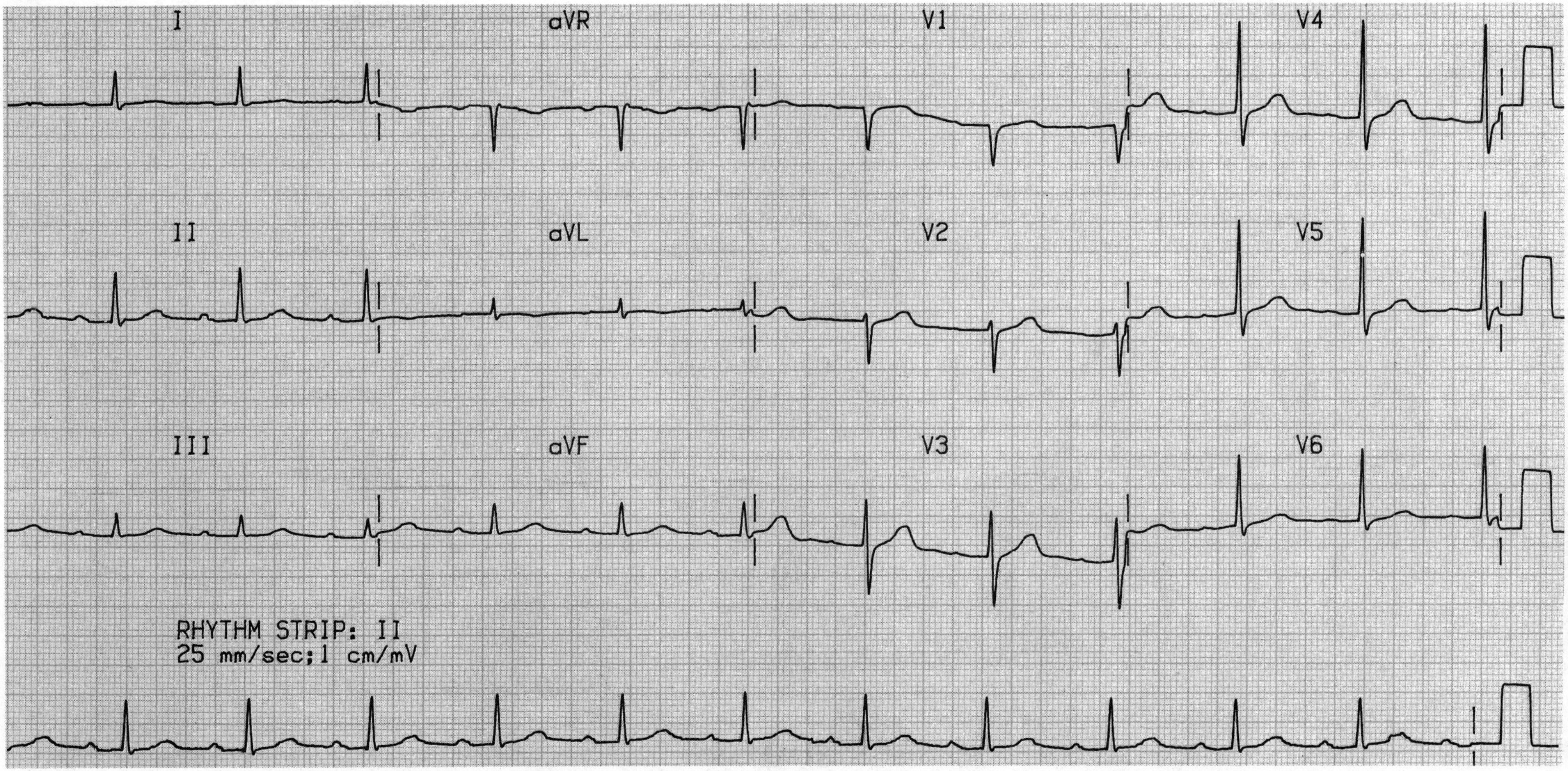

D-18

NARRATIVE INTERPRETATION

Rhythm: **Sinus with first-degree AV block**
Rate: **70**
Intervals: **PR 0.24, QRS 0.08, QT 0.36**
Axis: **+45 degrees**

Abnormalities

Prolonged PR interval.

Synthesis

Sinus rhythm. First-degree AV block. Otherwise within normal limits.

TEST ANSWERS: 1, 42.

Comment: This patient had clinical evidence of Lyme disease with a characteristic rash of erythema migrans. He also had evidence of Lyme carditis on the basis of first-degree AV block of new onset. Lyme carditis has been reported in 4 to 10 percent of cases of acute Lyme disease, with AV block the most common manifestation of cardiac involvement. Of patients who do develop conduction system disease, up to 98 percent will demonstrate first-degree AV block at some point in their illness. High-grade AV block may also develop and require insertion of a temporary pacemaker. The conduction abnormalities generally resolve over 1 to 2 weeks.

REFERENCES: Rubin (1992). Cox.

D-19

Clinical History

A 76-year-old woman admitted to the CCU.

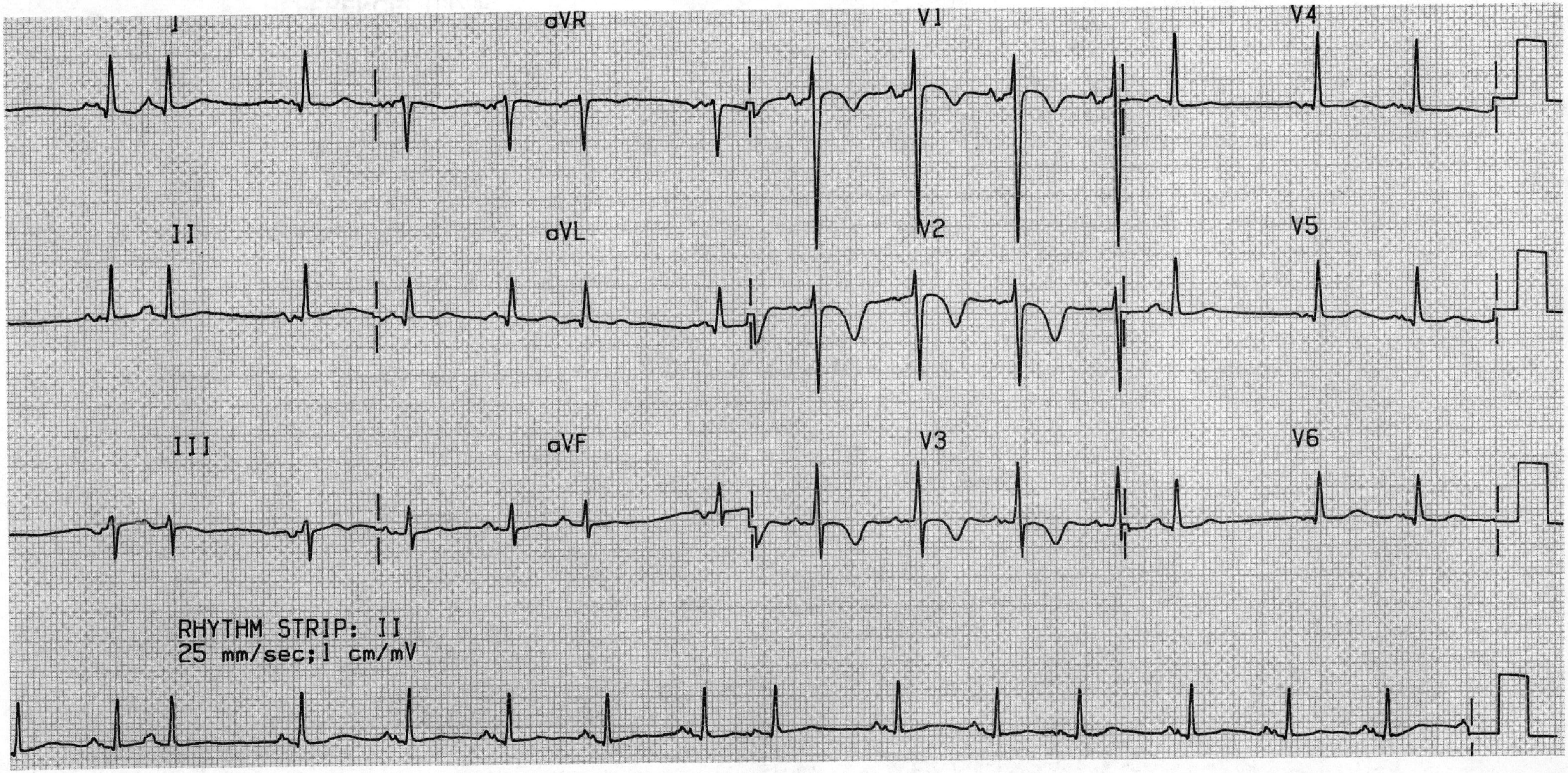

D-19

NARRATIVE INTERPRETATION

Rhythm:	**Sinus**
Rate:	**90**
Intervals:	**PR 0.16, QRS 0.08, QT 0.38**
Axis:	**+15 degrees**

Abnormalities
APCs. Abnormal P terminal force lead V1. ST segment straight with slight downward concavity leads V1–V3. T-wave inversion leads V1–V3.

Synthesis
Sinus rhythm. APCs. ST-T-wave abnormalities suggestive of recent myocardial injury. Left atrial abnormality.

TEST ANSWERS: 1, 10, 60, 100, (102).

Comment: This patient developed a non-Q-wave anterior wall MI. The configuration of the ST segment in leads V1–V3 suggests that these abnormalities are indicative of myocardial injury. It is difficult to differentiate recent injury from ischemia on the basis of a single electrocardiogram. However, the slight ST elevation and coving suggests that some degree of myocardial injury has occurred. A number of characteristic findings for left atrial enlargement also may be seen in this electrocardiogram. Note the abnormal P terminal force in lead V1, and the notched P waves and leftward P axis in the limb leads. Frequent APCs are also seen in this example.

REFERENCE: Hazen.

D-20

Clinical History

A 74-year-old asymptomatic woman scheduled for cataract surgery.

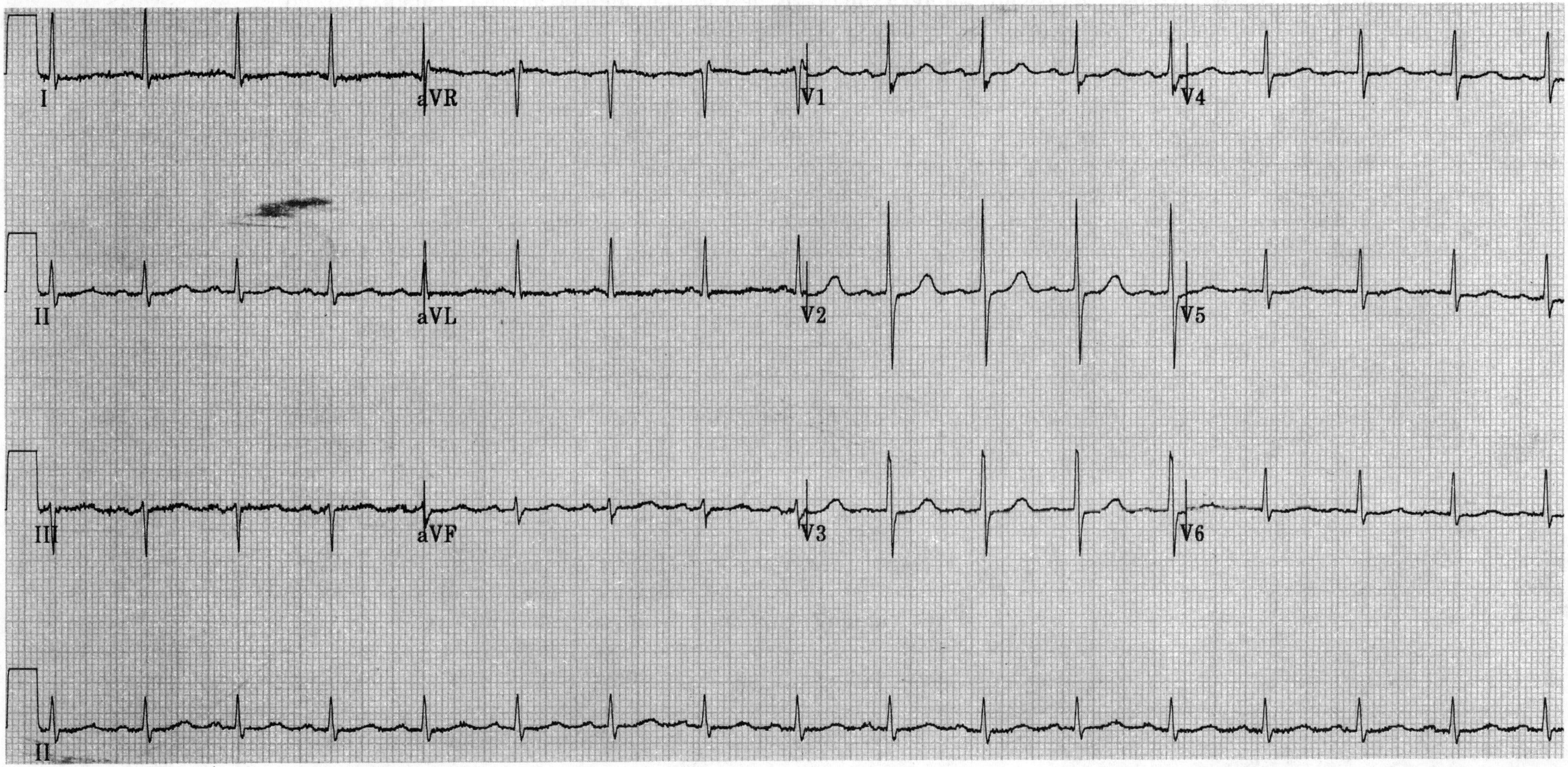

D-20

NARRATIVE INTERPRETATION

Rhythm: **Sinus**
Rate: **98**
Intervals: **PR 0.16, QRS 0.08, QT 0.36**
Axis: **0 degrees**

Abnormalities
R wave greater than S wave leads V1–V2. Flat T wave leads I, aVL.

Synthesis
Sinus rhythm. Tall R waves right precordial leads, probably within normal limits. Nonspecific T-wave abnormalities.

TEST ANSWERS: 1, 106.

Comment: This is a tracing with a difficult differential diagnosis. It is normal by the exclusion of abnormalities. Tall R waves in lead V1 with an R/S ratio greater than 1 are infrequent but may occur in about 1 percent of normal persons. An R/S ratio greater than 1 is more frequent in lead V2, where it is present in around 10 percent of normal persons. The differential diagnosis of this finding includes RVH, posterior wall MI, and misplacement of the chest leads. Other conditions that may produce tall R waves in the right precordial leads are RBBB, dextrocardia, and AV nodal bypass tract patterns. These should be easily excluded from observation of associated electrocardiographic findings. The differential diagnosis of posterior wall MI, RVH, and normal variants is more difficult. Clues for RVH are associated right axis deviation, low voltage in the limb leads, and right atrial abnormality, as well as an inverted T wave in lead V1. Findings suggesting posterior MI are an upright T wave in lead V1 and, most importantly, evidence of a concomitant inferior wall MI. In this example, the pattern is interpreted as a normal variant. Note that the tall R waves are quite narrow and are not diagnostic of a posterior wall MI. Minor T-wave abnormalities are present. The T wave is usually upright in leads I and aVL. The importance of a careful interpretation of the electrocardiogram in the context of a preoperative assessment must be emphasized.

REFERENCES: Zema (1990). Zema (1984). Goldberger I. Nestico. Perloff (1964). Chou p 57.

D-21

Clinical History

A 44-year-old man with 2 h of chest discomfort and diaphoresis.

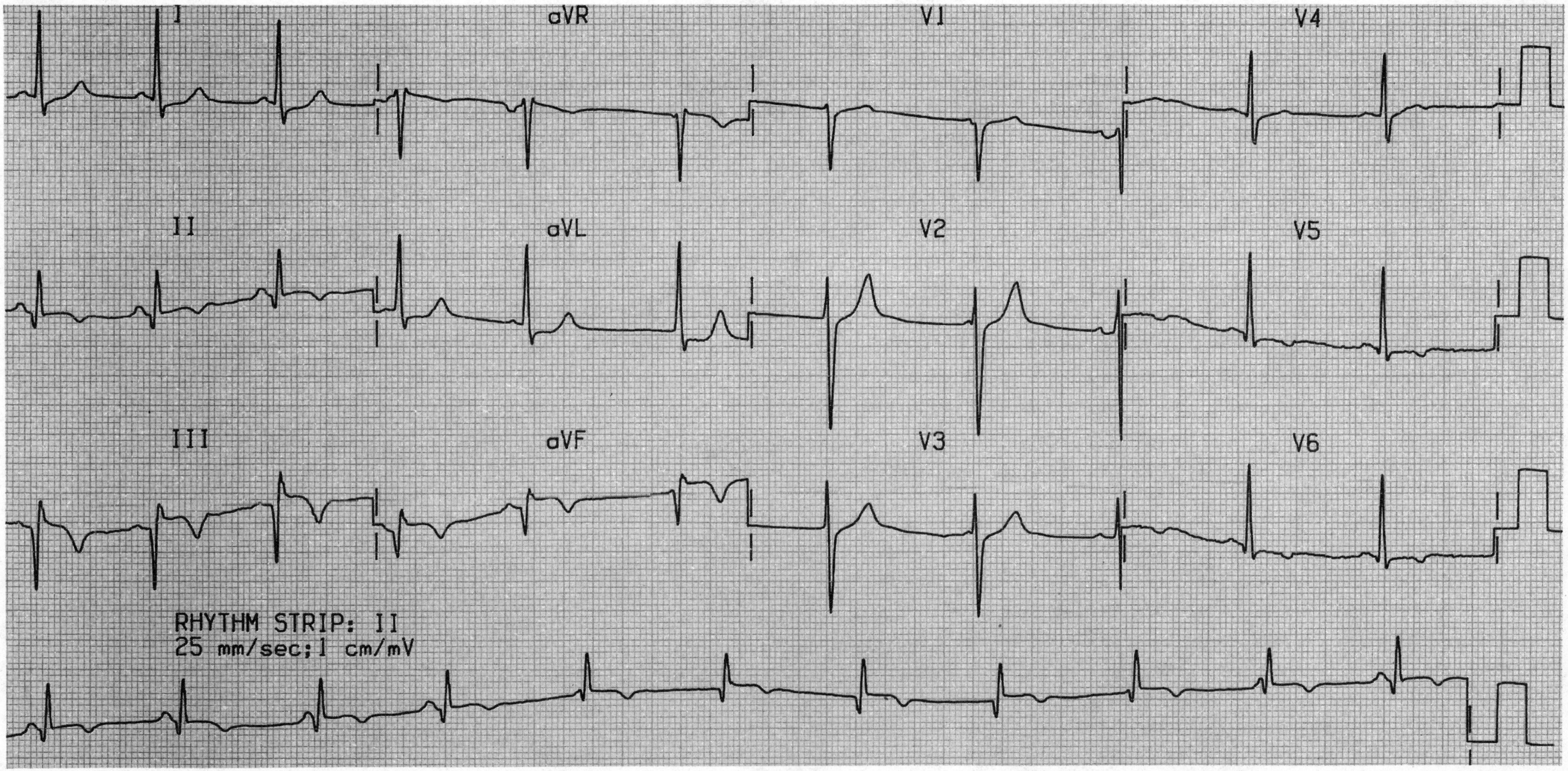

D-21

NARRATIVE INTERPRETATION

Rhythm:	**Sinus arrhythmia, AV junctional rhythm**
Rate:	**Sinus rate 65, AV junctional rate 63**
Intervals:	**PR 0.14, QRS 0.08, QT 0.40**
Axis:	**+15 degrees**

Abnormalities

Sinus rates vary by 0.16 s. AV dissociation. Junctional escape rhythm. Q waves leads II, III, aVF. ST elevation leads II, III, aVF, V5, V6. ST depression leads I, aVL. T-wave inversion leads II, III, aVF, V5, V6.

Synthesis

Sinus arrhythmia with AV junctional escape rhythm. Inferior wall MI with ST-T-wave abnormalities of acute myocardial injury. Isorhythmic AV dissociation.

TEST ANSWERS: 2, 22, 53, 91, 100.

Comment: This patient is experiencing an acute inferior wall MI. Profound vagal influences are commonly seen in this situation with a variety of rhythm manifestations including sinus bradyarrhythmias and first- or second-degree AV block. In this example, the sinus rate periodically slows from a sinus arrhythmia, which allows for a subsidiary pacemaker in the AV junction to emerge. A brief period of isorhythmic AV dissociation is seen where the sinus and junctional complexes occur nearly simultaneously but are unrelated to each other.

D-22

Clinical History

A 44-year-old man with 2 h of chest discomfort and diaphoresis. Right-sided precordial leads are presented for the patient in the previous ECG.

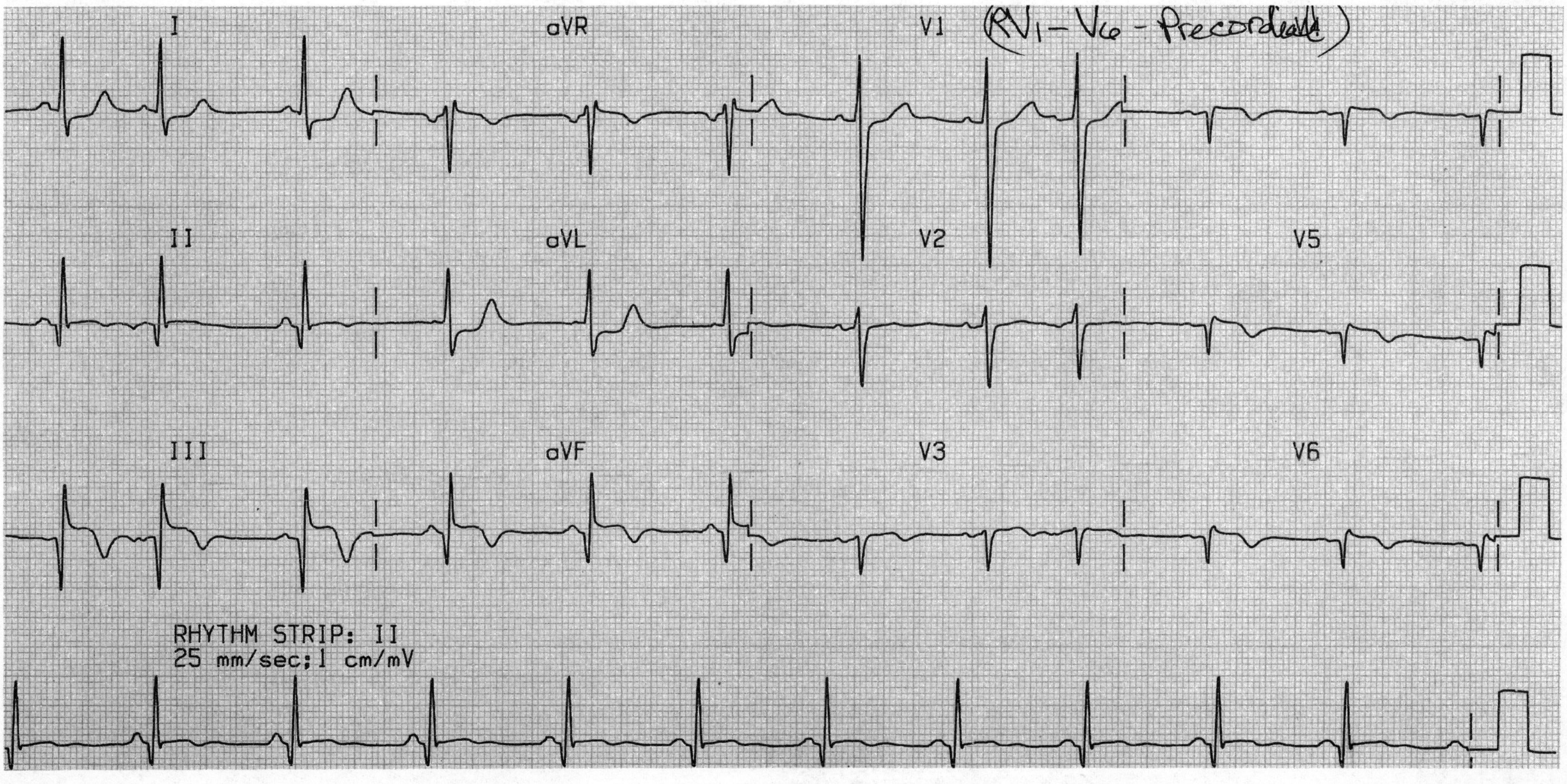

D-22

NARRATIVE INTERPRETATION

(Interpret and synthesize abnormalities of right precordial leads only, V2R–V6R)

Abnormalities

Q waves leads V4R, V5R, V6R. ST elevation leads V4R, V5R, V6R

Synthesis

ST elevation with Q waves in right precordial leads indicative of acute right ventricular MI.

TEST ANSWERS: not applicable

Comment: The performance of right precordial leads is extremely useful for any patient with acute inferior wall MI. This patient has an obvious inferior wall MI based on findings in the previous tracing. The right precordial leads presented here indicate a right ventricular infarction as well. ST elevation in the right precordial leads (particularly V4R) of 1 mm or more in a patient with inferior wall MI is indicative of right ventricular involvement. A QS or QR pattern in V4R is another useful sign of RV infarction.

REFERENCES: Robalino. Lopez-Sendon.

D-23

Clinical History

A 62-year-old man with palpitation. He is prescribed procainamide and digoxin.

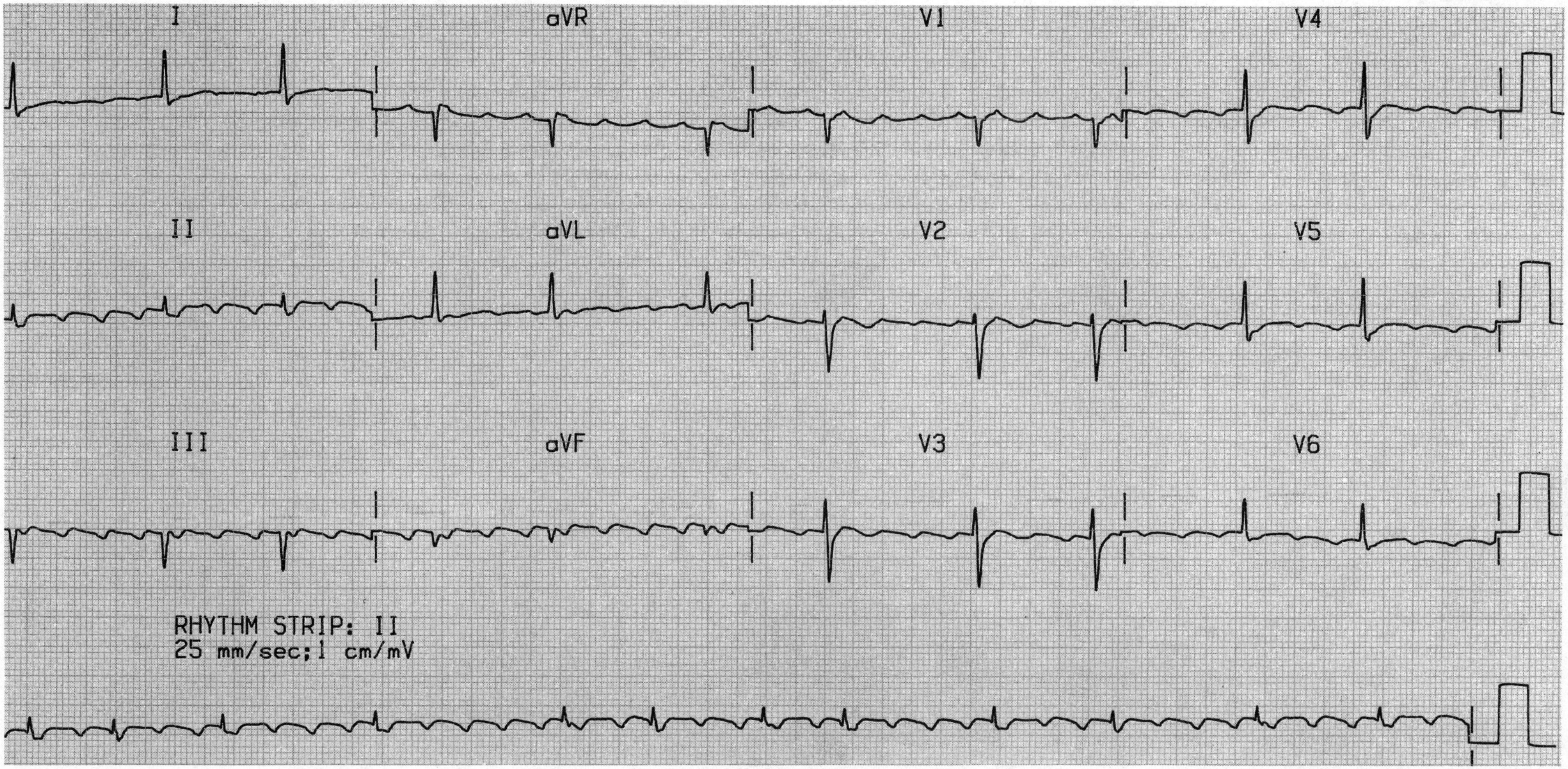

D-23

NARRATIVE INTERPRETATION

Rhythm: **Atrial flutter with variable AV conduction**
Rate: **Atrial 240, ventricular 64 (average)**
Intervals: **PR –, QRS 0.08, QT –**
Axis: **–15 degrees**

Abnormalities

Synthesis

Atrial flutter with variable AV conduction. Otherwise within normal limits.

TEST ANSWERS: 19, 51.

Comment: The differential diagnosis of the rhythm in this example should include atrial flutter and atrial tachycardia. The atrial rate in atrial flutter is generally between 250 and 350 beats per minute. Atrial tachycardia is characterized by slower atrial rates of 150 to 250 beats per minute. Flutter waves may be seen in leads II, III, and aVF; however, the atrial rate is somewhat less than expected for atrial flutter. The reason for this is the effect of procainamide, which acts to slow the atrial rate. Remember that in atrial tachycardia, the P waves are generally upright in leads II, III, and aVF, and there is an isoelectric baseline between the P waves. Classic atrial flutter should demonstrate a characteristic "sawtooth" appearance in these leads. The increased AV block in this example is a result of the effect of digoxin. Low T-wave voltage is suggested but cannot be accurately determined because of the superimposed flutter waves.

D-24

Clinical History

A 67-year-old man seen in preoperative evaluation.

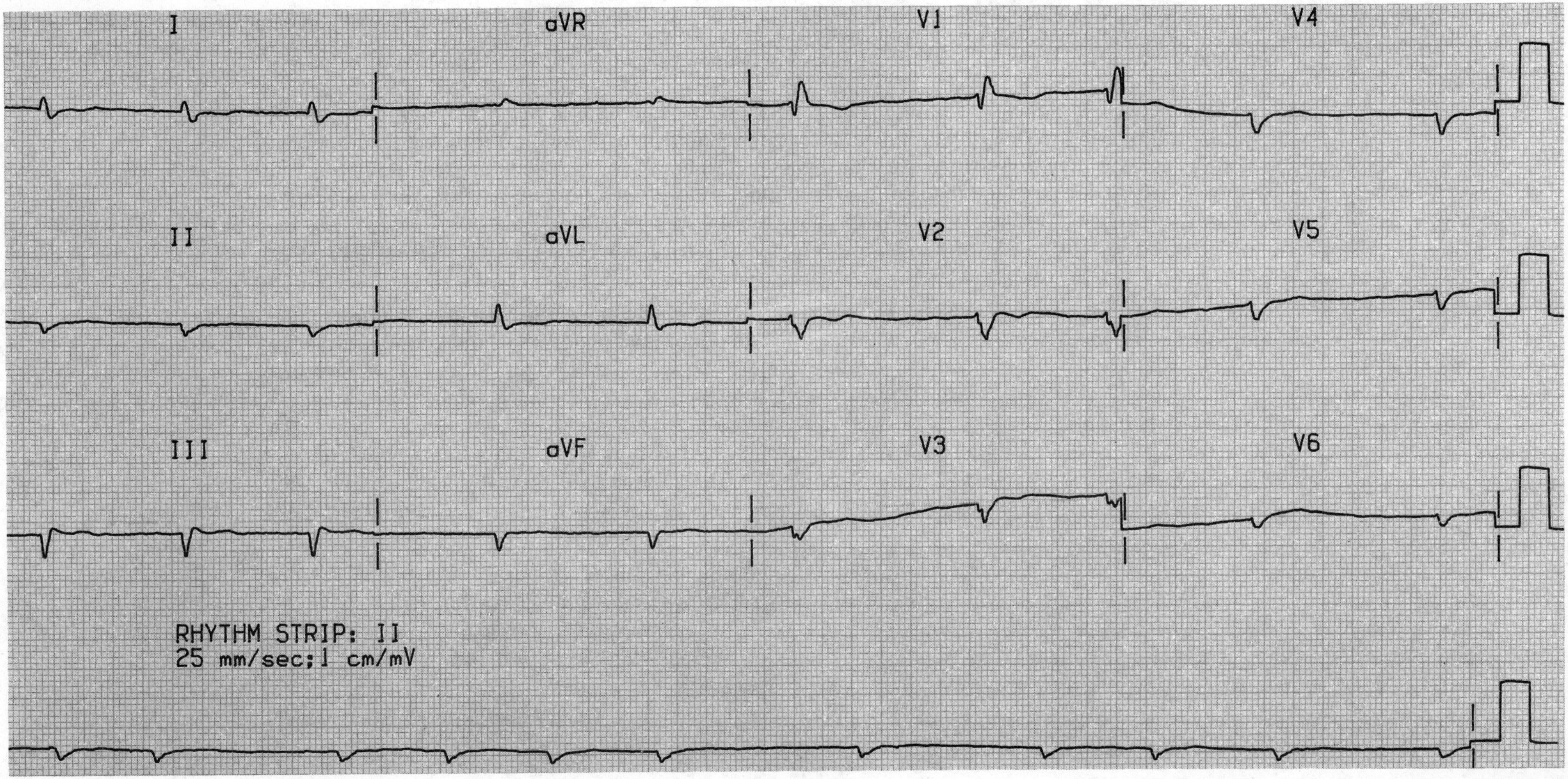

D-24

NARRATIVE INTERPRETATION

Rhythm: **Atrial fibrillation**
Rate: **63 (average)**
Intervals: **PR –, QRS 0.12, QT 0.42**
Axis: **−60 degrees**

Abnormalities

QRS voltage limb leads less than 6 mm. QRS voltage precordial leads less than 10 mm. Axis leftward of −30 degrees. QS waves leads II, III, aVF. Broad QRS and rSR′ pattern with T-wave inversion lead V1.

Synthesis

Atrial fibrillation with a controlled ventricular response. Low voltage limb and precordial leads. Inferior wall MI of indeterminate age. Left axis deviation. RBBB with associated ST-T-wave abnormalities.

TEST ANSWERS: 20, 51, 64, 67, 68, 70, 92, 104.

Comment: Low voltage may be caused by a number of entities including diffuse myocardial disease, pericardial effusion, myxedema, severe obesity, and chronic obstructive coronary disease. This patient had multiple reasons for low voltage including COPD, severe coronary heart disease with prior multiple myocardial infarctions, and a large anterior and posterior pericardial effusion. He had a prior inferior wall MI, which resulted in QS waves in leads II, III, and aVF. The left axis deviation is most likely related to the inferior wall MI. The low voltage and conduction abnormality in this example make it difficult to determine whether or not left anterior fascicular block is present as well.

D-25

Clinical History

An 86-year-old woman in the CCU.

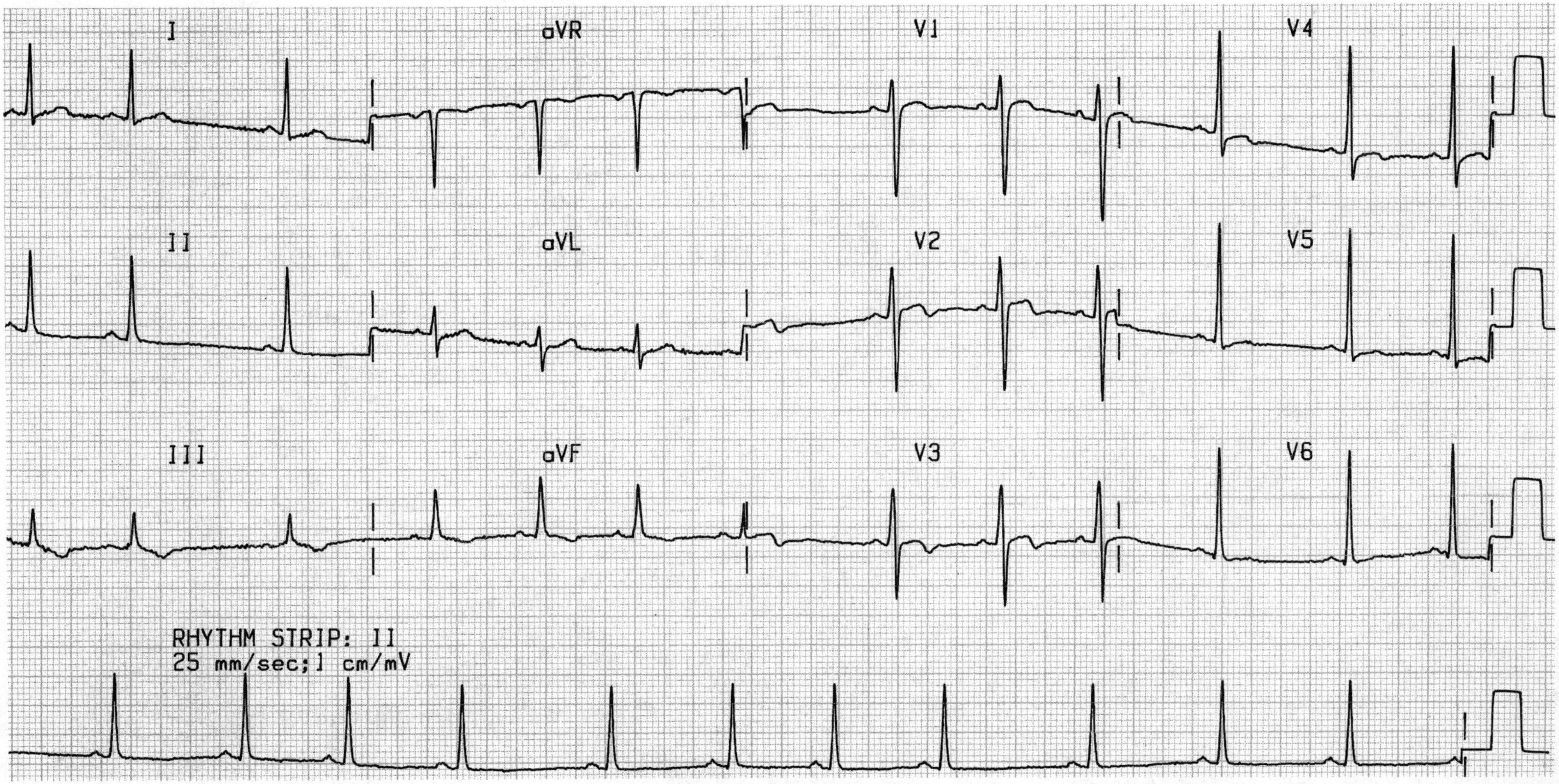

D-25

NARRATIVE INTERPRETATION

Rhythm: **Sinus with SA exit block**
Rate: **68**
Intervals: **PR 0.14, QRS 0.08, QT 0.36**
Axis: **+60 degrees**

Abnormalities

Gradual shortening of PP interval with abrupt lengthening of PP interval on rhythm strip. ST elevation leads V1–V4. Flat T wave leads II, V6. T-wave inversion leads III, aVF, V2–V4.

Synthesis

Sinus rhythm. Sinoatrial exit block. Nonspecific ST-T-wave abnormalities.

TEST ANSWERS: 1, 8, 106.

Comment: This is an interesting tracing in that normal sinus rhythm is seen only in the last three complexes of the rhythm strip. Prior to these complexes there are two sequences of four complexes that demonstrate shortening of the PP interval followed by a slight pause. The likely mechanism of this sequence is second-degree SA exit block, type I.

D-26

Clinical History

A 78-year-old asymptomatic man.

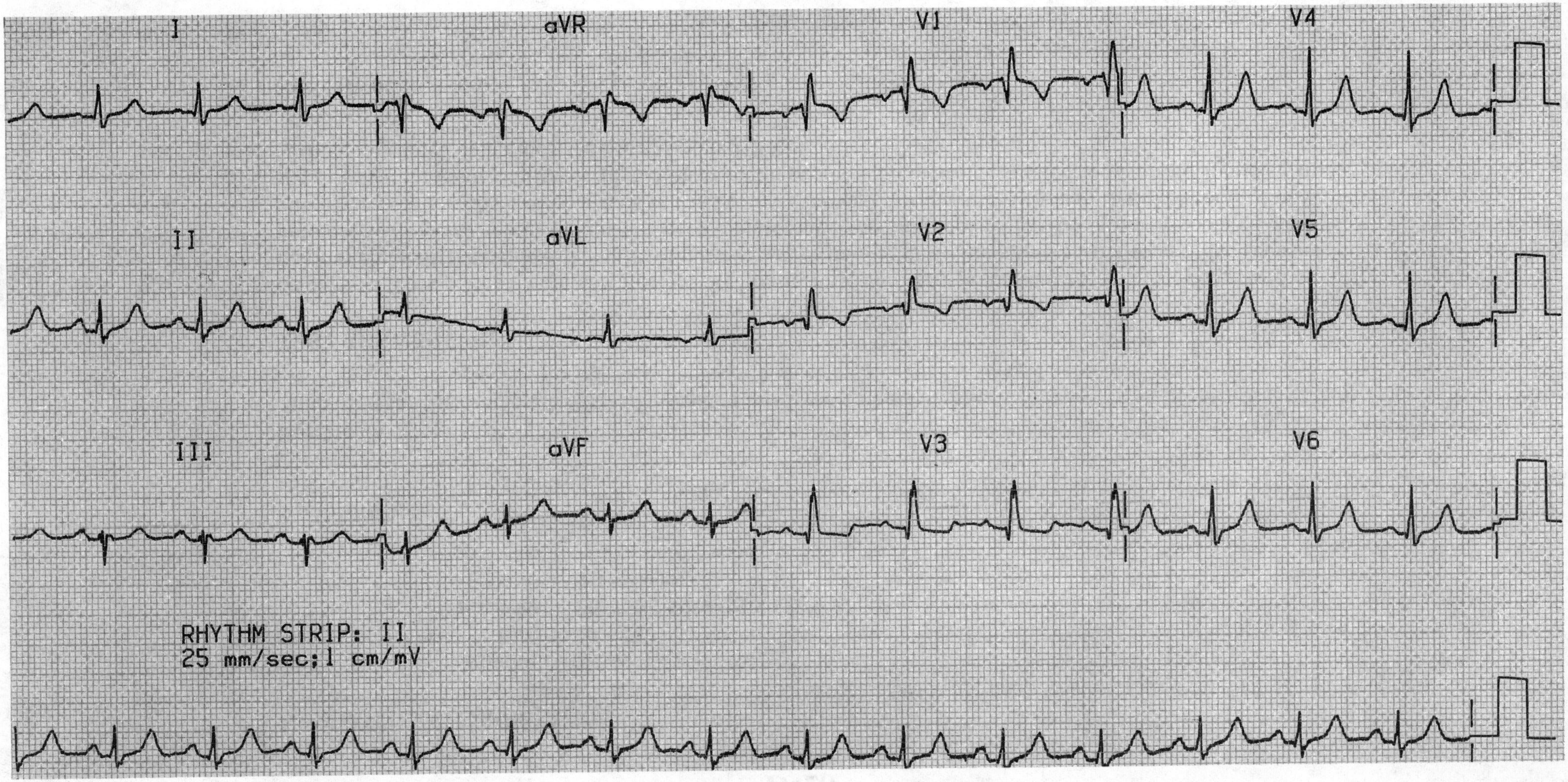

D-26

NARRATIVE INTERPRETATION

Rhythm:	**Sinus**
Rate:	**90**
Intervals:	**PR 0.16, QRS 0.10, QT 0.32**
Axis:	**+15 degrees**

Abnormalities
rSR′ pattern with T-wave inversion leads V1–V2.

Synthesis
Sinus rhythm. Incomplete RBBB. Associated ST-T-wave abnormalities.

TEST ANSWERS: 1, 71, 104.

Comment: This patient demonstrates an rSR′ pattern in the right precordial leads. It is diagnosed as incomplete RBBB because the QRS duration is less than 0.12 s. Incomplete RBBB may be seen in patients with atrial septal defect. In most cases, however, incomplete RBBB is not associated with underlying cardiac disease and does not indicate an adverse prognosis. Although the likelihood of progression to complete RBBB is higher than in the general population, studies indicate no increase in cardiac mortality in persons with incomplete RBBB.

REFERENCE: Liao.

D-27

Clinical History

A 78-year-old woman admitted to the CCU with coronary heart disease and hypertension.

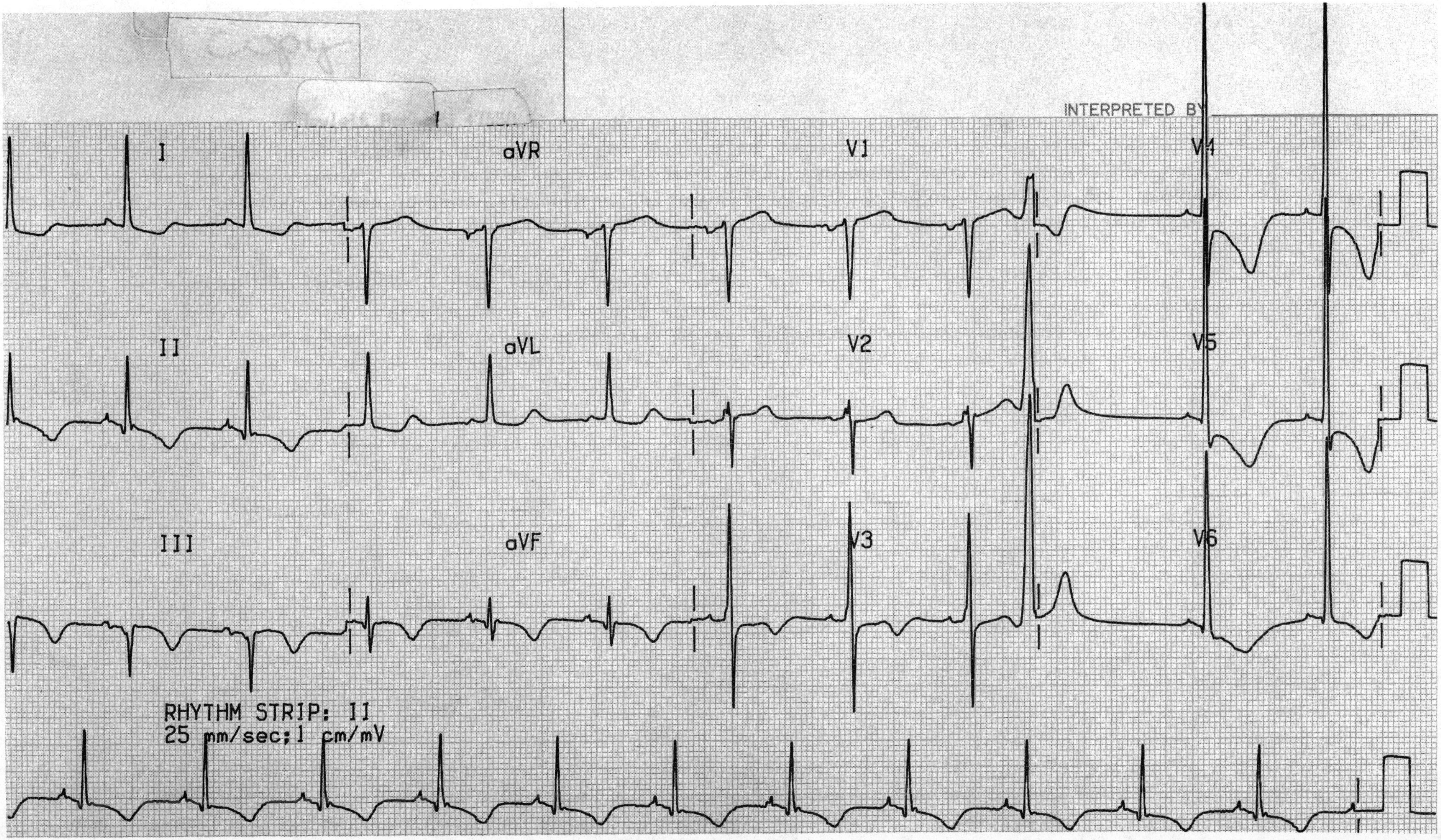

D-27

NARRATIVE INTERPRETATION

Rhythm: **Sinus**
Rate: **68**
Intervals: **PR 0.16, QRS 0.08, QT 0.46**
Axis: **0 degrees**

Abnormalities

VPC. ST depression leads I, II, aVL, V3–V6. T-wave inversion leads II, III, aVF, V3–V6. Abnormal P terminal force lead V1. SV2 + RV5 greater than 35. QS lead III, with small Q waves leads II, aVF. Prolonged QTc.

Synthesis

Sinus rhythm. VPC. LVH. Left atrial abnormality. ST-T-wave abnormalities suggestive of myocardial ischemia. Probable inferior wall MI of indeterminate age. Prolongation of QTc interval.

TEST ANSWERS: 1, 26, 60, 78, (92), 102, 109.

Comment: This patient had marked cardiomegaly and extensive coronary heart disease confirmed at cardiac catheterization. A prior inferior wall MI had occurred, although diagnostic Q waves in the inferior leads are not evident on the present tracing. It should be noted that even small Q waves would not normally be expected in the inferior leads with this relatively leftward axis. The small Q waves in leads II and aVF, accompanied by a QS in lead III, as well as the T-wave abnormalities in these leads suggest an inferior wall MI. An additional finding in this example is QT prolongation, which is frequently associated with coronary heart disease.

REFERENCE: Witham.

D-28

Clinical History

An 87-year-old woman with sepsis.

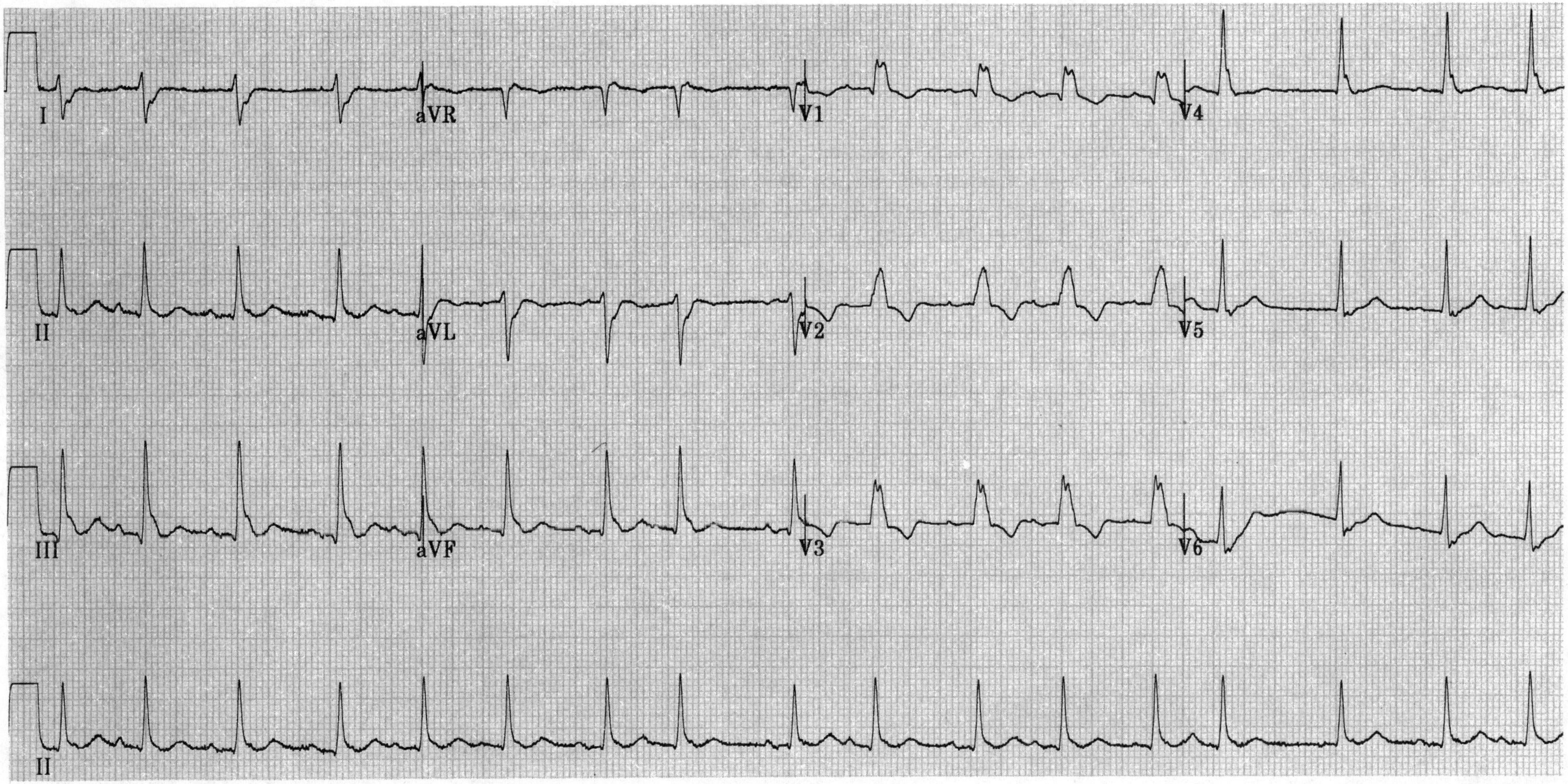

D-28

NARRATIVE INTERPRETATION

Rhythm:	**Multifocal atrial rhythm**
Rate:	**98**
Intervals:	**PR variable, QRS 0.14, QT 0.34**
Axis:	**+105 degrees**

Abnormalities

Irregular rhythm with variable P-wave morphologies. Axis rightward of +100 degrees. Broad QRS with rsR′ pattern and T-wave inversion leads V1–V3.

Synthesis

Multifocal atrial rhythm. RBBB. Associated ST-T-wave changes. Right axis deviation. Left posterior fascicular block.

TEST ANSWERS: 13, 65, 70, 73, 104.

Comment: This electrocardiogram demonstrates a chaotic, or multifocal, atrial rhythm. Note the differing P-wave morphologies and variable PR intervals. By definition, if the heart rate were greater than 100 beats per minute, the rhythm would be classified as multifocal atrial tachycardia. Multifocal atrial rhythm is differentiated from sinus rhythm with frequent APCs by virtue of the fact that there appears to be no clear sinus mechanism. RBBB is evident in the right precordial leads. A marked right axis is also present, which in the absence of RVH is indicative of left posterior fascicular block.

D-29

Clinical History

A 61-year-old woman with severe dyspnea.

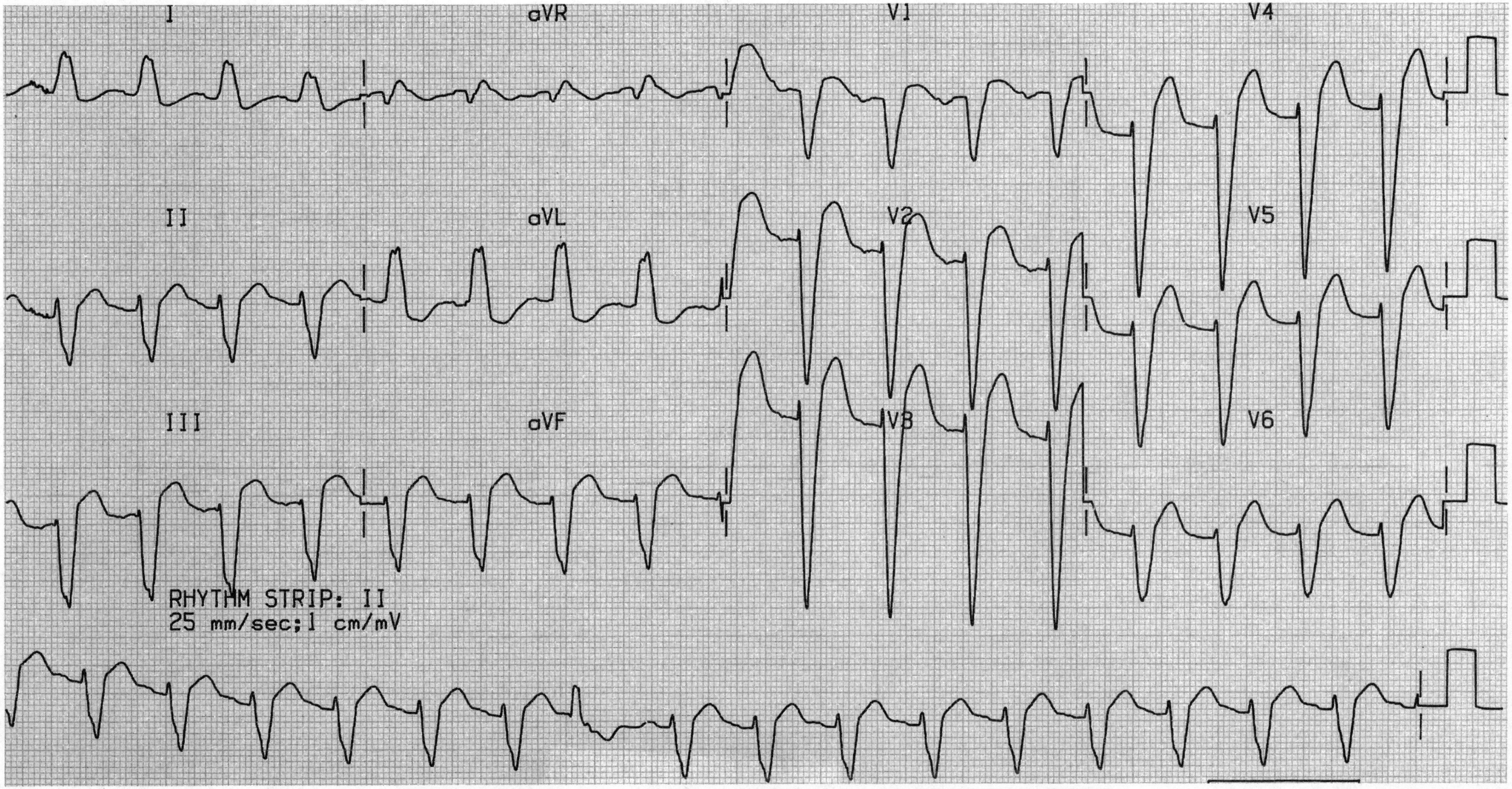

D-29

NARRATIVE INTERPRETATION

Rhythm: **Sinus**
Rate: **100**
Intervals: **PR 0.20, QRS 0.18, QT 0.36**
Axis: **−60 degrees**

Abnormalities

Prolonged QRS with broad, slurred R wave leads I, aVL, with ST depression and T-wave inversion leads I, aVL. Axis leftward of −30 degrees. S wave lead V3 greater than 25 mm. VPC.

Synthesis

Sinus rhythm. VPC. LBBB with associated ST-T-wave abnormalities. Left axis deviation. Probable LVH.

TEST ANSWERS: 1, 26, 64, 74, (78), 104.

Comment: This is an interesting tracing in that LVH would be suspected clinically in this patient with massive cardiomegaly, but this is not readily apparent on the electrocardiogram. One study found that additional criteria for LVH in the presence of LBBB had high specificity (SV3 greater than 25). Because of the difficulty in diagnosing LVH with LBBB, this has been categorized as "probable." Note also in this example that measuring the PR interval was quite difficult. The first beat after the VPC on the rhythm strip was helpful in this regard.

REFERENCE: Kafka.

D-30

Clinical History

A 75-year-old man who is asymptomatic seen on routine examination. His pacemaker has a special programming function.

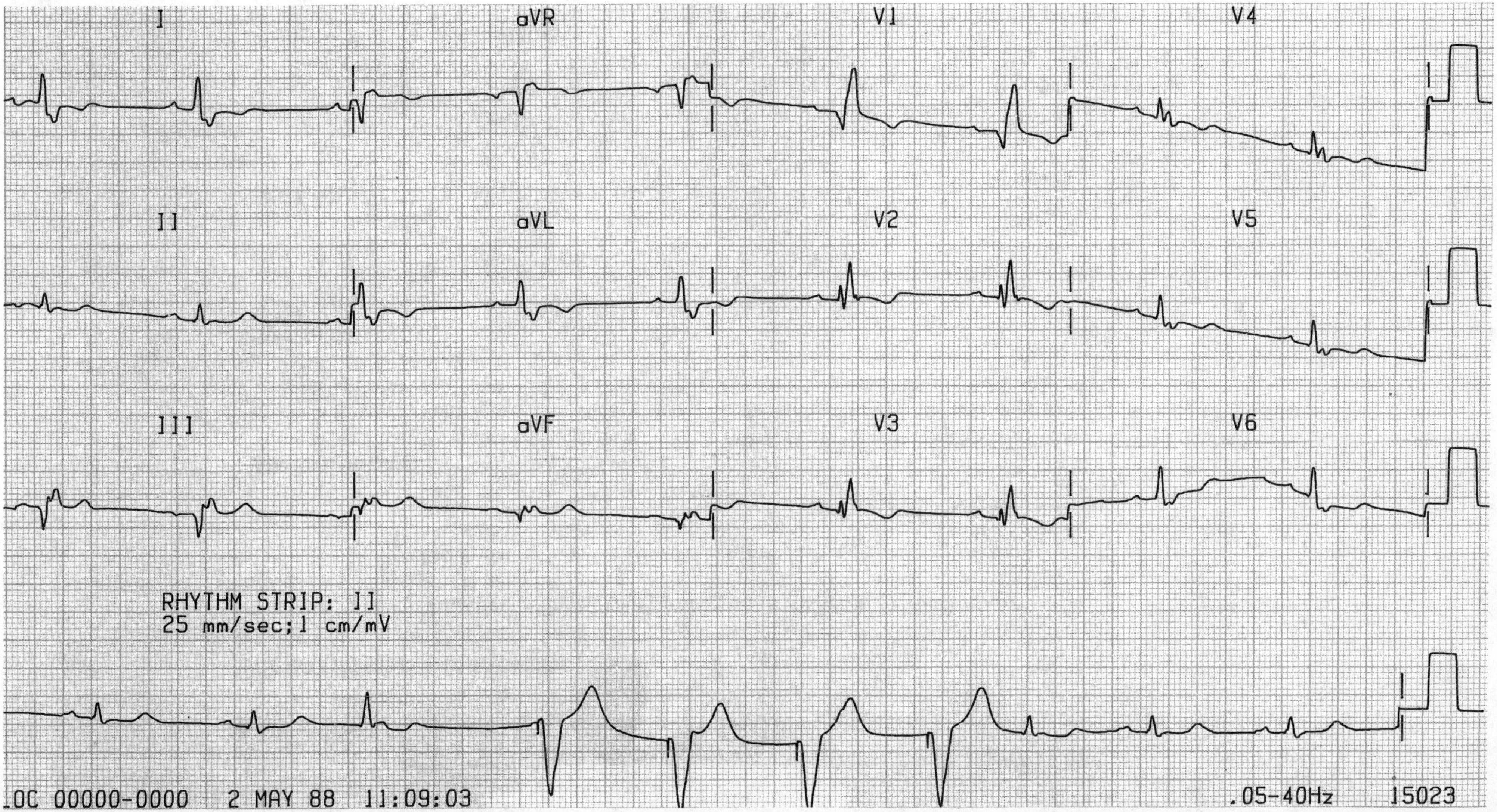

D-30

NARRATIVE INTERPRETATION

Rhythm: **Sinus bradycardia with first-degree AV block**
Rate: **55**
Intervals: **PR 0.21, QRS 0.16, QT 0.42**
Axis: **0 degrees**

Abnormalities

Slow heart rate. Prolonged PR interval. Broad QRS complex with rSR′ pattern V1–V3 with T-wave inversion. VPC. Ventricular pacemaker firing on demand with appropriate capture, escape rate of 50 (escape interval of 1200 ms), and pacing rate of 72 (pacing interval of 833 1/3 ms).

Synthesis

Sinus bradycardia with first-degree AV block. RBBB with associated ST-T-wave changes. VPC. Ventricular pacemaker functioning on demand with appropriate sensing and pacing function. Pacing interval different from escape interval demonstrating hysteresis function.

TEST ANSWERS: 3, 26, 35, 42, 70, 104.

Comment: This is an excellent example of why it is mandatory that one knows the characteristics of a pacemaker before commenting on potential malfunction. If one were unaware of the hysteresis function (escape interval programmed at a longer interval than the pacing interval), it would be appropriate to consider a sensing malfunction of the pacemaker. Instead, this tracing demonstrates normal pacemaker function. When a ventricular premature beat interrupted the sinus mechanism and induced a pause of at least 1200 ms (heart rate of 50), the pacemaker fired at a pacing rate of 72. Hysteresis is used to maintain AV synchrony for as long as possible, while pacing at a higher rate when the pacemaker engages. One should not make a diagnosis of inferior wall MI in this patient despite a deep Q wave in lead III and a small Q wave in lead aVF. A significant Q wave in lead II is mandatory for confirmation of this diagnosis.

REFERENCE: Garson.

D-31

Clinical History

A 73-year-old man with chest discomfort.

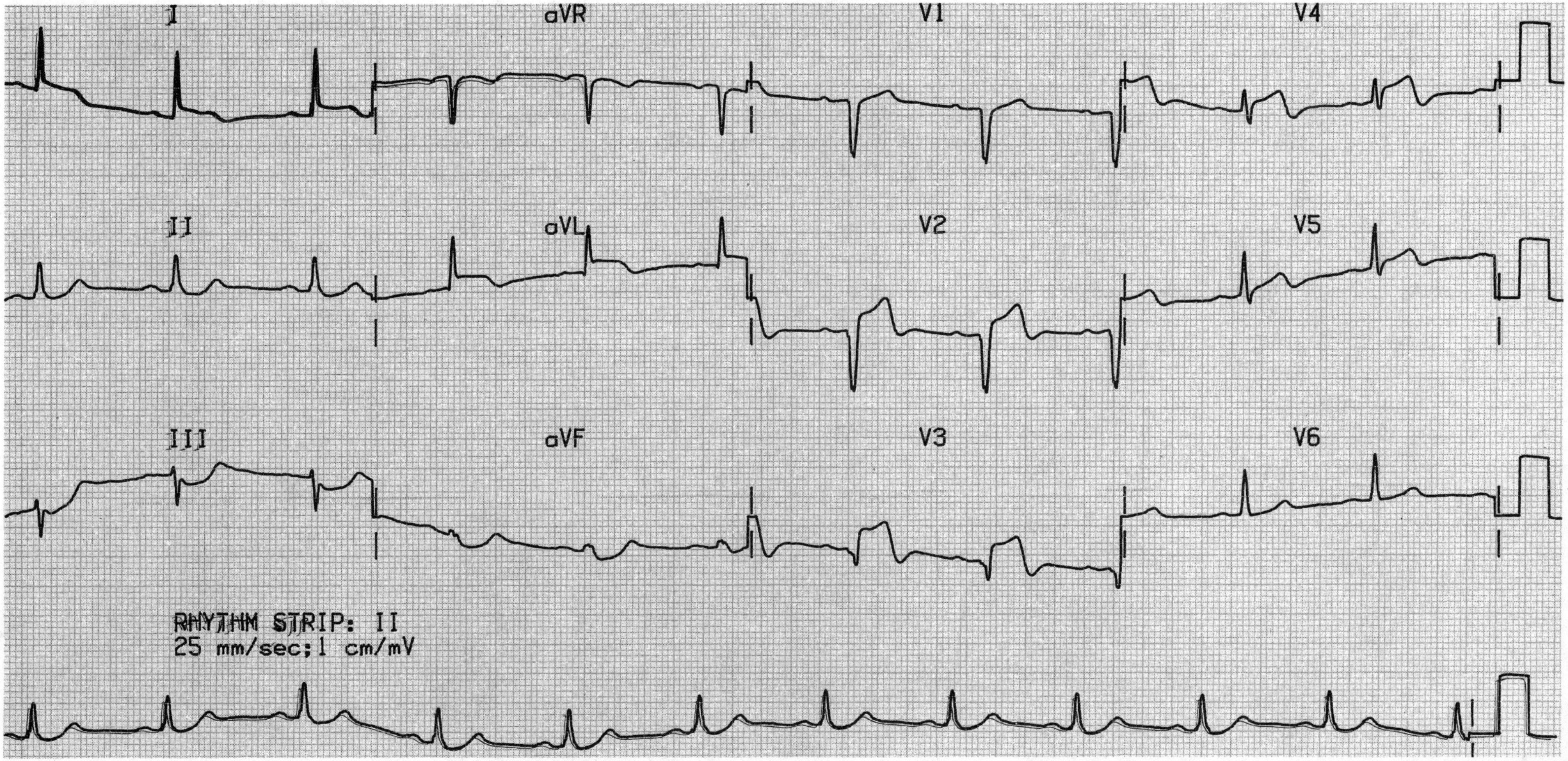

D-31

NARRATIVE INTERPRETATION

Rhythm: **Sinus**
Rate: **68**
Intervals: **PR 0.20, QRS 0.08, QT 0.36**
Axis: **+15 degrees**

Abnormalities

ST elevation leads I, aVL, V2–V5. ST depression leads II, III, aVF. T-wave inversion leads V2–V5. Q waves leads V2–V3.

Synthesis

Sinus rhythm. Anteroseptal and lateral (anterolateral) wall MI, with ST-T-wave abnormalities suggesting acute myocardial injury. ST-T-wave abnormalities in leads II, III, aVF suggesting either reciprocal changes or myocardial ischemia.

TEST ANSWERS: 1, 81, 85, (89), 100, 101.

Comment: This patient sustained a large MI involving the anteroseptal and lateral (anterolateral) segments of the left ventricle. Note the additional ST depression in the inferior leads. The significance of this finding has not been resolved. Some investigators have found that reciprocal ST depression in anterior MI does not reflect additional inferior ischemia and is simply an electrical phenomenon. In contrast, others have determined that this finding reflects more extensive anterior infarction.

REFERENCES: Ferguson. Haraphongse.

D-32

Clinical History

A 71-year-old man with chest discomfort in the CCU.

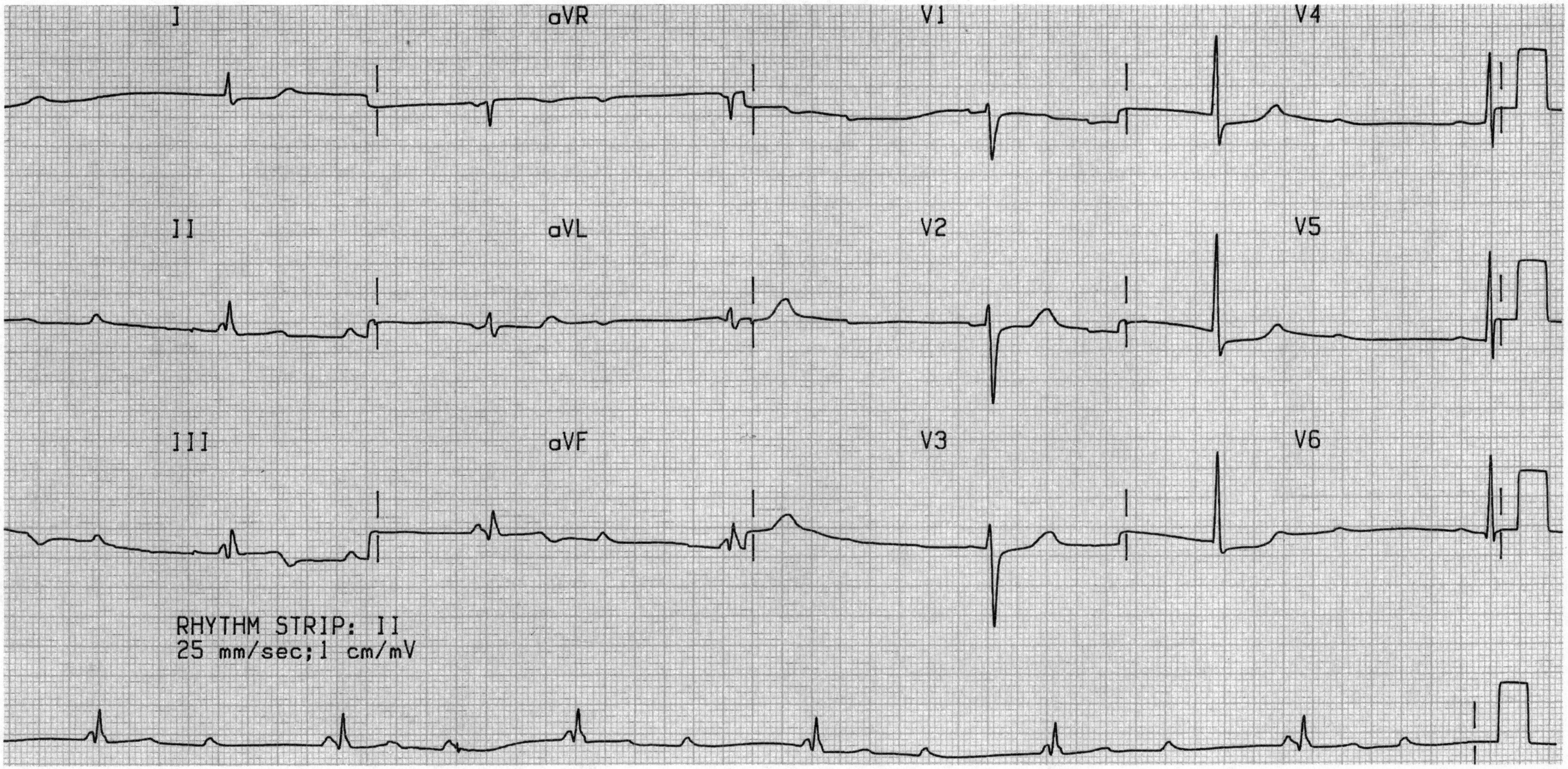

D-32

NARRATIVE INTERPRETATION

Rhythm:	**Sinus rhythm with complete AV block, AV junctional escape rhythm**
Rate:	**Atrial rate 74, junctional rate 36**
Intervals:	**PR –, QRS 0.08, QT 0.48**
Axis:	**+60 degrees**

Abnormalities

P waves fail to conduct to ventricles. ST elevation leads III, aVF. Straight ST segment lead II. ST depression leads I, aVL, V2–V6. T-wave inversion leads III, aVF.

Synthesis

Sinus rhythm with complete AV block. AV dissociation. AV junctional escape rhythm. Inferior wall MI with ST abnormalities suggestive of acute myocardial injury. ST abnormalities in leads I, aVL, V2–V6 consistent with myocardial ischemia or reciprocal changes.

TEST ANSWERS: 1, 22, 47, 53, 91, 100, 101.

Comment: The reader might initially mistake this tracing for sinus rhythm with some form of 2:1 AV block. However, the P waves that appear before half of the QRS complexes are of normal configuration and are too close to be normally conducted. On careful analysis, the "PR intervals" vary and it can then be seen that the sinus rate is approximately twice that of the AV junctional escape rate. This gives the appearance of 2:1 AV conduction, but in fact, there is AV dissociation. Note that this patient has early ST changes of an acute inferior wall MI. Patients with inferior wall infarction may develop transient high-grade heart block as a result of profound vagotonia. In general, temporary pacemaker therapy is required only if the escape rate is so slow that there is hemodynamic compromise.

REFERENCES: Feigl. Berger.

D-33

Clinical History

A 74-year-old woman with palpitations.

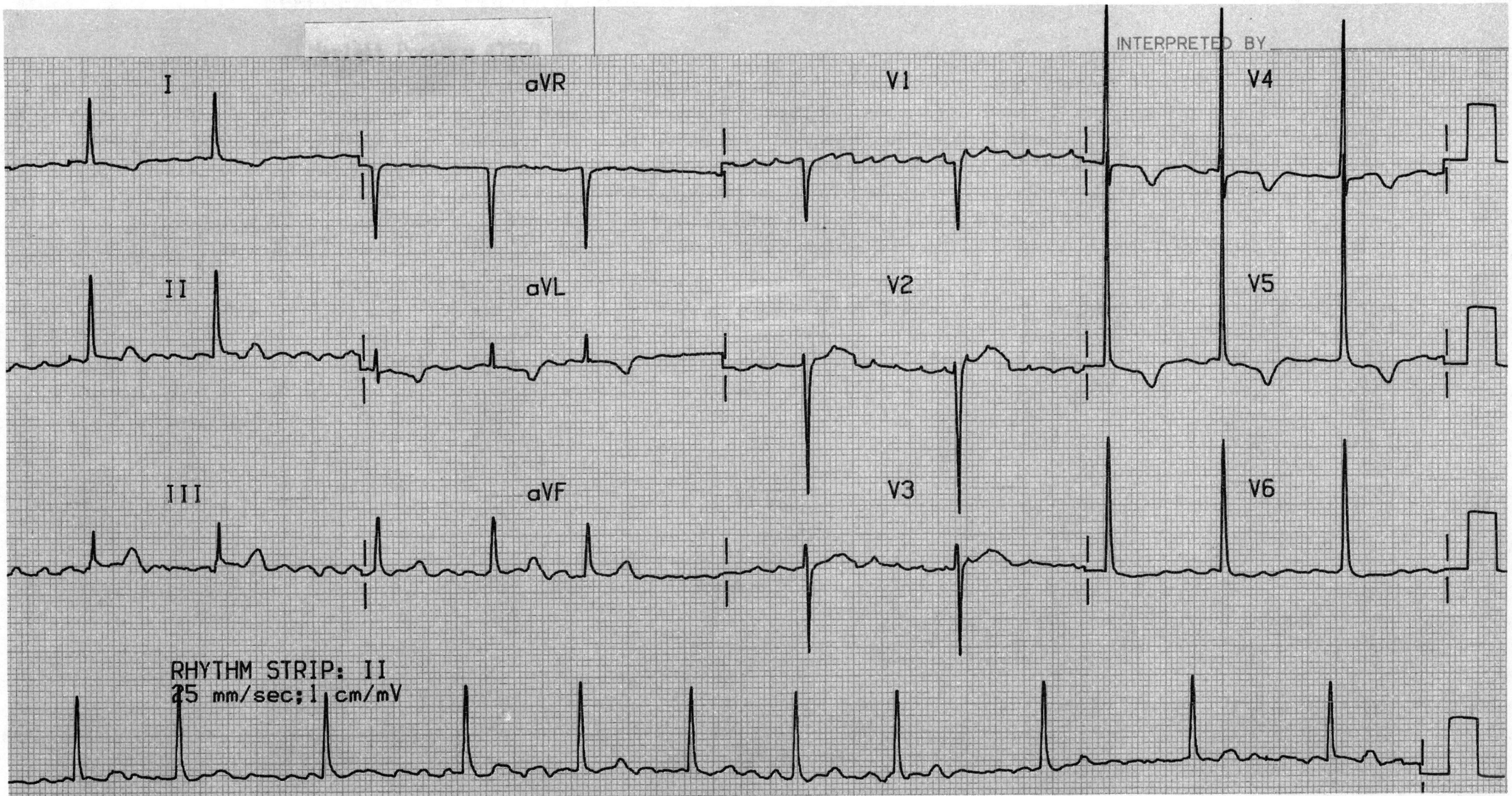

D-33

NARRATIVE INTERPRETATION

Rhythm: **Atrial fibrillation**
Rate: **75 (average)**
Intervals: **PR –, QRS 0.08, QT 0.40**
Axis: **+45 degrees**

Abnormalities

ST depression leads I, V4–V6. T-wave inversion leads I, aVL, V4–V5. Flat T wave lead V6. SV2 + RV5 greater than 35.

Synthesis

Atrial fibrillation with a controlled ventricular response. LVH. Associated ST-T-wave abnormalities.

TEST ANSWERS: 20, 51, 78, 103.

Comment: Atrial fibrillation is an extremely common arrhythmia estimated to occur in 0.4 percent of the adult population. Most patients with atrial fibrillation have organic heart disease. Causes include coronary heart disease, congestive heart failure, hypertensive heart disease, valvular heart disease, and hyperthyroidism. The Framingham study reported that the presence of LVH on the electrocardiogram was strongly associated with the development of atrial fibrillation. Initial therapy is directed at controlling the ventricular rate, usually with digoxin. Additional therapeutic interventions may then be considered, such as anticoagulation and cardioversion via electrical or chemical means (see following two tracings).

REFERENCES: Kannel (1982). Pritchett.

D-34

Clinical History

A 74-year-old woman in the CCU who has been treated with digoxin and quinidine.

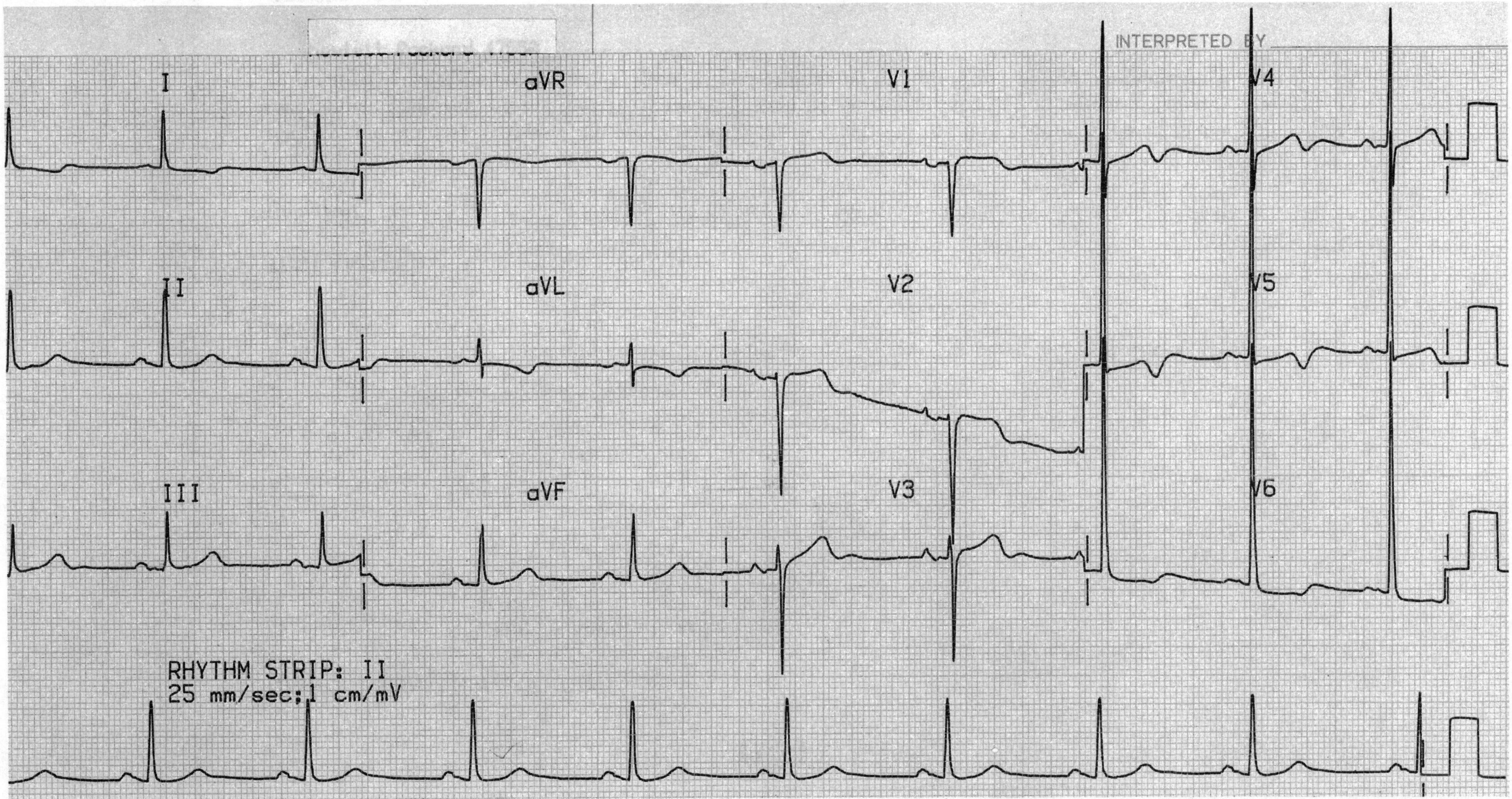

D-34

NARRATIVE INTERPRETATION

Rhythm: **Sinus bradycardia**
Rate: **54**
Intervals: **PR 0.20, QRS 0.08, QT 0.42**
Axis: **+60 degrees**

Abnormalities

Slow heart rate. Abnormal P terminal force lead V1. ST depression leads I, V5–V6. T-wave inversion leads I, aVL, V4–V6. Prominent U waves. SV2 + RV5 greater than 35.

Synthesis

Sinus bradycardia. Left atrial abnormality. LVH by voltage criteria. Associated nonspecific ST-T-wave abnormalities. Prominent U waves.

TEST ANSWERS: 3, 60, 78, 103, (106), 110.

Comment: The patient in the previous tracing has been treated with digoxin and quinidine, with resumption of sinus rhythm. The QT interval is not prolonged; however, U waves have become more prominent, which is probably secondary to the effect of quinidine. This is not reflective of quinidine toxicity. Quinidine is a type I antiarrhythmic agent that acts on the fast sodium channel of the cell membrane. The drug affects the His-Purkinje system by depressing the action potential velocity and automaticity, decreasing conduction velocity, and prolonging the refractory period. Quinidine also has anticholinergic properties (see next tracing).

REFERENCE: Lepeshkin.

D-35

Clinical History

A 74-year-old patient treated with digoxin and quinidine for control of paroxysmal atrial fibrillation.

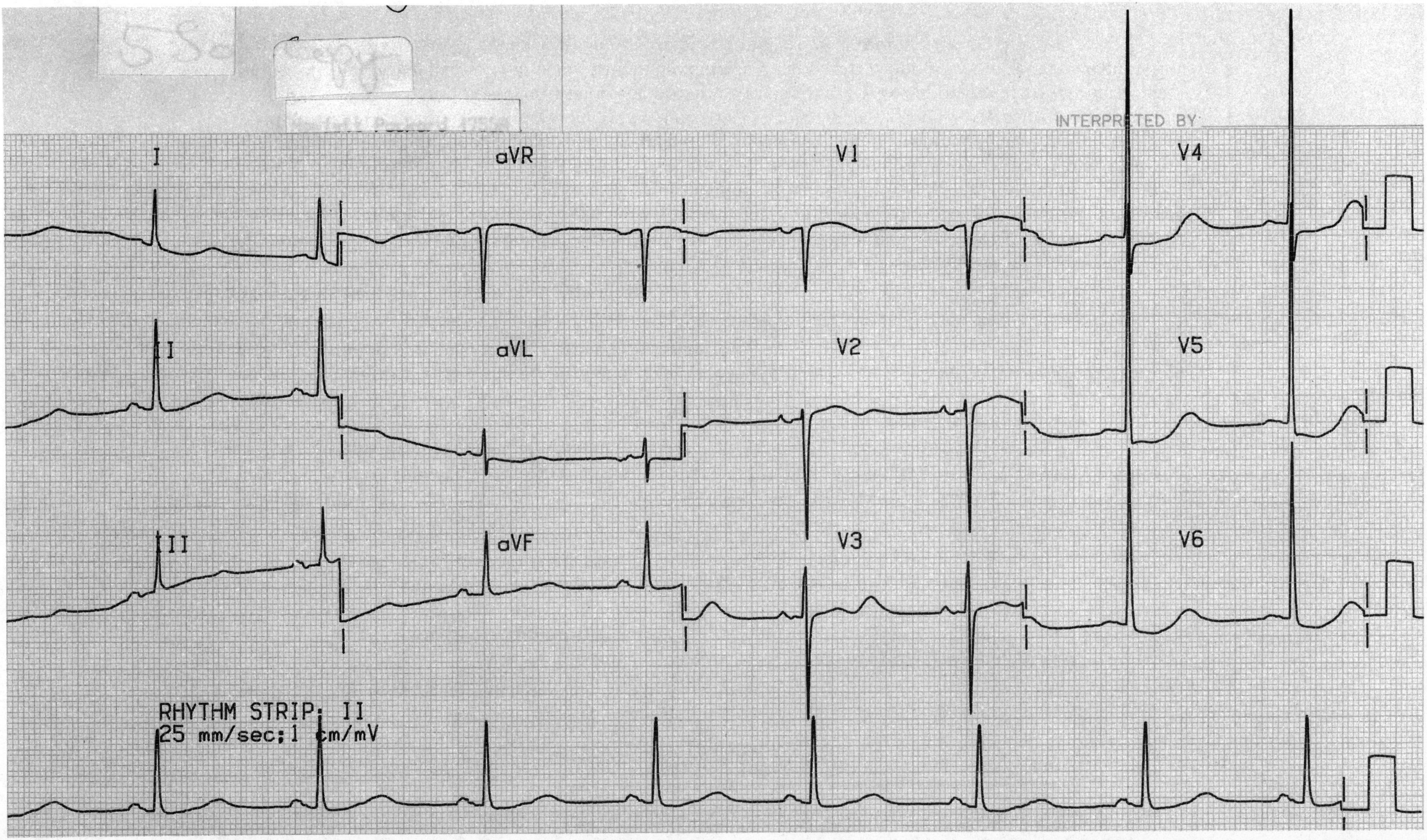

D-35

NARRATIVE INTERPRETATION

Rhythm:	**Sinus bradycardia**
Rate:	**47**
Intervals:	**PR 0.20, QRS 0.08, QT –**
Axis:	**+60 degrees**

Abnormalities

Slow heart rate. Abnormal P terminal force lead V1. ST depression leads I, II, aVL, aVF, V4–V6. SV2 + RV5 greater than 35. QT-QU prolongation.

Synthesis

Sinus bradycardia. Left atrial abnormality. Prolonged QTc (QU) interval. LVH by voltage criteria. Diffuse, associated nonspecific ST-T-wave abnormalities.

TEST ANSWERS: 3, 60, 78, 103, (106), 109.

Comment: This tracing demonstrates many of the electrocardiographic effects of excessive quinidine. Quinidine normally will induce T-wave flattening and slight prolongation of the QT interval. Prominent U waves are also often seen. Marked QT prolongation reflects a toxic effect of quinidine. Additional toxic effects may include widening of the QRS interval, atrial slowing, and AV block. Compared with the previous tracing, the QT interval now appears considerably more prolonged, with more prominent ST depression that reflects quinidine toxicity. The true QT interval is difficult to measure, as it is merged with the U wave. Note, however, that in the previous tracing the T wave appeared distinct, particularly in the left precordial leads. That is not true in the current example. It is important to recognize quinidine-induced QT prolongation because it may predispose to torsades de pointes.

REFERENCES: Friedman pp 331–332. Stratman.

D-36

Clinical History

A 68-year-old asymptomatic man with congestive heart failure.

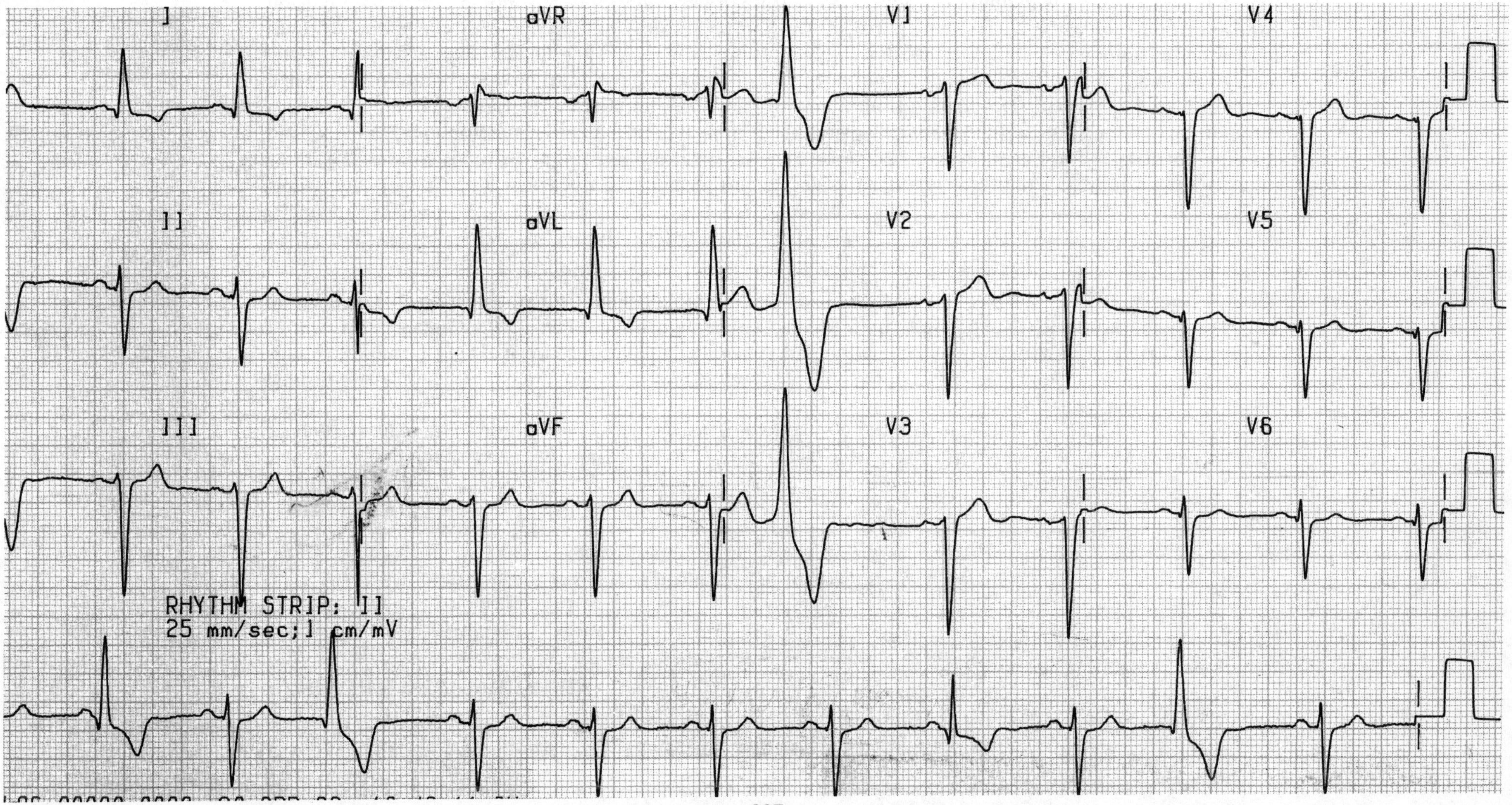

D-36

NARRATIVE INTERPRETATION

Rhythm:	**Sinus**
Rate:	**72**
Intervals:	**PR 0.16, QRS 0.12, QT 0.36**
Axis:	**−45 degrees**

Abnormalities
VPCs. Fusion complexes. Axis leftward of −30 degrees. Prolonged QRS duration. R wave aVL equals 15 mm. T-wave inversion leads I, aVL. R wave leads V1–V3 less than 3 mm.

Synthesis
Sinus rhythm. VPCs. Fusion complexes. Left axis deviation. LVH by voltage criteria. Poor R-wave progression. Nonspecific T-wave abnormalities associated with ventricular hypertrophy or conduction abnormality or both. Intraventricular conduction delay.

TEST ANSWERS: 1, 26, 56, 64, 66, 76, 78, (103), (104), 106.

Comment: This tracing is a good example of fusion beats. Frequent VPCs are present on the rhythm strip. Because of slight variability of the relatively late coupling interval, some of the ventricular complexes have the opportunity to superimpose with the impulse derived from the sinus node. The first and third wide complex beats of the rhythm strip demonstrate a morphology intermediate between the normal sinus configuration and that of the VPCs. Note that the third wide complex beat is the most narrow and similar to the native beat. This is because the ventricular depolarization occurs somewhat later than the previous fusion beat and demonstrates a longer PR interval. Thus, there is a greater opportunity for normal conduction before the ventricular ectopic beat occurs and simultaneously depolarizes the ventricle. The intraventricular conduction delay and poor R-wave progression are most likely secondary to LVH. Left anterior fascicular block should not be diagnosed in the presence of an intraventricular conduction delay of this degree.

REFERENCE: Marriott and Conover pp 190–193.

D-37

Clinical History

A 59-year-old man with dyspnea.

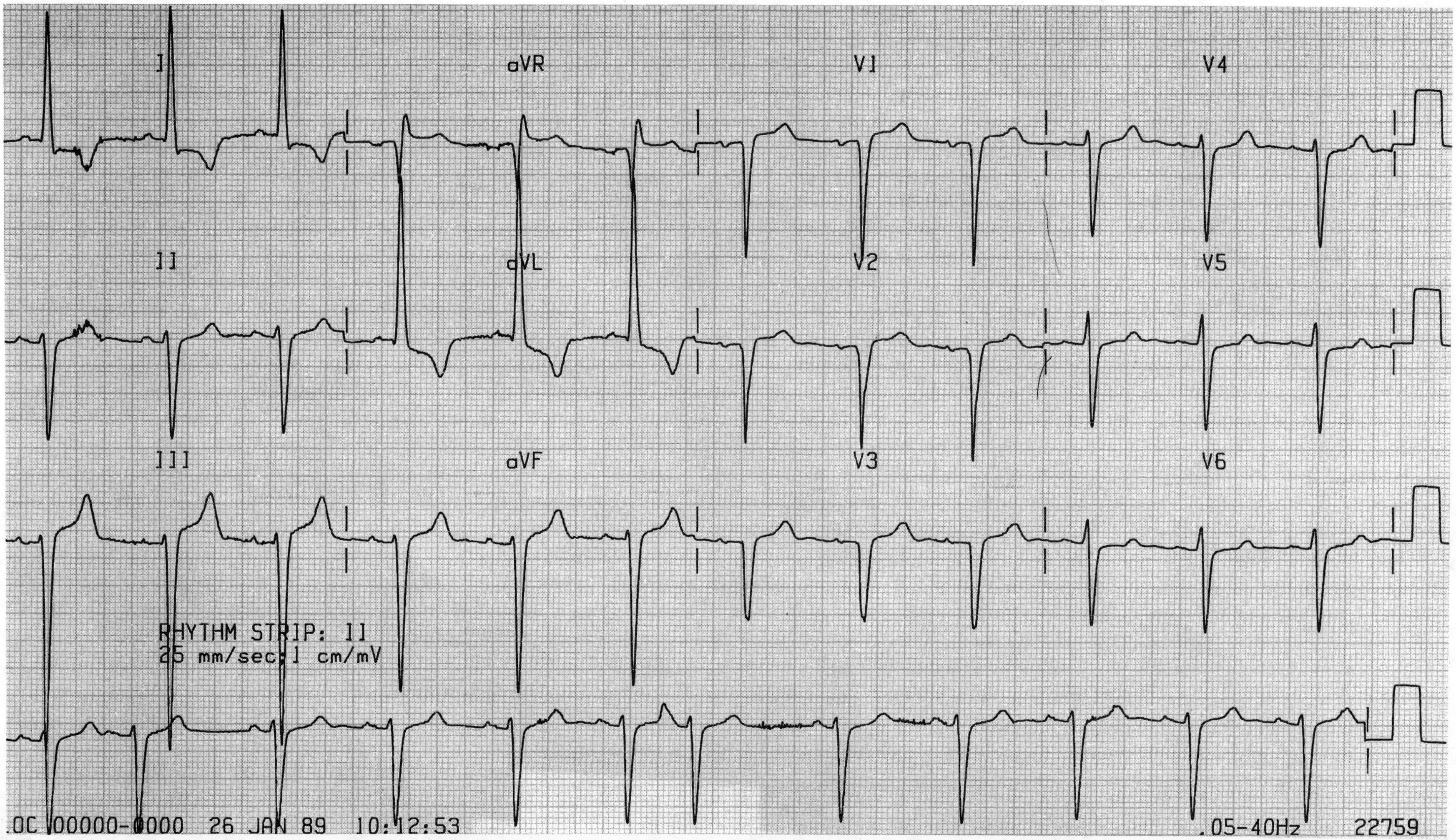

D-37

NARRATIVE INTERPRETATION

Rhythm:	**Sinus**
Rate:	**70**
Intervals:	**PR 0.16, QRS 0.10, QT 0.40**
Axis:	**−45 degrees**

Abnormalities
Axis leftward of −30 degrees. R wave aVL greater than 13. S wave III + precordial voltage greater than 30. ST depression leads I, aVL. T-wave inversion leads I, aVL. QS waves leads V1–V3. APC.

Synthesis
Sinus rhythm. APCs. Left axis deviation. Left anterior fascicular block. LVH by voltage criteria with associated ST-T-wave abnormalities. Possible anteroseptal wall MI of indeterminate duration.

TEST ANSWERS: 1, 10, 64, 72, (82), 103.

Comment: This patient had marked cardiomegaly secondary to a dilated cardiomyopathy. Precordial voltage criteria for LVH are absent because of the loss of R forces in the lateral precordial leads and left axis deviation from the left anterior fascicular block (LAFB). In contrast, limb-lead voltage criteria for LVH are present. The diagnosis of anteroseptal wall MI cannot be made definitively in the presence of LVH, particularly with coexistent LAFB. Both can cause a pseudoinfarction pattern. In general, this diagnosis should not be made unless there is supporting clinical or electrocardiographic evidence. In the author's opinion, when QS waves are present in the right precordial leads in a patient with LVH, it is reasonable to comment on the potential diagnosis of anteroseptal MI so as not to mislead the reader that it is absent.

REFERENCES: Gertsch. Goldberger I. Farnham.

D-38

Clinical History

A 78-year-old woman admitted for elective colon surgery. She has a history of hypertension and congestive heart failure. Medications include digoxin, a diuretic and ACE inhibitor.

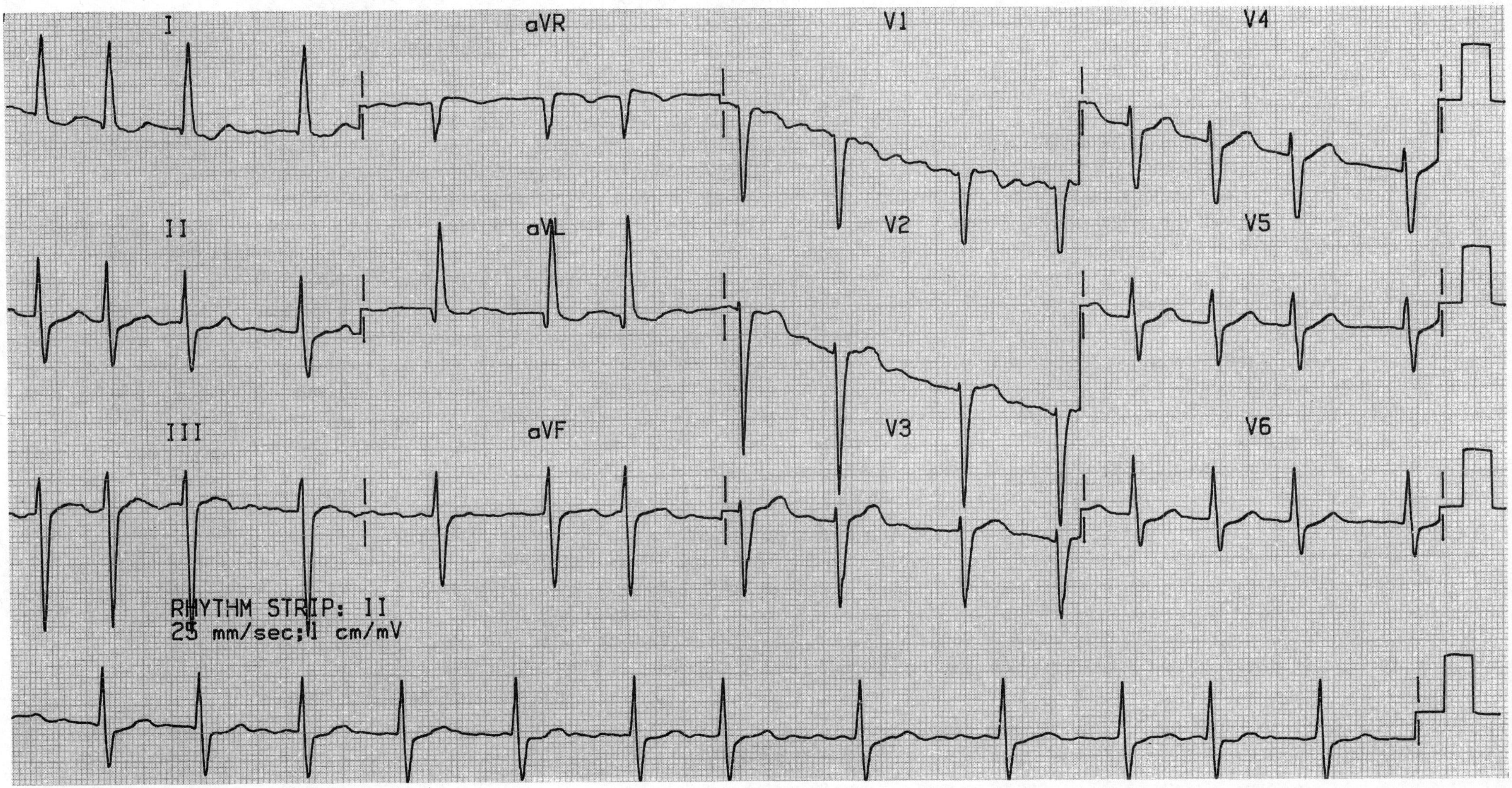

D-38

NARRATIVE INTERPRETATION

Rhythm: **Atrial fibrillation**
Rate: **75 (average)**
Intervals: **PR –, QRS 0.12, QT 0.40**
Axis: **−15 degrees**

Abnormalities
Prolonged QRS duration. R wave aVL greater than 11. R-wave voltage V1–V3 less than 3 mm. ST depression leads I, aVL, V6.

Synthesis
Atrial fibrillation with a controlled ventricular response. LVH. Intraventricular conduction delay. Poor R-wave progression. ST-T-wave abnormalities associated with LVH.

TEST ANSWERS: 20, 51, 66, 76, 78, 103.

Comment: This patient had marked cardiomegaly secondary to long-standing hypertension and mitral insufficiency. The increased limb-lead voltage, intraventricular conduction delay, and poor R-wave progression are all secondary to LVH. Incomplete LBBB cannot be diagnosed because of the persistence of septal Q waves in leads I and aVL. The axis is at the leftward limits of normal but remains slightly positive in lead II and does not demonstrate left axis deviation. Consideration of left anterior fascicular block would not be applicable in the presence of an intraventricular conduction delay. Remember also that atrial fibrillation with a ventricular response of this rate is not truly physiologic and is a result of treatment with digoxin.

D-39

Clinical History

A 55-year-old man with severe chest discomfort.

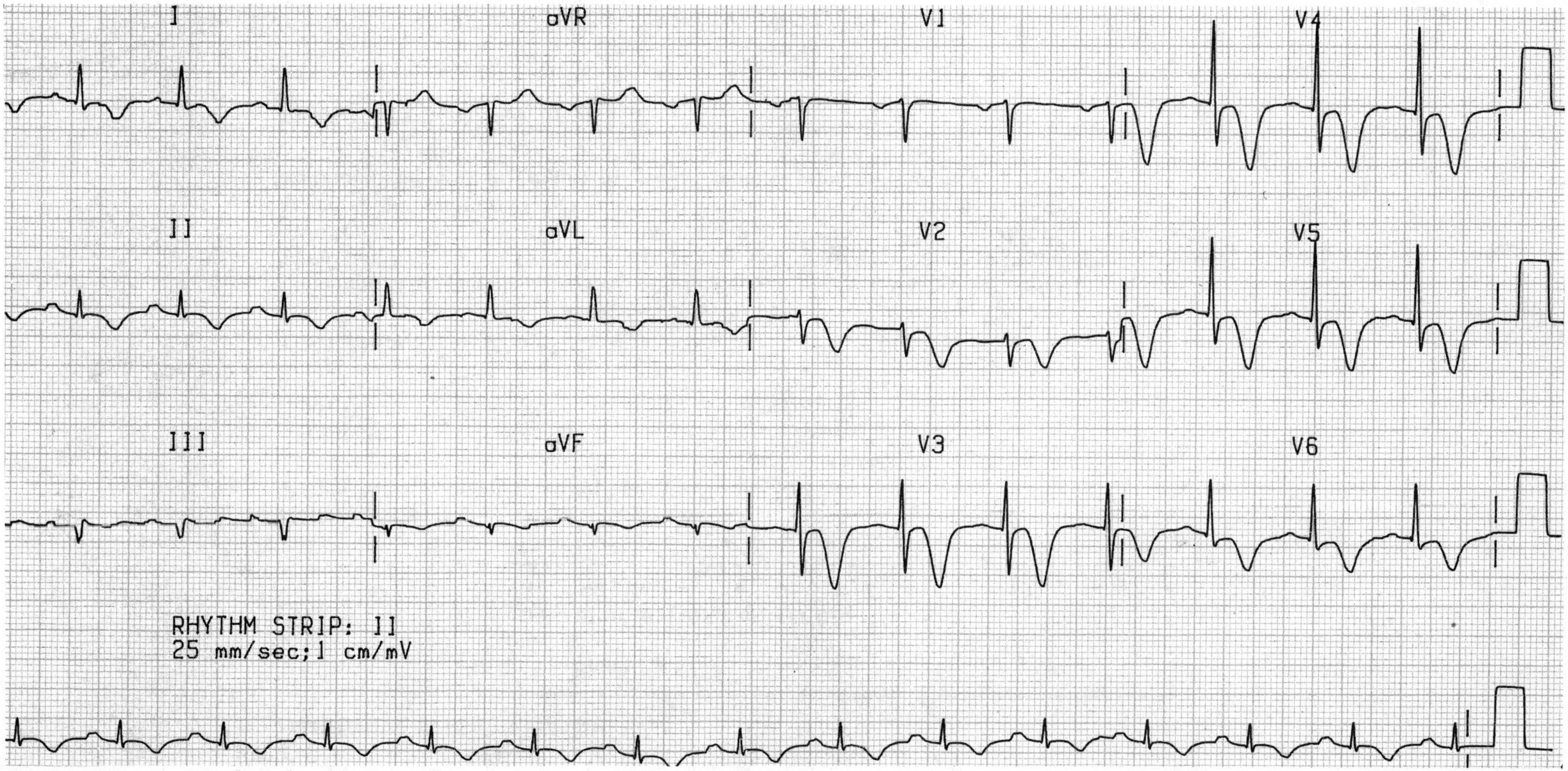

D-39

NARRATIVE INTERPRETATION

Rhythm:	**Sinus**
Rate:	**84**
Intervals:	**PR 0.20, QRS 0.08, QT 0.36**
Axis:	**−15 degrees**

Abnormalities
T-wave inversion leads I, II, III, aVL, aVF, V2–V6.

Synthesis
Sinus rhythm. T-wave inversions suggestive of myocardial ischemia.

TEST ANSWERS: 1, 102.

Comment: This patient presented with profound, diffuse T-wave inversion. This pattern has anatomic significance. In patients with unstable angina, new T-wave inversion in the anterior precordial leads has been found to be predictive of a critical lesion in the proximal left anterior descending coronary artery. In the author's experience, when the T-wave inversion also involves the inferior and lateral leads, the lesion may be more distal and involve ischemia of primarily the apex of the heart.

REFERENCES: Haines. de Zwaan.

D-40

Clinical History

A 45-year-old asymptomatic man.

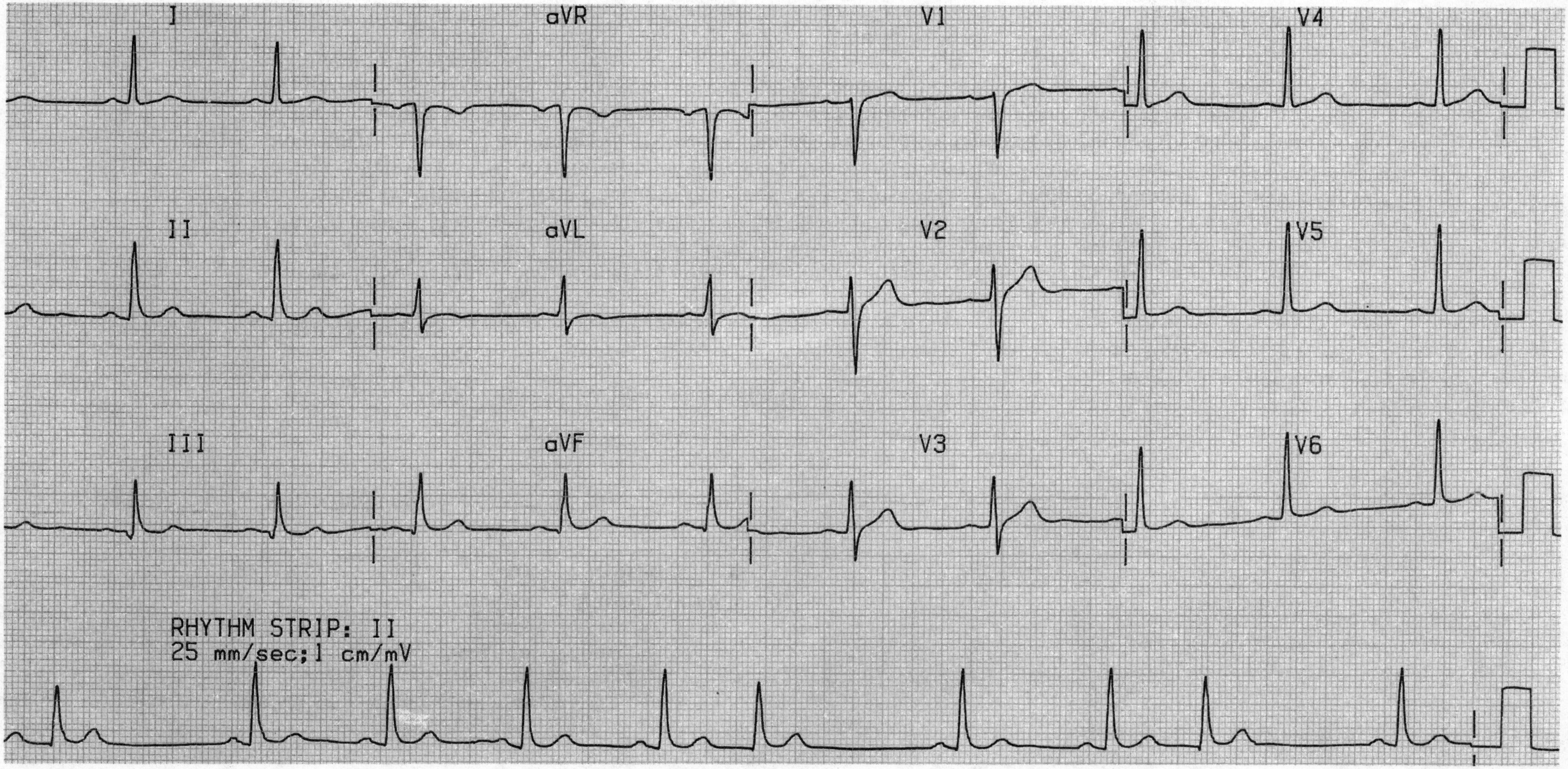

D-40

NARRATIVE INTERPRETATION

Rhythm: **Sinus**
Rate: **65**
Intervals: **PR 0.20, QRS 0.08, QT 0.40**
Axis: **+45 degrees**

Abnormalities

JPCs.

Synthesis

Sinus rhythm. JPCs. Otherwise within normal limits.

TEST ANSWERS: 1, 25.

Comment: Supraventricular premature complexes, either atrial or junctional, are frequently found in normal persons. Both atrial and junctional premature complexes generally have a constant coupling interval related to the previous sinus beat. Unlike ventricular premature complexes, a fully compensatory pause is usually not found because the sinus node is reset via retrograde conduction. In this example, junctional rather than atrial premature complexes are diagnosed because of absent P waves in the premature beats. The retrograde P wave is "buried" in the QRS. On close inspection the ST segment of the premature beats is slightly elevated owing to the influence of the retrograde P wave. Premature atrial or junctional complexes are generally benign but may be the initiators of repetitive supraventricular tachyarrhythmias.

TEST E

E-1

Clinical History

A 77-year-old man with lightheadedness.

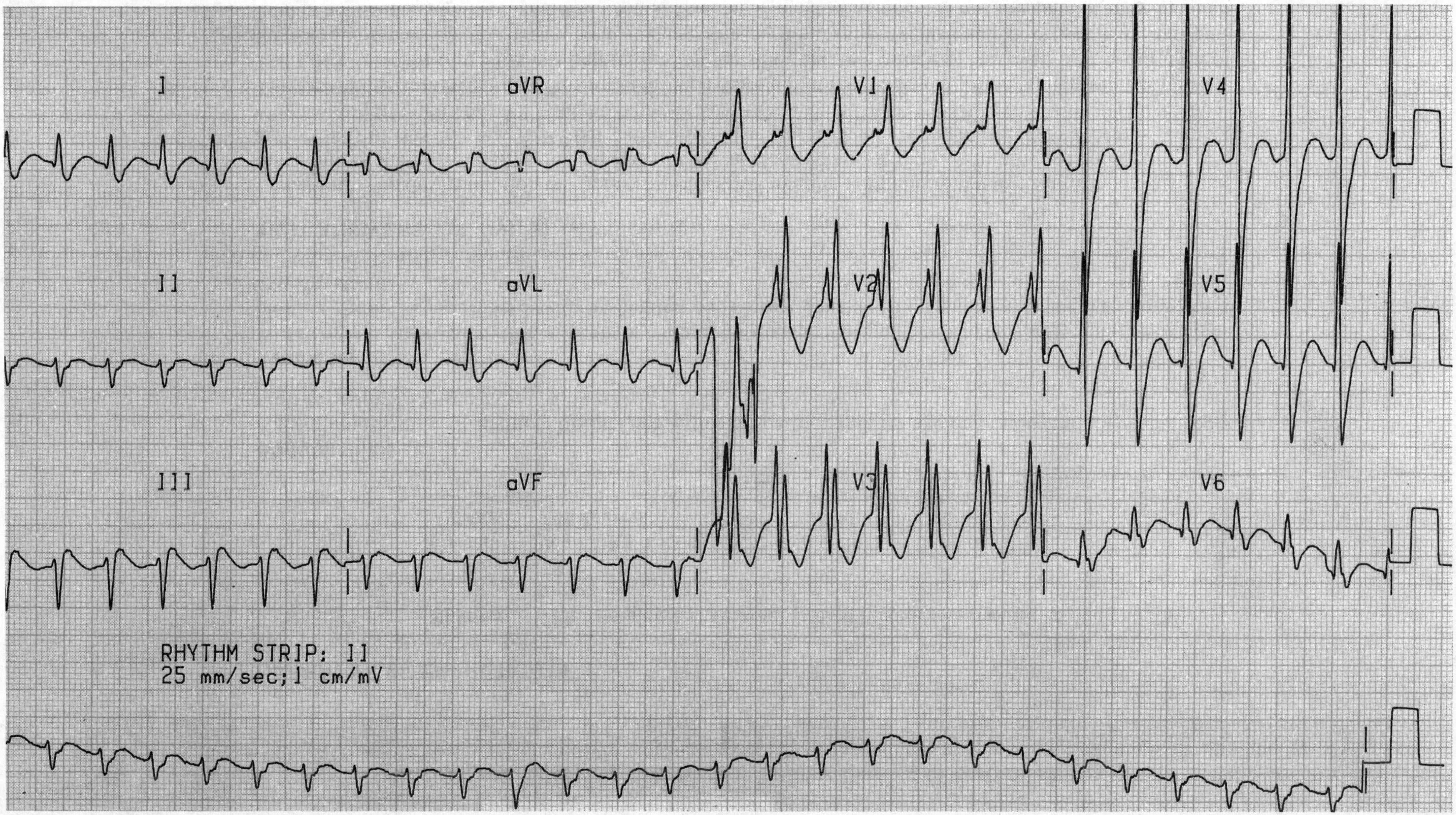

E-1

NARRATIVE INTERPRETATION

Rhythm: **Wide complex tachycardia, probably supraventricular in origin**
Rate: **158**
Intervals: **PR –, QRS 0.13, QT 0.32**
Axis: **−45 degrees**

Abnormalities

Axis leftwards of −30 degrees. Broad QRS with rsR′ pattern and T-wave inversion leads V1–V3. Aberrantly conducted complex on rhythm strip.

Synthesis

Wide complex tachyarrhythmia, probably supraventricular in origin. Single aberrantly conducted complex on rhythm strip. RBBB with associated ST-T-wave changes. Left anterior fascicular block. Left axis deviation.

TEST ANSWERS: 18, (19), 50, 64, 70, 72, 104.

Comment: The differentiation of supraventricular tachycardia with aberrancy and ventricular tachycardia is one of the most challenging aspects of clinical electrocardiography. A number of conflicting clues are present in this tracing. A RBBB pattern is present in lead V1, but it is not classic in this lead for aberrancy (although lead V2 is highly suggestive). In contrast, the left axis favors ventricular ectopy. The rate of 168 somewhat favors ventricular tachycardia, but the finding is neither sensitive nor specific. The QRS duration of 0.13 is not helpful in distinguishing the two entities. The even longer duration of the tenth complex of the rhythm strip suggests the rhythm is supraventricular in origin, with that particular beat more aberrant than the others. It must also be remembered that the patient may have an underlying conduction abnormality that is unaltered by the tachyarrhythmia. This indeed turns out to be the case in this example (see next tracing). If one makes a very careful search in lead aVF, tiny, notched P waves can be seen before and after the QRS, which suggests the rhythm is atrial flutter with 2:1 AV conduction.

REFERENCES: Wellens. Kremers (1988). Stewart. Tchou. Akhtar. Steinman.

E-2

Clinical History

A 77-year-old man with a history of atrial fibrillation and atrial flutter. He is treated with digoxin.

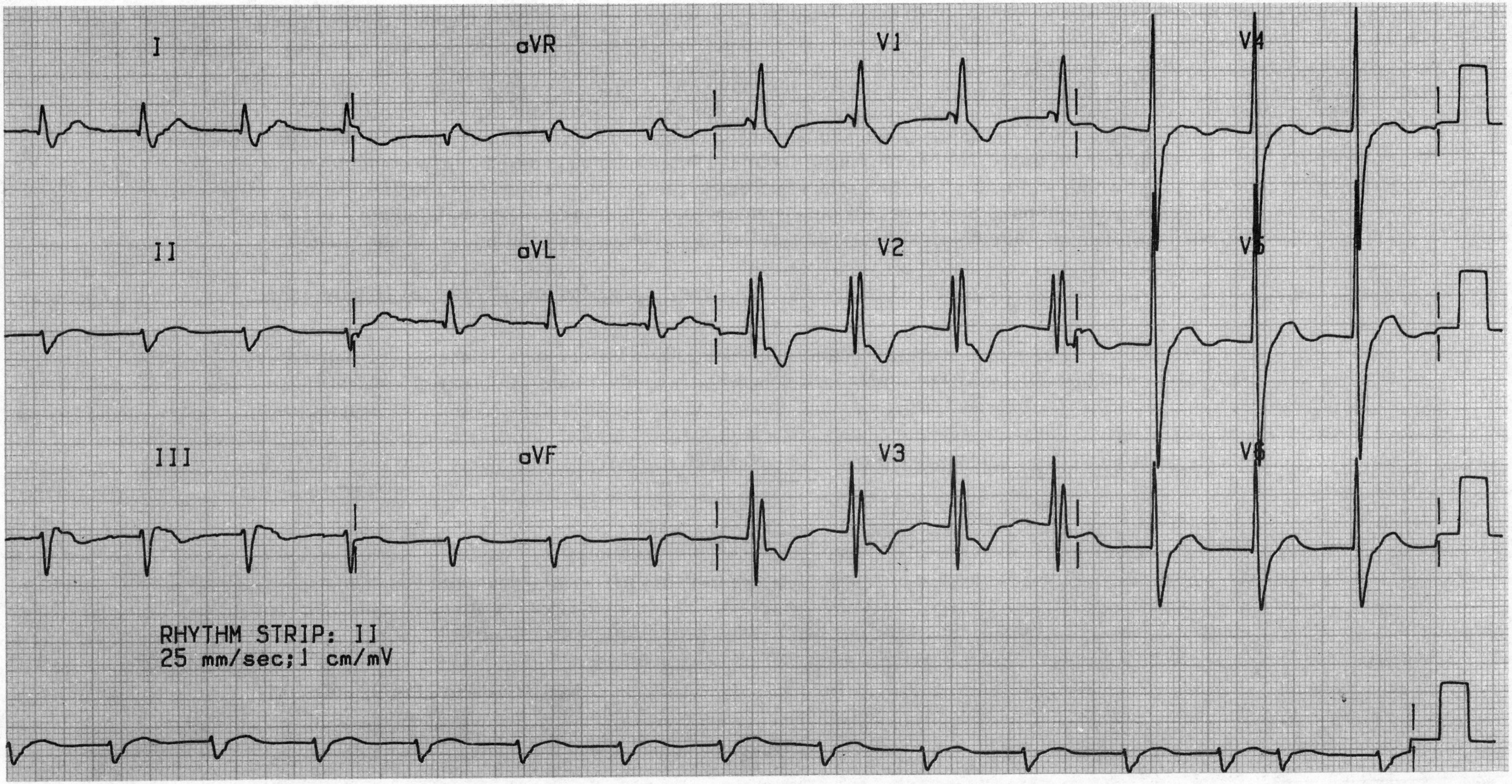

E-2

NARRATIVE INTERPRETATION

Rhythm: **Atrial fibrillation, accelerated AV junctional rhythm**
Rate: **82**
Intervals: **PR –, QRS 0.13, QT 0.38**
Axis: **−45 degrees**

Abnormalities

Axis leftward of −30 degrees. Broad QRS with rsR′ pattern and T-wave inversion leads V1–V3.

Synthesis

Atrial fibrillation. Period of high-grade AV block with accelerated AV junctional rhythm. RBBB with associated ST-T-wave changes. Left anterior fascicular block. Left axis deviation.

TEST ANSWERS: 20, 23, 46, 64, 70, 72, 104.

Comment: When comparing this tracing with the previous electrocardiogram, one can now determine that the wide complex tachyarrhythmia was secondary to an underlying conduction abnormality and not to ventricular tachycardia. The present electrocardiogram also demonstrates the result of too vigorous treatment with digoxin. The underlying rhythm is atrial fibrillation, evident in only the final three complexes of the rhythm strip. The remainder of the tracing demonstrates an accelerated AV junctional rhythm secondary to digitalis toxicity. The degree of AV block is considered high-grade and not complete because there is evidence of intact AV conduction toward the end of the rhythm strip.

REFERENCE: Kastor (1967).

E-3

Clinical History

A 56-year-old man with profound diaphoresis and dyspepsia.

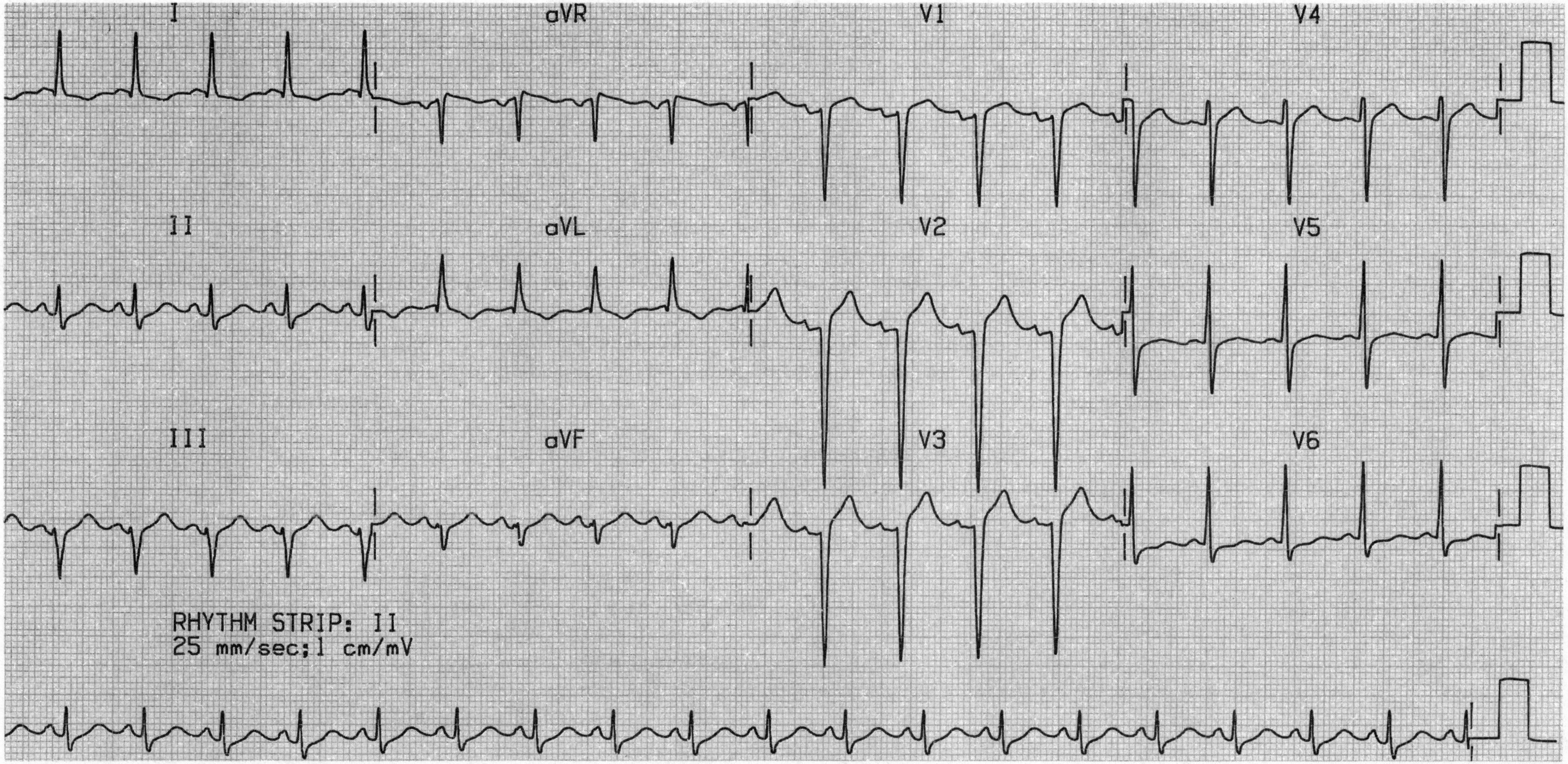

E-3

NARRATIVE INTERPRETATION

Rhythm: **Sinus tachycardia**
Rate: **110**
Intervals: **PR 0.14, QRS 0.08, QT 0.36**
Axis: **−15 degrees**

Abnormalities

Rapid heart rate. ST elevation leads V1–V4. ST depression leads I, aVL, V6. T-wave inversion leads I, aVL. R wave V1–V3 less than 3 mm. SV2 + RV5 greater than 35.

Synthesis

Sinus tachycardia. Nonspecific ST-T-wave abnormalities. Possible ST-T-wave abnormalities of acute myocardial injury V1–V6. Poor R-wave progression. Possible anteroseptal wall MI of indeterminate age.

TEST ANSWERS: 4, 66, 78, (82), (100), (101), (102), (103), 106.

Comment: This tracing illustrates the need in many cases for serial tracings to accurately make an electrocardiographic diagnosis. The ST-T-wave abnormalities in the precordial leads are nonspecific but could be representative of early acute myocardial injury. Until a more precise electrocardiographic diagnosis can be made, it is acceptable to categorize the ST-T-wave changes as nonspecific while mentioning the potential for a more ominous condition. Using the algorithm proposed by Zema, the poor R-wave progression is suggestive of an anteroseptal wall MI. Diagnostic Q waves, however, are not present. Poor R-wave progression may also be secondary to LVH. A number of hours after admission, the diagnosis for this patient became clear (see next tracing).

REFERENCES: Zema (1982). James.

E-4

Clinical History

A 56-year-old man admitted to the CCU.

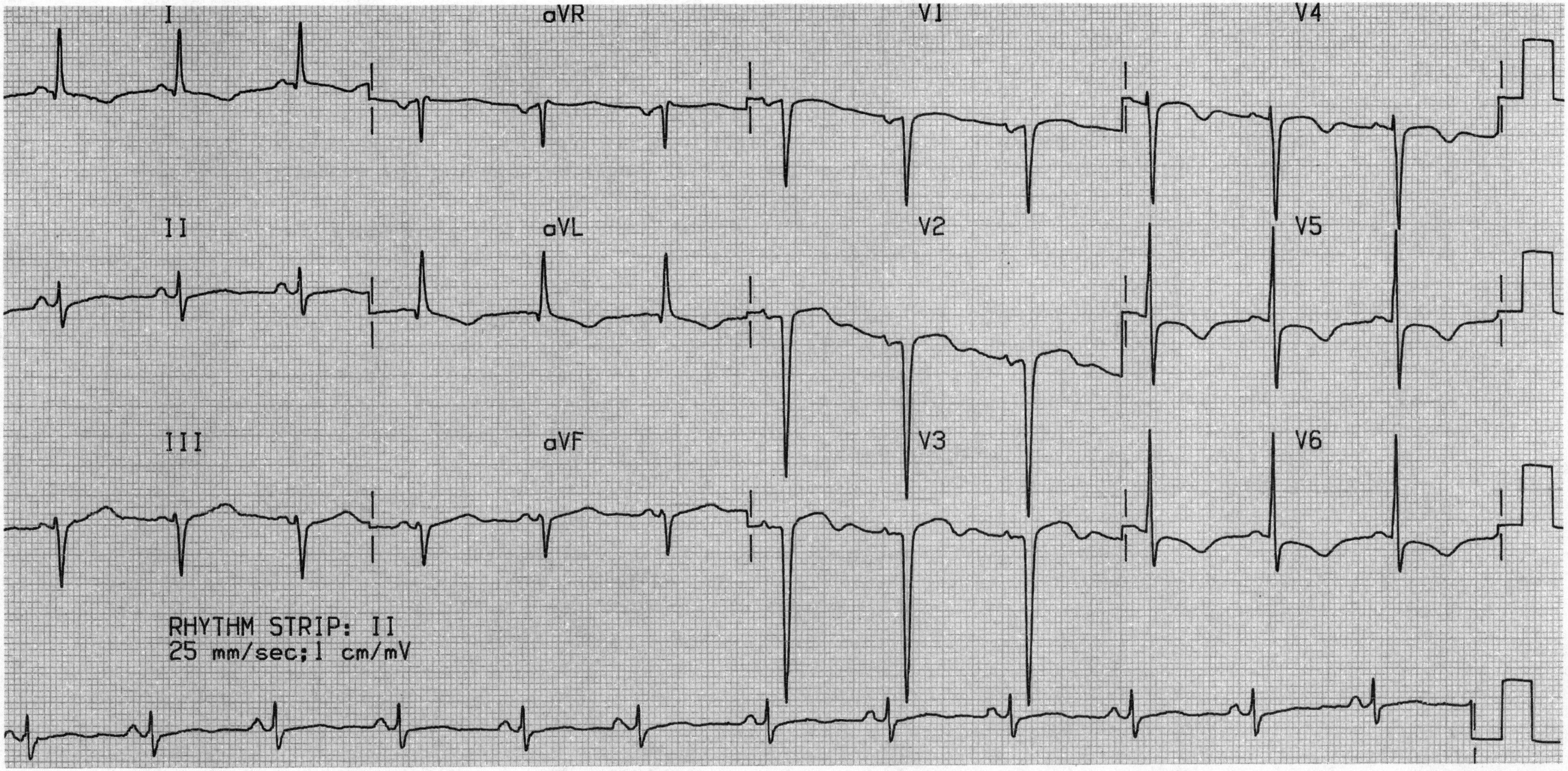

E-4

NARRATIVE INTERPRETATION

Rhythm:	**Sinus**
Rate:	**72**
Intervals:	**PR 0.16, QRS 0.08, QT 0.46**
Axis:	**−30 degrees**

Abnormalities
ST elevation leads V1–V4. ST depression leads I, aVL, V5–V6. T-wave inversion leads I, aVL, V3–V6. QS waves leads V1–V3. Loss of R wave V4. QT prolongation for heart rate. SV2 + RV5 greater than 35.

Synthesis
Sinus rhythm. Anterior (anteroseptal) wall MI with ST-T-wave abnormalities of recent myocardial injury. ST-T-wave abnormalities in leads I, aVL, V5–V6, suggestive of myocardial ischemia. Prolongation of QTc interval. LVH.

TEST ANSWERS: 1, 78, (81), 83, 100, 101, 109.

Comment: This represents the follow-up to the previous tracing. The reason for the nonspecific ST-T-wave abnormalities is now clear. The infarction may be considered anterior because of ST abnormalities and a loss of the R wave in lead V4. The septum is also most likely involved in view of the ST findings and tiny R wave in lead V1. Additional leads with ST-T-wave abnormalities suggest ischemia without Q-wave infarction in that area of the myocardium. The QT interval is also now prolonged, a frequent finding in myocardial ischemia. The actual QT interval is a bit difficult to determine because of superimposition of the U wave. Even so, the QT interval is most likely prolonged.

REFERENCES: Chou p 178. Schweitzer (1992). Simonson.

E-5

Clinical History

A 66-year-old woman seen in routine follow-up for chronic dyspnea.

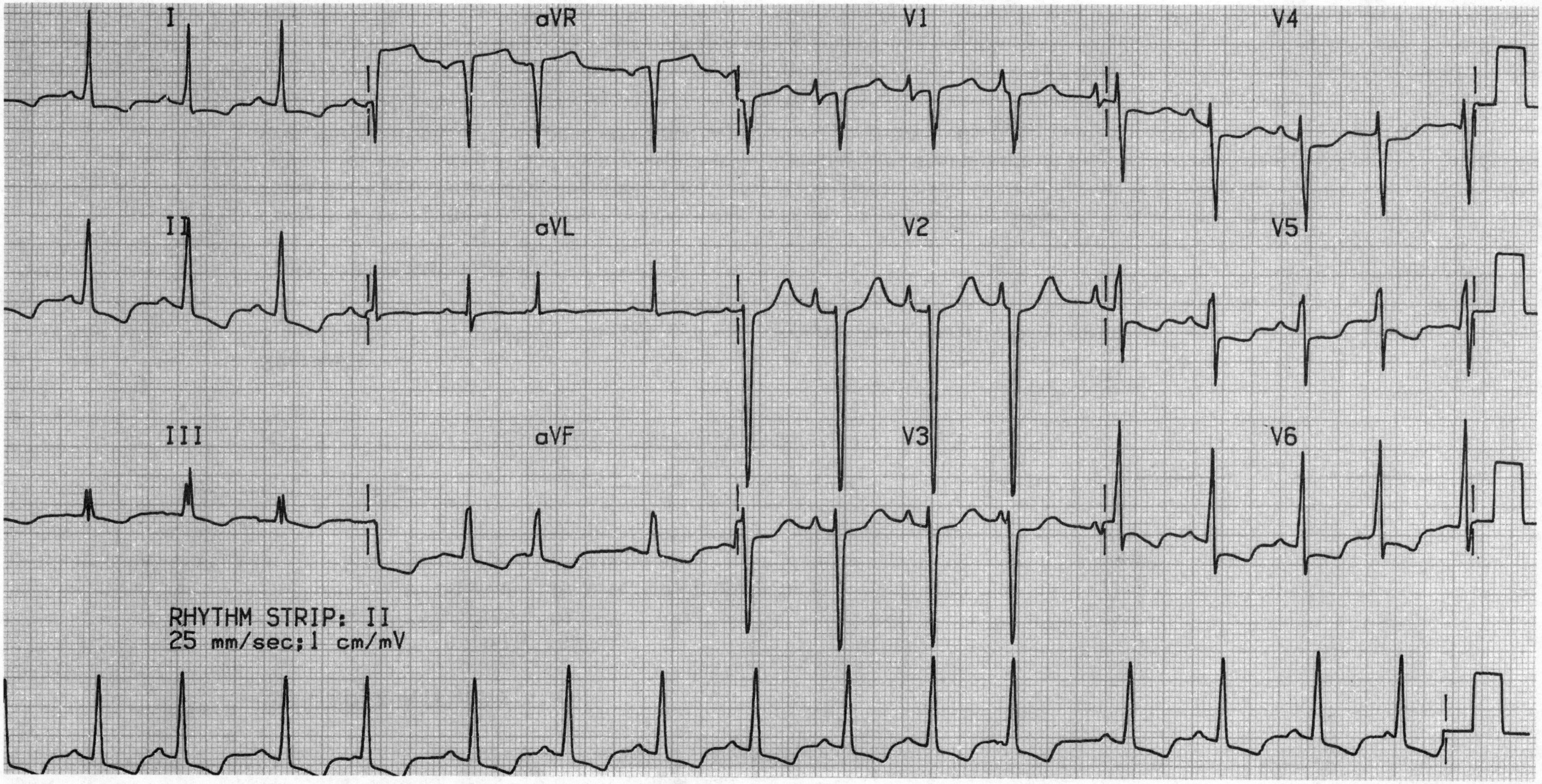

E-5

NARRATIVE INTERPRETATION

Rhythm:	**Sinus**
Rate:	**92**
Intervals:	**PR 0.16, QRS 0.08, QT 0.36**
Axis:	**+40 degrees**

Abnormalities

JPCs. Diphasic P wave with tall initial component and abnormal P terminal force lead V1. ST depression leads I, II, III, aVF, V4–V6. T-wave inversion leads I, II, III, aVF, V5–V6. SV2 + RV5 greater than 35.

Synthesis

Sinus rhythm. JPCs. LVH. Associated ST-T-wave abnormalities. Biatrial enlargement.

TEST ANSWERS: 1, 25, 61, 78, 103.

Comment: This patient had four-chamber dilatation on the basis of an idiopathic cardiomyopathy. LVH is evident without electrocardiographic criteria for RVH. Because left ventricular forces predominate, criteria for combined left and right ventricular hypertrophy are often absent on the electrocardiogram even in the presence of anatomic combined ventricular hypertrophy. Both left and right atrial enlargement is present as seen in lead V1.

E-6

Clinical History

A 61-year-old woman with a history of mitral valve replacement and atrial fibrillation. She is prescribed digoxin.

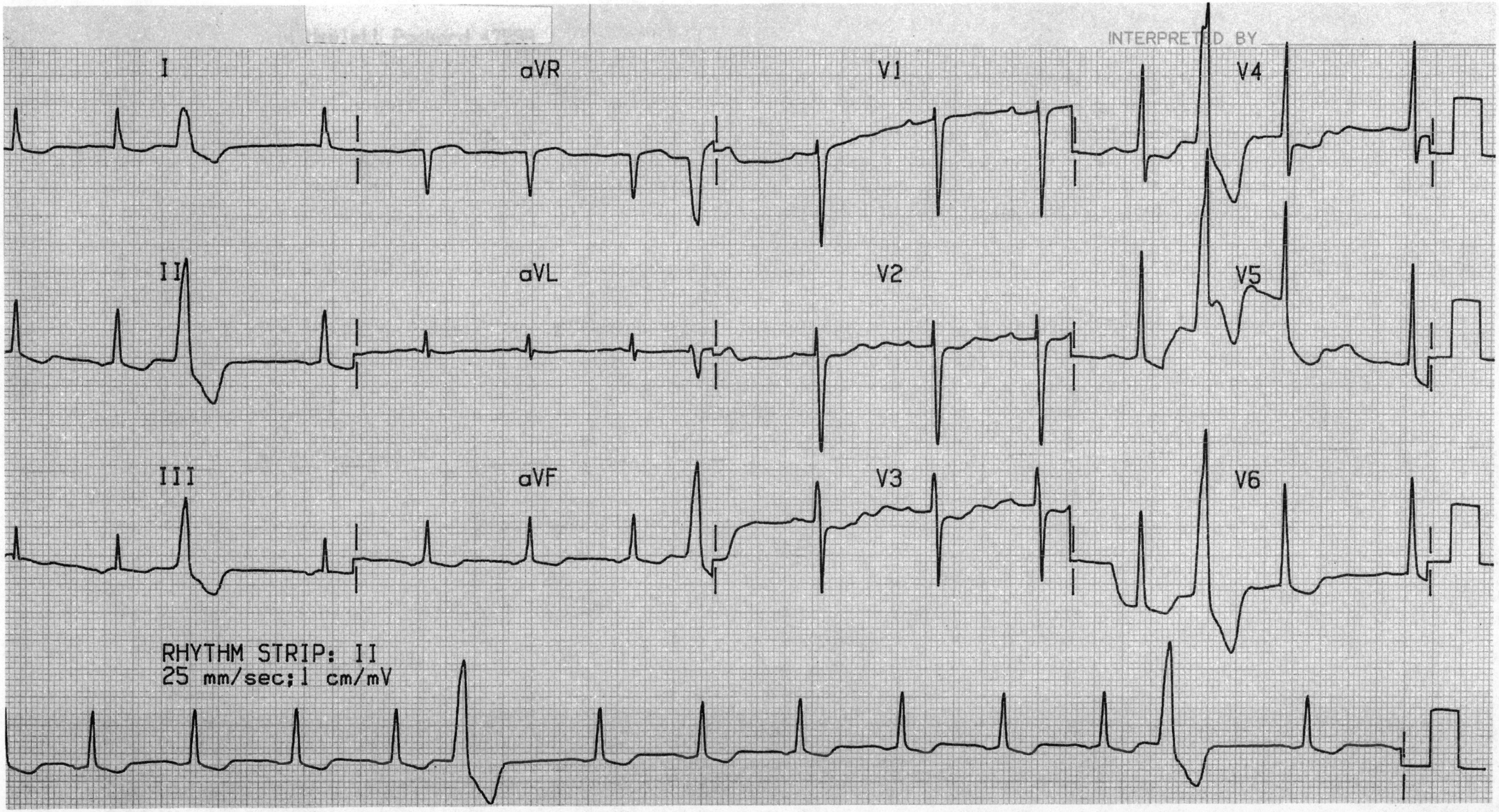

E-6

NARRATIVE INTERPRETATION

Rhythm: **Ectopic atrial rhythm**
Rate: **84**
Intervals: **PR 0.20, QRS 0.08, QT 0.32**
Axis: **+60 degrees**

Abnormalities

Inverted P waves leads II, III, aVF. VPCs. Interpolated VPC. ST depression leads I, II, III, aVL, aVF, V2–V6.

Synthesis

Ectopic atrial rhythm. VPCs. Interpolated VPC. Diffuse, nonspecific ST abnormalities.

TEST ANSWERS: 9, 26, 58, 106.

Comment: On careful inspection, inverted P waves can be seen in leads II, III, and aVF, which implies a pacemaker focus outside the sinus node. It cannot be determined with certainty whether this focus is AV junctional with a considerable degree of antegrade block or is derived from an ectopic atrial site. It would be unusual, however, for an accelerated AV junctional rhythm to have a PR interval of 0.20 s. Digoxin toxicity may present with suppression of normal pacemakers and enhancement of others, and it is likely that this tracing represents a "dig toxic" rhythm. The most common digitalis-induced arrhythmias are ventricular in origin, and this tracing demonstrates frequent VPCs. Note also an interpolated VPC sandwiched between two supraventricular beats.

REFERENCES: Smith. Saner. Fisch.

E-7

Clinical History

A 92-year-old woman with dyspnea.

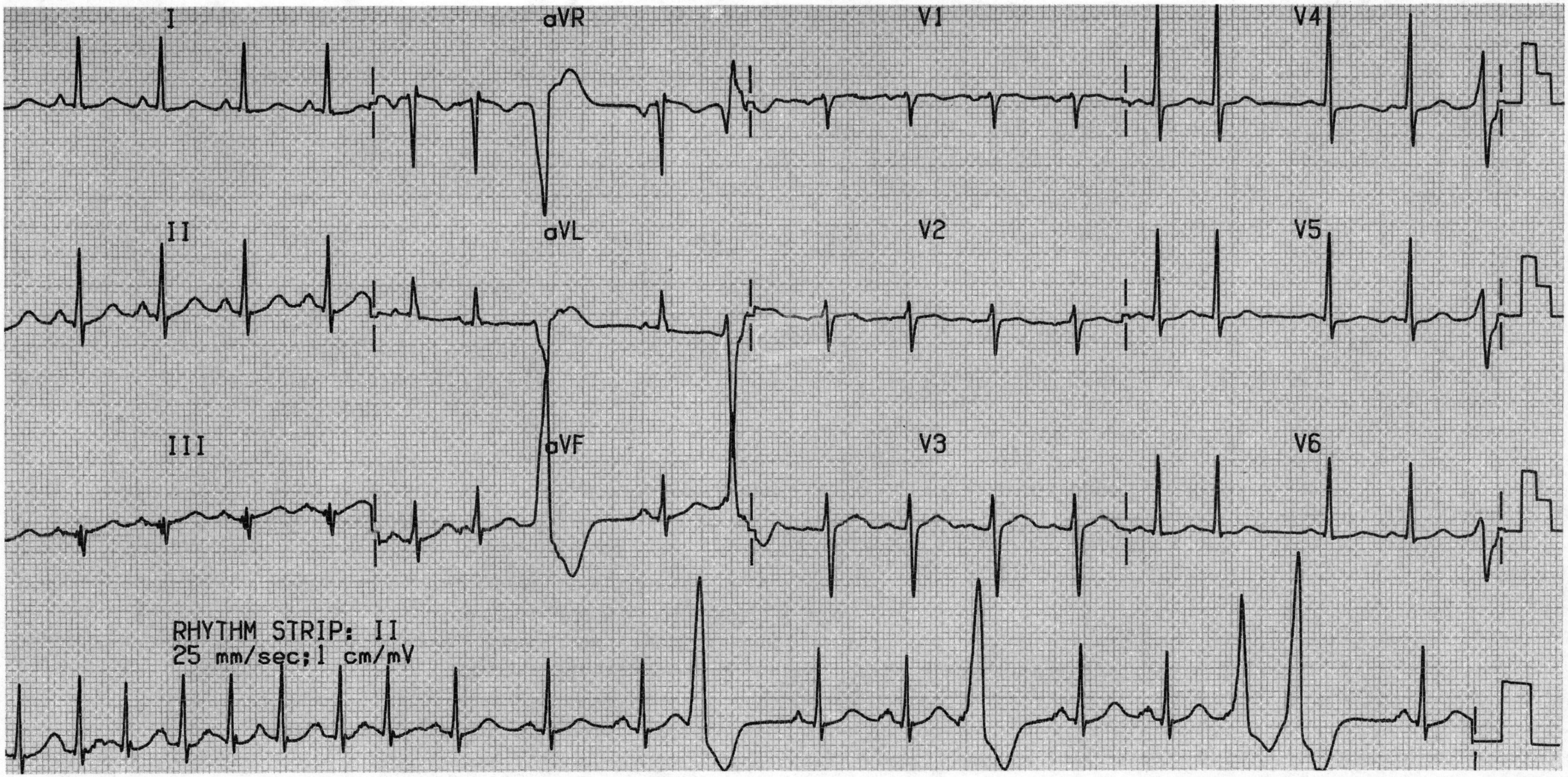

E-7

NARRATIVE INTERPRETATION

Rhythm: **Sinus tachycardia, multifocal atrial tachycardia (MAT)**
Rate: **Sinus rate 104, rate of MAT 180**
Intervals: **PR 0.16, QRS 0.08, QT 0.34**
Axis: **+15 degrees**

Abnormalities
Rapid heart rate. APCs. VPCs, multiform. Paired VPCs. SV2 + RV5 greater than 35. ST depression leads I, aVL, V5–V6.

Synthesis
Sinus tachycardia. APCs. VPCs, multiform. Paired VPCs. Multifocal atrial tachycardia on rhythm strip. LVH by voltage criteria. Associated ST abnormalities.

TEST ANSWERS: 4, 10, 14, 27, 28, 78, 103.

Comment: On first glance, the general QRST morphology of this electrocardiogram appears nearly normal, although there are a number of rhythm disturbances present. On closer inspection, the chest leads are seen to be recorded at one-half standard and demonstrate increased voltage for LVH. APCs are demonstrated by the fifth and fifteenth beats of the 12-lead tracing. Frequent VPCs are noted on the rhythm strip, both multiform and in pairs. A run of MAT is also present on the rhythm strip. It is initially difficult to differentiate this from atrial fibrillation. However, there are deformities of the T waves that suggest superimposed P waves rather than fibrillatory waves.

E-8

Clinical History

A 79-year-old man with palpitations and lightheadedness. He takes no medications.

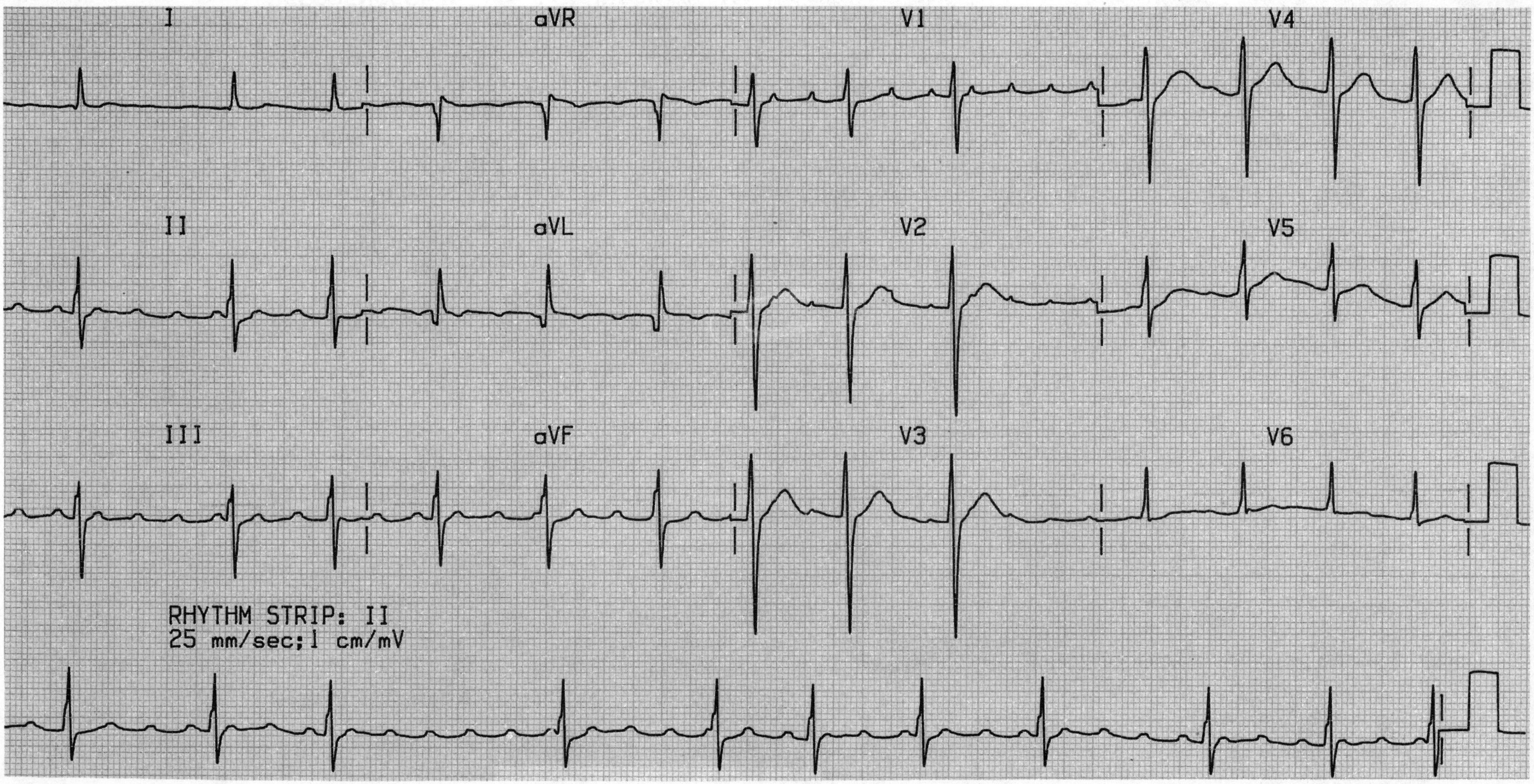

E-8

NARRATIVE INTERPRETATION

Rhythm:	**Atrial tachycardia with variable AV conduction**
Rate:	**Atrial 210, ventricular 62 (average)**
Intervals:	**PR –, QRS 0.10, QT 0.40**
Axis:	**−15 degrees**

Abnormalities
Rapid atrial rate with variable conduction.

Synthesis
Atrial tachycardia with variable AV conduction. Otherwise within normal limits.

TEST ANSWERS: 17, 51.

Comment: Atrial tachycardia with block is considered a characteristic arrhythmia of digitalis toxicity. This arrhythmia may also result from pulmonary, coronary, or valvular heart disease. Atrial tachycardia with block should be differentiated from atrial flutter with block. The atrial rate in atrial tachycardia is between 150 and 250, whereas the atrial rate in atrial flutter is usually greater than 250. Atrial flutter should also demonstrate characteristic flutter waves, which are inverted in leads II, III and aVF. Atrial tachycardia has an isoelectric baseline between the P waves. Remember that at atrial rates greater than 200, 2:1 AV conduction is an expected physiologic response of the AV node. Conduction ratios greater than 2:1 imply a nonphysiologic response secondary to either intrinsic conduction disease or the effect of pharmacologic agents.

REFERENCES: Bar (*Am J Cardiol*). Keefe. Manolis.

E-9

Clinical History

A 60-year-old man in the CCU.

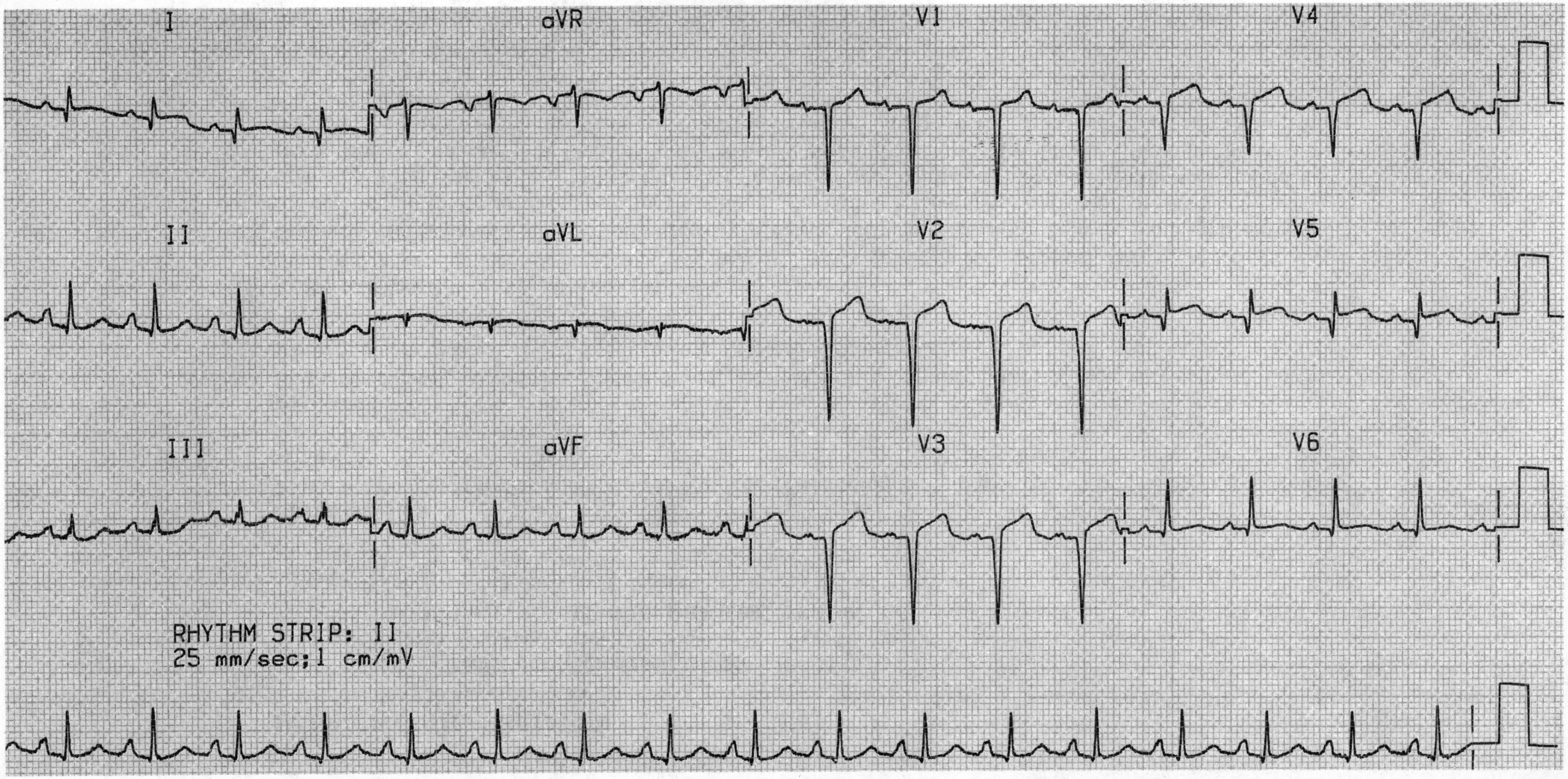

E-9

NARRATIVE INTERPRETATION

Rhythm: **Sinus tachycardia**
Rate: **105**
Intervals: **PR 0.18, QRS 0.08, QT 0.30**
Axis: **+75 degrees**

Abnormalities

Rapid heart rate. Q waves leads I, aVL, V1–V6. ST elevation leads I, aVL, V1–V6. ST depression leads III, aVF.

Synthesis

Sinus tachycardia. Extensive anterior and lateral MI with ST abnormalities of acute myocardial injury. ST depression in leads III, aVF suggesting myocardial ischemia.

TEST ANSWERS: 4, 87, 89, 100, 101.

Comment: This patient suffered an extensive MI secondary to occlusion of the proximal left anterior descending coronary artery. The abnormalities in the lateral leads reflect occlusion of this artery proximal to a large diagonal vessel that supplied the lateral wall of the left ventricle. Sinus tachycardia in the setting of acute MI may be a response to discomfort and anxiety. Alternatively, the rapid heart rate may be a compensatory mechanism to maintain cardiac output in the presence of extensive loss of functioning myocardium.

E-10

Clinical History

An 84-year-old man seen in a clinic with chronic dyspnea on exertion. Medications include digitalis and diuretics.

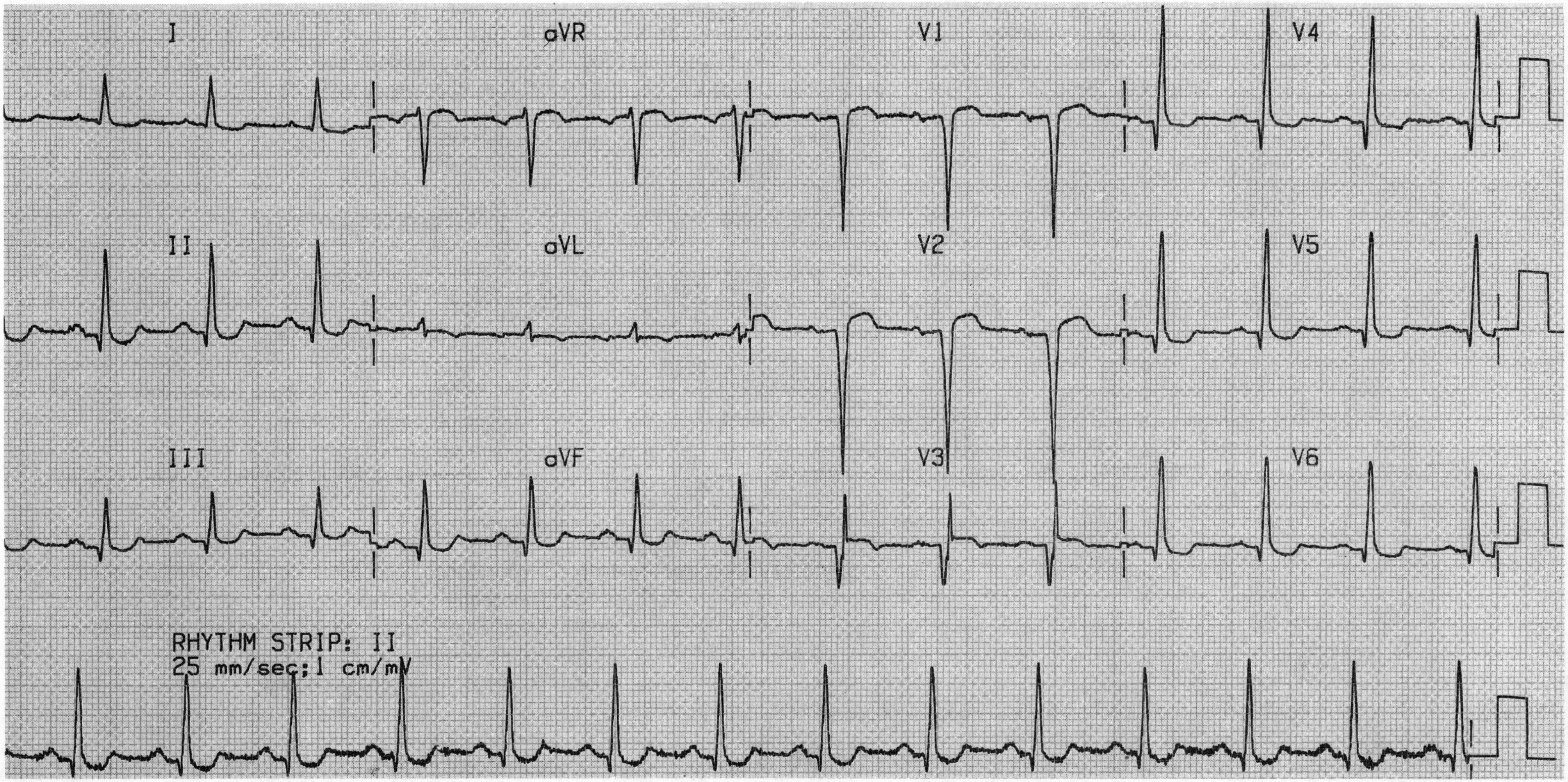

E-10

NARRATIVE INTERPRETATION

Rhythm: **Sinus**
Rate: **82**
Intervals: **PR 0.20, QRS 0.10, QT 0.32**
Axis: **+60 degrees**

Abnormalities

QS leads V1–V2. Q waves leads V3–V4. ST depression leads I, II, III, aVF, V4–V6. ST elevation leads V1–V3. T-wave inversion leads aVL, V3. Biphasic T waves leads I, V4–V6. SV2 + RV5 greater than 35.

Synthesis

Sinus rhythm. LVH. Anterior wall MI of indeterminate age. ST elevation suggestive of ventricular aneurysm. Nonspecific ST-T-wave abnormalities.

TEST ANSWERS: 1, 78, (82), 84, 95, (103), 106.

Comment: This tracing demonstrates the coexistence of LVH and prior anterior MI. LVH may produce poor R-wave progression or even a QS pattern in leads V1–V3 and mimic anteroseptal MI. The QR pattern in lead V3 in this tracing, however, cannot be ascribed to LVH alone and points to the additional diagnosis of anterior wall infarction. It is difficult to confirm whether the septum is involved. The ST elevation seen in lead V3 also suggests formation of a ventricular aneurysm when combined with the clinical history. The diffuse ST-T-wave abnormalities are likely to be a combination of factors from LVH, anterior wall MI, and digitalis effect and are therefore listed as nonspecific in this example. The effect of digitalis is also suggested by a relatively short QT interval.

E-11

Clinical History

A 60-year-old asymptomatic man seen for an insurance physical. He takes no medications.

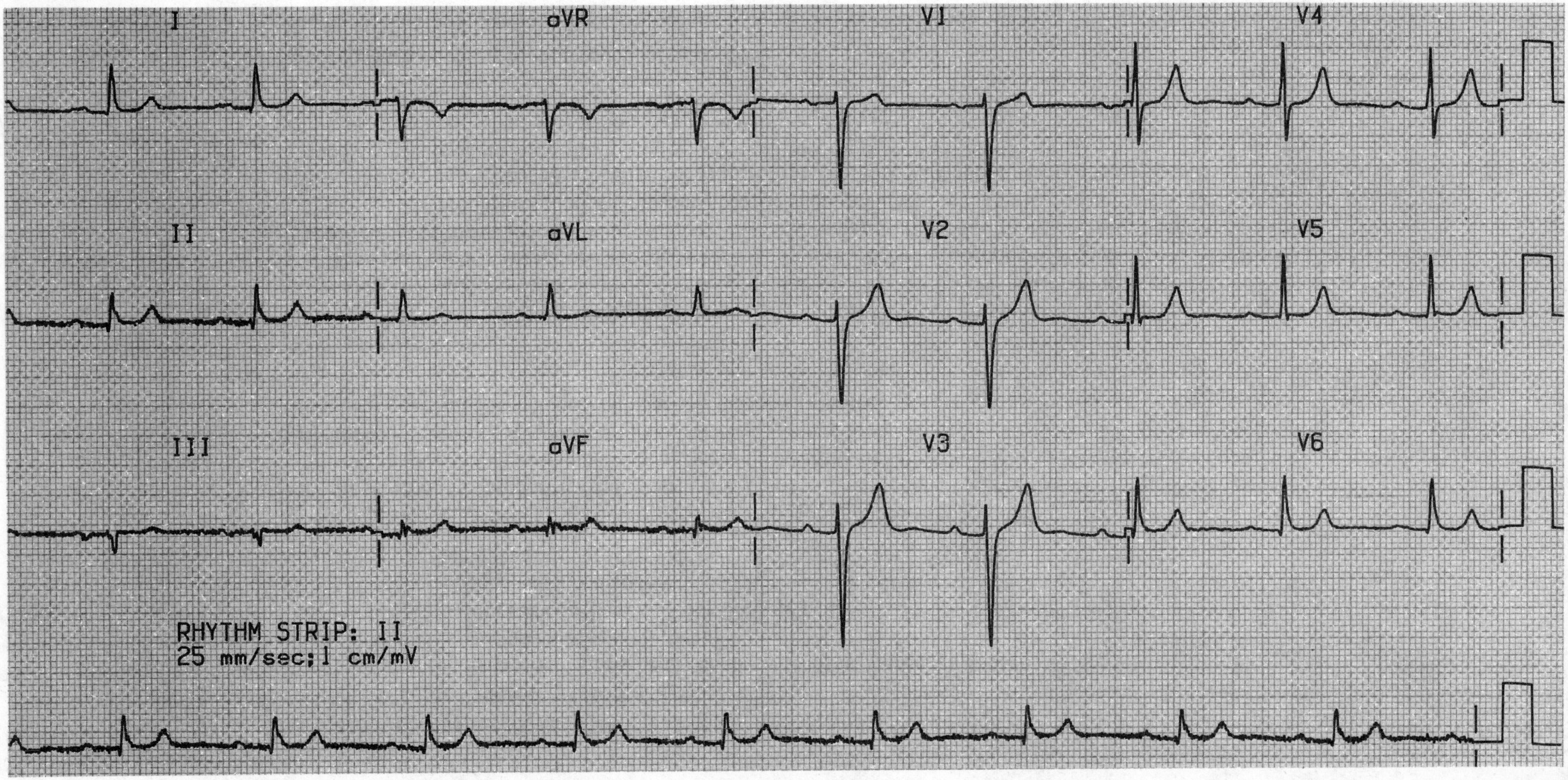

E-11

NARRATIVE INTERPRETATION

Rhythm: **Sinus bradycardia with first-degree AV block**
Rate: **58**
Intervals: **PR 0.24, QRS 0.08, QT 0.38**
Axis: **0 degrees**

Abnormalities
Slow heart rate. Prolonged PR interval.

Synthesis
Sinus bradycardia. First-degree AV block. Otherwise within normal limits.

TEST ANSWERS: 3, 42.

Comment: First-degree AV block is diagnosed when the PR interval is prolonged beyond 0.20 s. This may be observed in completely healthy persons. In a review of a number of series, there was found to be a 0.6 percent prevalence of first-degree AV block in healthy servicemen. The long-term prognosis of first-degree AV block was analyzed in one study of 3983 healthy men. In the 30 years of follow-up, there was no difference in mortality compared with that in persons without first-degree AV block. A number of medications may prolong the PR interval, including digoxin, verapamil, and diltiazem. Acute prolongation of the PR interval may also be seen in inferior wall MI or acute rheumatic fever.

REFERENCES: Mymin. Barrett. Chung p 281.

E-12

Clinical History

A 91-year-old man with congestive heart failure.

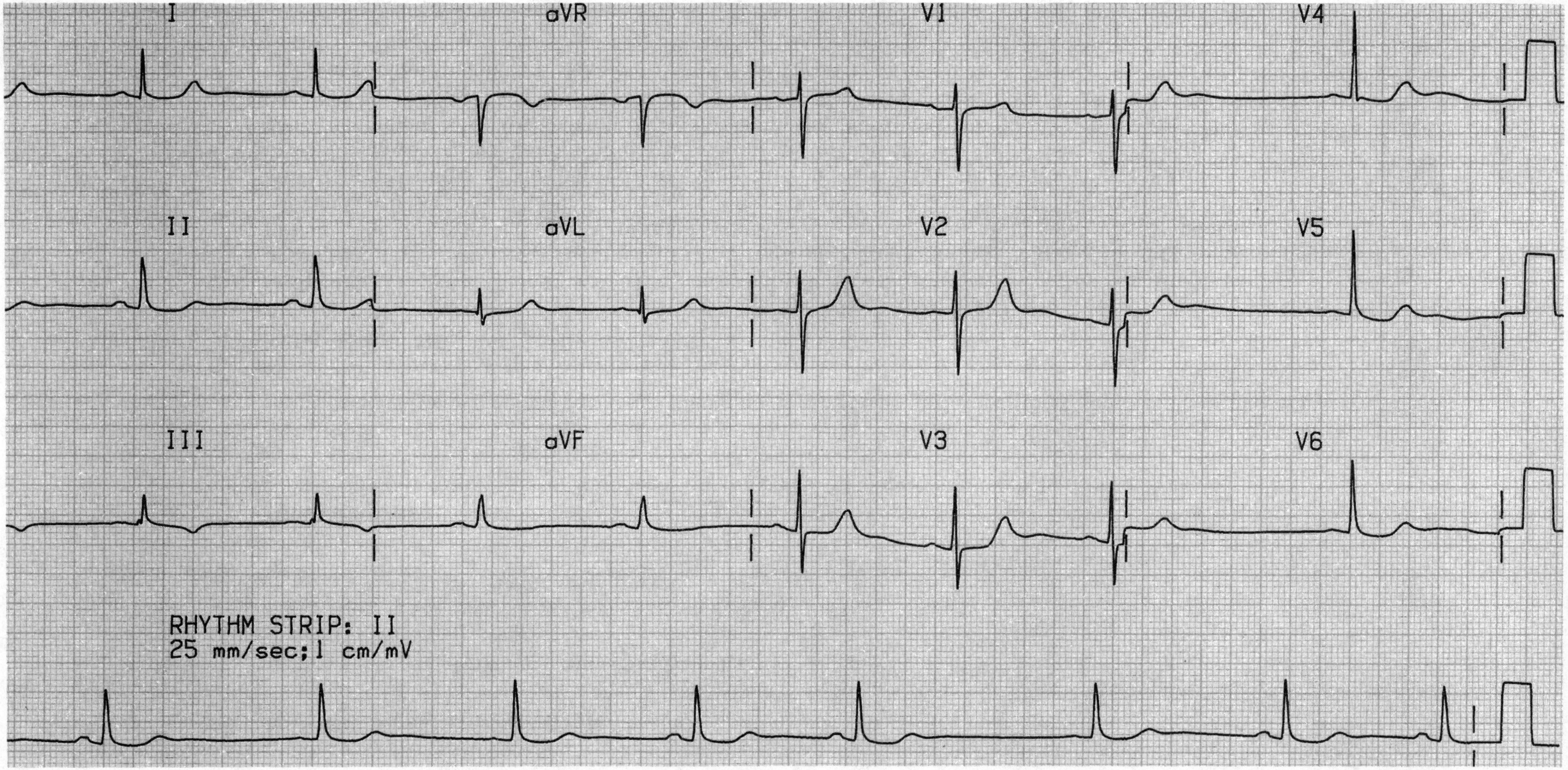

E-12

NARRATIVE INTERPRETATION

Rhythm: **Sinus bradycardia**
Rate: **55**
Intervals: **PR 0.16, QRS 0.08, QT 0.44**
Axis: **+45 degrees**

Abnormalities

Slow heart rate. Sinus pause. Junctional escape beats. ST depression leads I, II, aVF, V4–V6.

Synthesis

Sinus bradycardia with sinus pause and junctional escape beats. Nonspecific ST-segment abnormalities.

TEST ANSWERS: 3, 7, 24, 106.

Comment: The basic rhythm is sinus bradycardia with periodic sinus pauses. The intrinsic sinus rate is approximately 55 beats per minute and the rate of the escape rhythm is approximately 46 beats per minute. The differential diagnosis of this rhythm would include sinus arrhythmia with wandering atrial pacemaker to the AV junction. This is not a correct diagnosis as there is little variation in the PP interval and there is a rather abrupt pause in the sinus rate on the rhythm strip. First-degree SA block is also possible; however, this cannot be diagnosed on the surface electrocardiogram. The escape rate of 46 beats per minute also suggests an escape focus in the AV junction rather than a gradual shift in the pacemaker. The likely cause of this patient's rhythm disturbance was digoxin, which was also responsible for the nonspecific ST changes.

E-13

Clinical History

A 58-year-old man in the CCU with recurrent chest pain. A temporary ventricular pacemaker was placed earlier in his hospital course for symptomatic bradyarrhythmias.

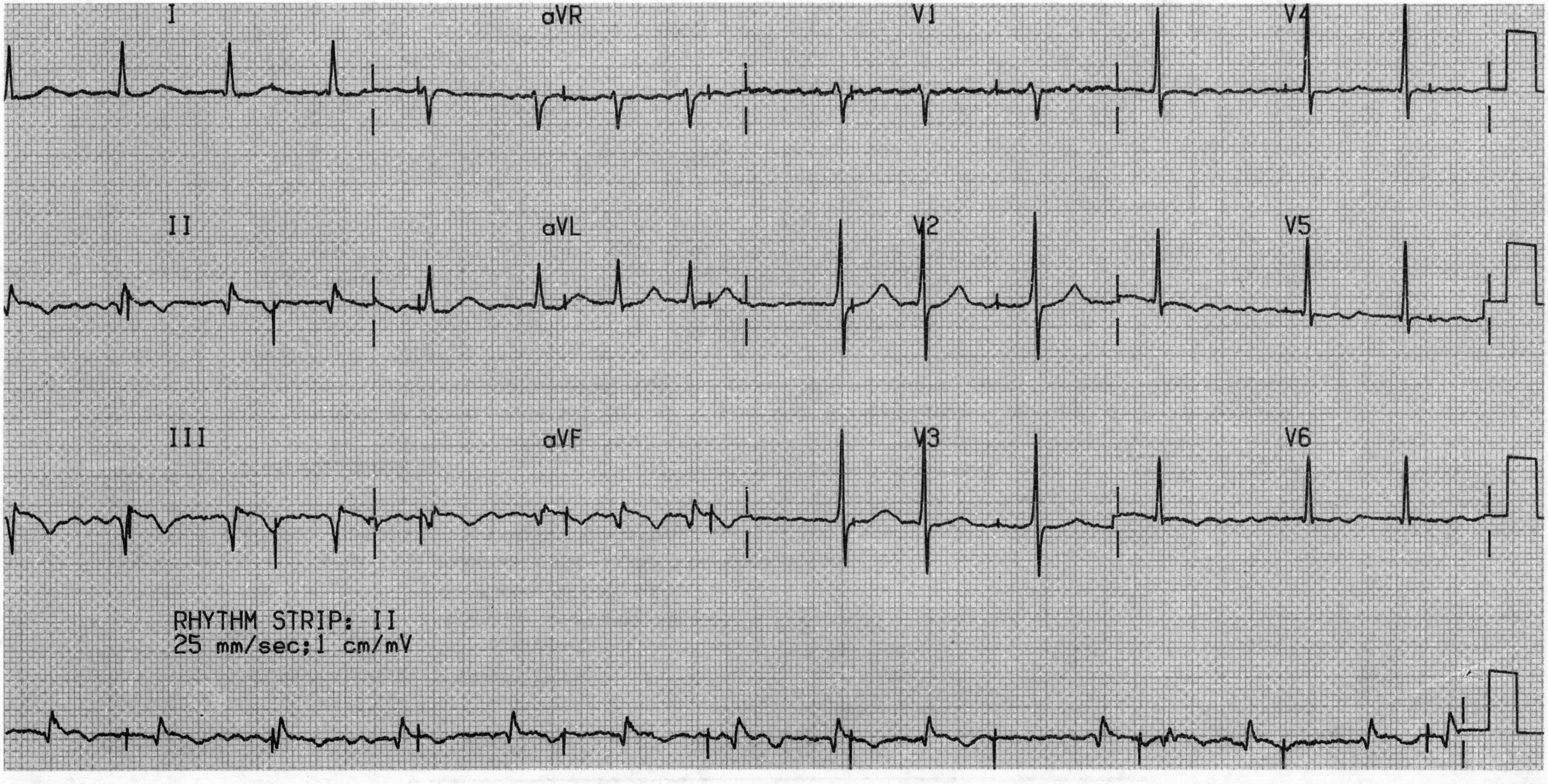

E-13

NARRATIVE INTERPRETATION

Rhythm: **Atrial fibrillation**
Rate: **75 (average)**
Intervals: **PR –, QRS 0.08, QT 0.38**
Axis: **−15 degrees**

Abnormalities

Q waves leads II, III, aVF. ST elevation leads II, III, aVF. ST depression leads aVL, V2. T-wave inversion leads II, III, aVF, V4–V6. Tall R wave with R greater than S and upright T wave lead V2. Pacemaker complexes at rate of 60 beats per minute with no relation to QRS complex. No pacemaker capture of ventricle.

Synthesis

Atrial fibrillation with a controlled ventricular response. Acute inferior wall and posterior wall MI with ST-T-wave abnormalities of acute myocardial injury. Pacemaker malfunction, failure to sense QRS complex. Pacemaker malfunction, failure to capture ventricle.

TEST ANSWERS: 20, 39, 40, 51, 91, 93, 100.

Comment: This electrocardiogram demonstrates an acute inferior and probable posterior wall MI. The Q waves and ST-T-wave abnormalities of the acute inferior wall are fairly obvious; however, the posterior wall involvement is more subtle. Note the tall R wave in lead V2 with slight ST depression. In the presence of a concomitant inferior wall infarction, these findings suggest posterior wall MI as well. Two separate forms of pacemaker malfunction are also present in this electrocardiogram. The pacemaker clearly fails to sense the native rhythm and is firing at a set rate of 60 beats per minute. Failure to capture is easily diagnosed on the rhythm strip. The first, fifth, and seventh pacemaker stimuli occur far enough outside the refractory period of the ventricle to produce capture. It is conceivable that the other pacemaker complexes fall in the refractory period and might not produce ventricular capture. In this patient, the pacemaker wire had slipped out of position.

REFERENCES: Nestico. Huey. Chaitman.

E-14

Clinical History

A 72-year-old man with a harsh systolic murmur.

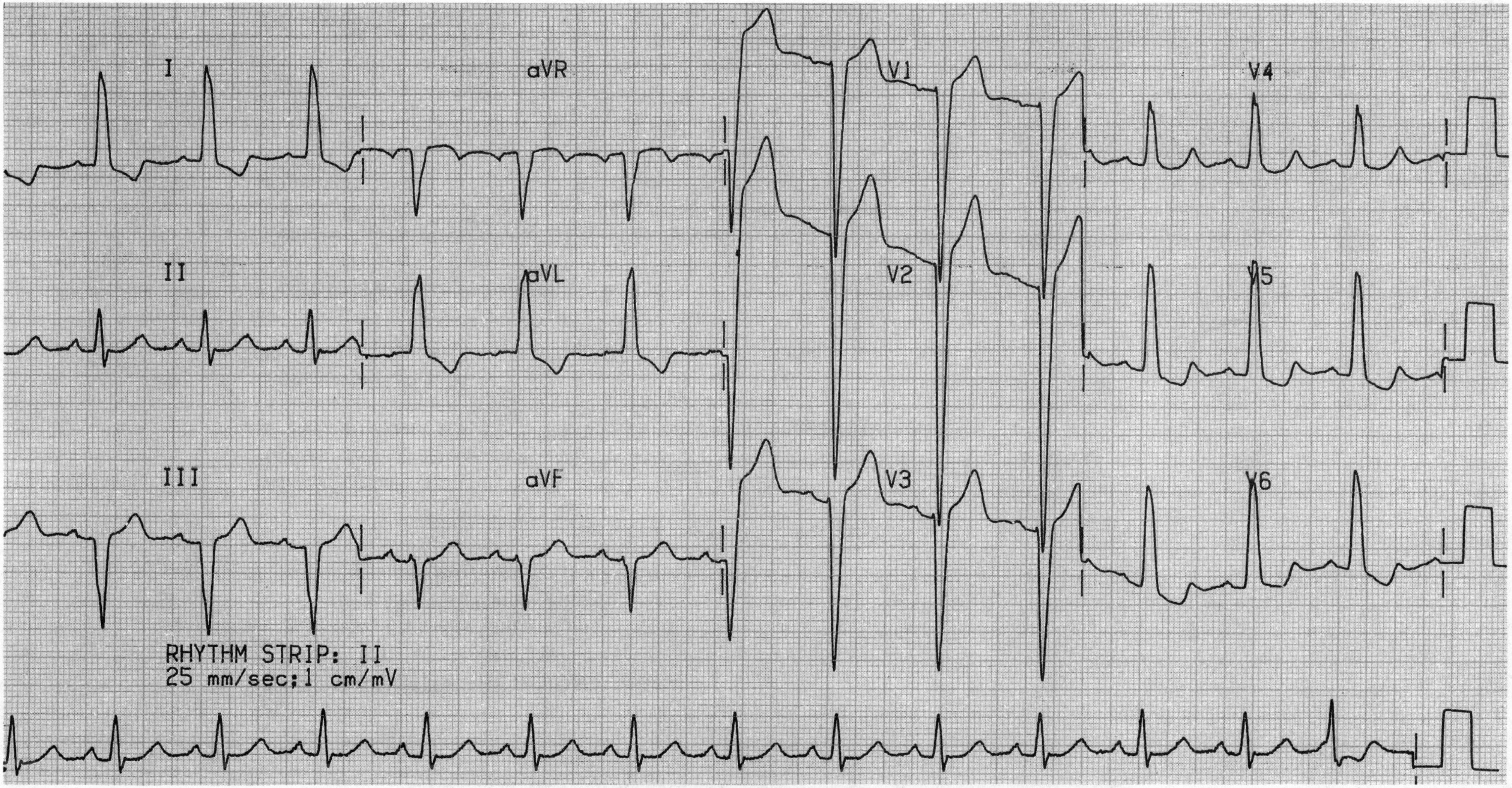

E-14

NARRATIVE INTERPRETATION

Rhythm: **Sinus**
Rate: **82**
Intervals: **PR 0.18, QRS 0.12, QT 0.38**
Axis: **−15 degrees**

Abnormalities

Broad, slurred QRS leads I, aVL, V5–V6. ST depression leads I, aVL, V4–V6. T-wave inversion leads I, aVL. Biphasic T waves leads V5, V6. SV2 + RV5 greater than 45.

Synthesis

Sinus rhythm. LBBB. Associated ST-T-wave abnormalities. Probable LVH.

TEST ANSWERS: 1, 74, (78), (103), 104.

Comment: The diagnosis of LVH in the presence of LBBB is problematic. One of the more reliable criteria has been SV2 + RV5 greater than 45, which was reported in one study to have a sensitivity of 86 percent and a specificity of 100 percent for the diagnosis of LVH. The ST-T-wave abnormalities in this example are related to both ventricular hypertrophy and the conduction abnormality. It is reasonable to consider LVH as "probable" in the presence of complete LBBB. It should be noted that the great majority of patients with LBBB have anatomic LVH. This patient indeed had marked LVH secondary to aortic stenosis.

REFERENCE: Klein RC.

E-15

Clinical History

A 59-year-old diabetic woman admitted to the CCU.

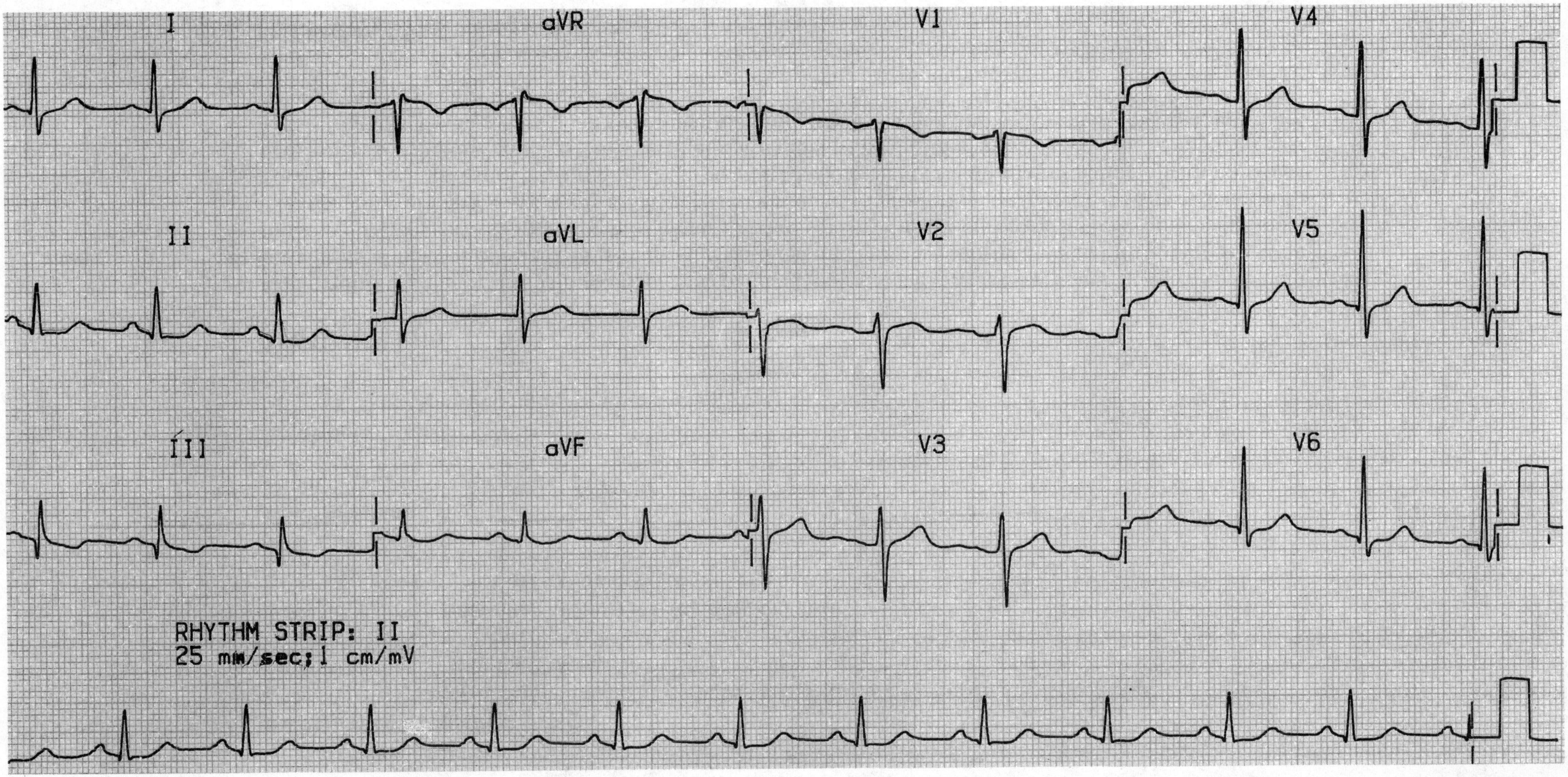

E-15

NARRATIVE INTERPRETATION

Rhythm: **Sinus**
Rate: **72**
Intervals: **PR 0.16, QRS 0.08, QT 0.40**
Axis: **+60 degrees**

Abnormalities

Slight ST depression leads II, aVF, V6.

Synthesis

Sinus rhythm. Nonspecific ST abnormalities.

TEST ANSWERS: 1, 106.

Comment: It is important to remember that patients may have extensive coronary heart disease with little or no abnormalities on the resting electrocardiogram. The ST abnormalities in this tracing are quite minor. Nevertheless, this patient was found to have severe, diffuse coronary disease on angiography. The presence of ST-T-wave abnormalities has been found to have prognostic relevance in patients with coronary heart disease. One large study of nearly 10,000 patients found that in patients with coronary heart disease, the presence of ST-T-wave abnormalities was an independent predictor of reduced survival. Importantly, in patients with this electrocardiographic finding and no coronary disease, it did not have an independent effect on survival.

REFERENCES: Crenshaw. Joy.

E-16

Clinical History

A 74-year-old man with lightheadedness.

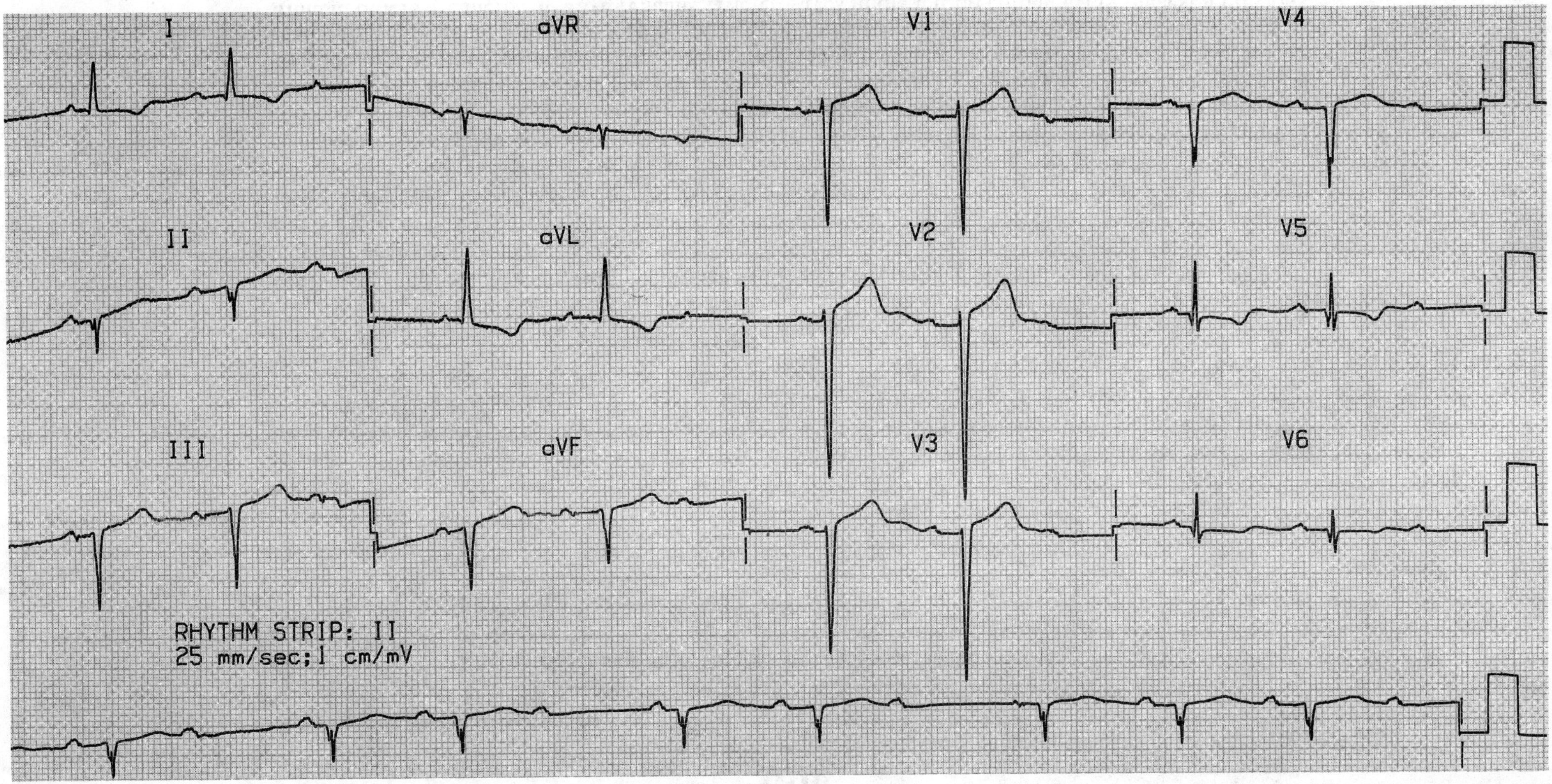

E-16

NARRATIVE INTERPRETATION

Rhythm: **Sinus with second-degree AV block, Mobitz type I**
Rate: **75**
Intervals: **PR variable, QRS 0.08, QT 0.40**
Axis: **−45 degrees**

Abnormalities

Variable PR intervals with periodic failure to conduct. Atrial escape complex on rhythm strip. Axis leftward of −30 degrees. Abnormal Q wave leads V5–V6. SV2 + RV5 greater than 35 mm. T wave inverted leads I, aVL, V5–V6. ST depression leads aVL, V5–V6. R wave less than 3 mm leads V1–V3. Prolonged QTc interval.

Synthesis

Sinus rhythm. Second-degree AV block, Mobitz type I (Wenckebach). Atrial escape complex on rhythm strip. Poor R-wave progression. Left axis deviation. Left anterior fascicular block. LVH. Associated ST-T-wave abnormalities. Probable inferolateral MI of indeterminate age. Possible anterior wall MI of indeterminate age. Prolonged QTc.

TEST ANSWERS: 1, 43, 64, 66, 72, 78, (84), (92), 103, 109.

Comment: The rhythm is easily identified as sinus with a Wenckebach pattern. Note that the ninth P wave on the rhythm strip has a different configuration than the others and is likely an atrial escape complex that emerged following the pause. Left axis deviation with left anterior fascicular block is present. It is more difficult to confirm whether a concomitant inferior wall MI is present. This is suggested by the notched S wave in lead II. A small Q wave in lead II appears in some of the complexes, while in others a "micro" R wave remains. The Q waves in the left precordial leads suggest a previous MI. Prior anterior wall MI is also possible on the basis of reverse R-wave progression in leads V1–V4. This is also difficult to confirm in the presence of LVH and left axis deviation. The QTc interval is slightly prolonged.

REFERENCES: Zema (*J Electrocardiol* 12:3, 1979; 12:11, 1979; 13:135, 1980). DePace. Warner (*Am J Cardiol* 52:690, 1983).

E-17

Clinical History

A 67-year-old man taking verapamil for hypertension.

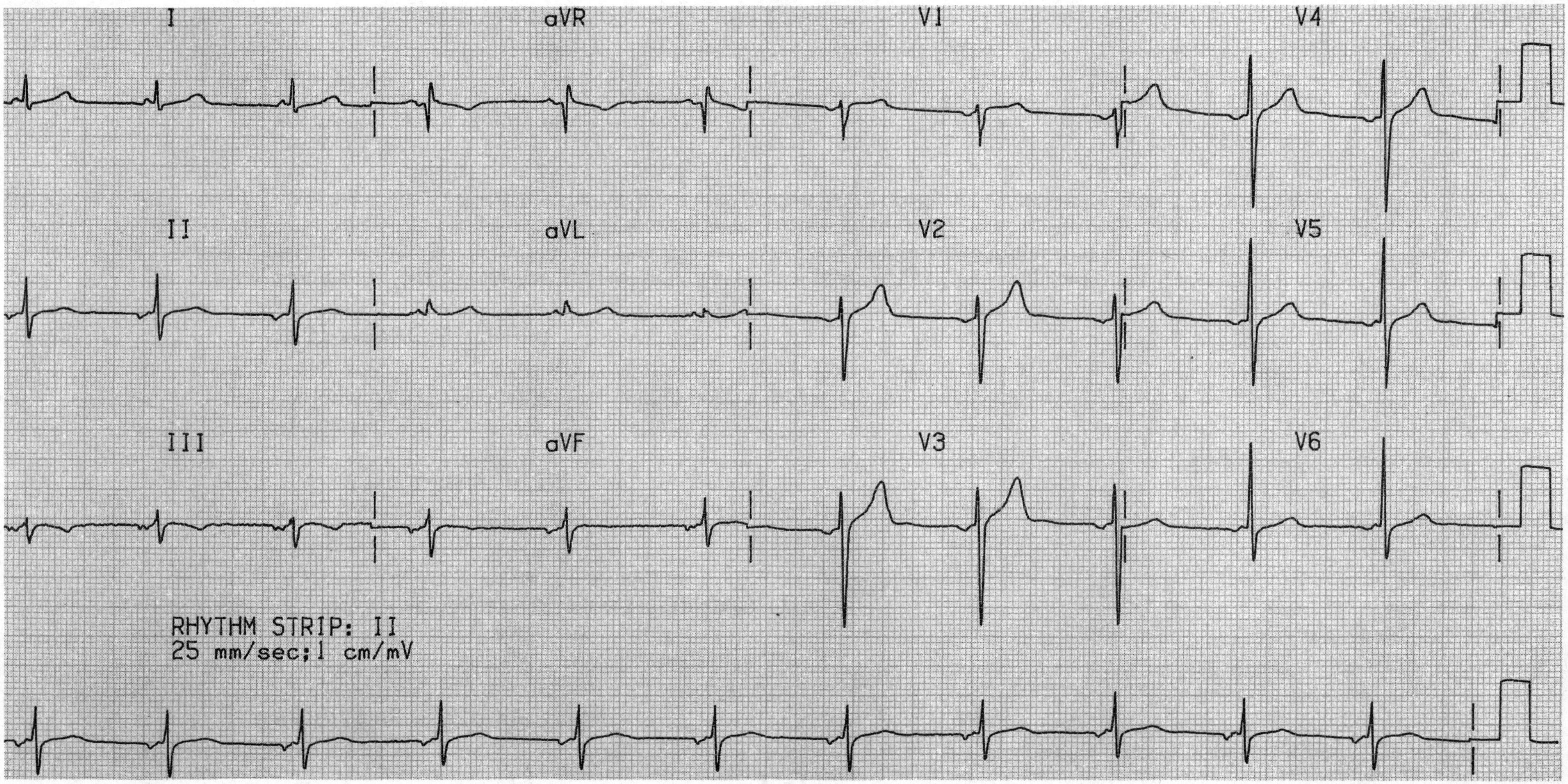

E-17

NARRATIVE INTERPRETATION

Rhythm: **AV junctional rhythm**
Rate: **65**
Intervals: **PR 0.11, QRS 0.08, QT 0.36**
Axis: **−15 degrees**

Abnormalities

Inverted P wave leads II, III, aVF with short PR interval.

Synthesis

AV junctional rhythm. Otherwise within normal limits.

TEST ANSWERS: 21, (23).

Comment: This patient had suppression of the sinus node induced by verapamil, which allowed a subsidiary pacemaker in the AV junctional tissue to become dominant. Without first knowing the intrinsic sinus rate, it is not possible to determine whether this rhythm is an escape rhythm induced by sinus node depression or whether the AV junctional rhythm usurps control because of enhanced automaticity. For this reason, this example is simply characterized as "AV junctional rhythm" rather than accelerated or escape rhythm. It would not be incorrect, however, to classify this rhythm as "accelerated" because the rhythm is at a slightly faster rate than is normally expected for the AV junction.

E-18

Clinical History

A 29-year-old woman with a history of rheumatic fever.

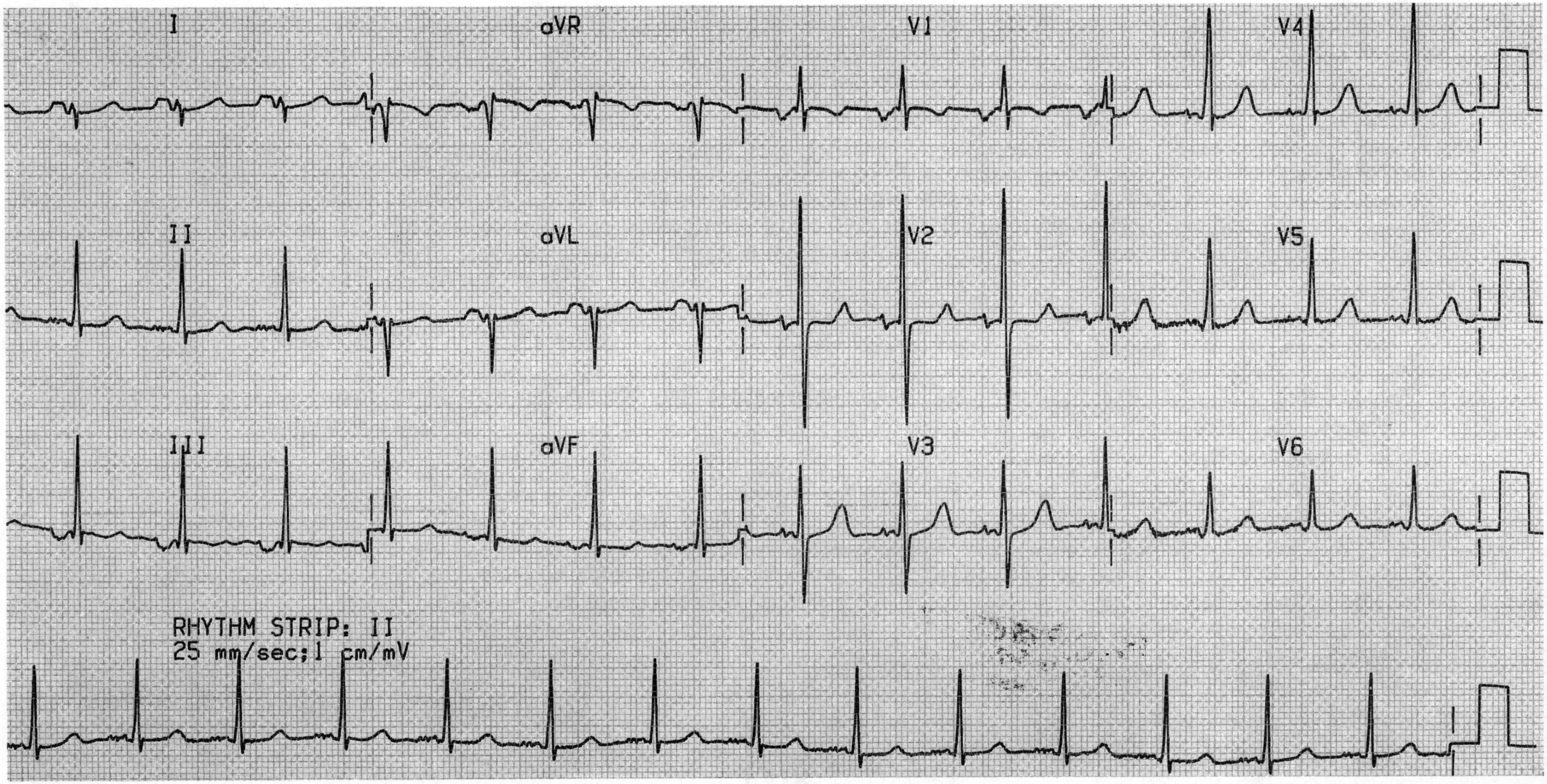

E-18

NARRATIVE INTERPRETATION

Rhythm: **Sinus**
Rate: **84**
Intervals: **PR 0.16, QRS 0.08, QT 0.38**
Axis: **+110 degrees**

Abnormalities
Axis rightward of +90 degrees. Abnormal P terminal force lead V1. Tall R waves leads V1–V2.

Synthesis
Sinus rhythm. Left atrial abnormality. Right axis deviation. RVH.

TEST ANSWERS: 1, 60, 65, 79.

Comment: This electrocardiogram demonstrates the characteristic findings of a patient with long-standing mitral stenosis. There is a markedly abnormal P terminal force in V1 and a broad, notched P wave in lead II. Right axis deviation and tall R waves in the right precordial leads are indicative of RVH, a result of the increased right-sided pressures seen in critical mitral stenosis.

E-19

Clinical History

An 89-year-old woman with congestive heart failure. Medications include digoxin.

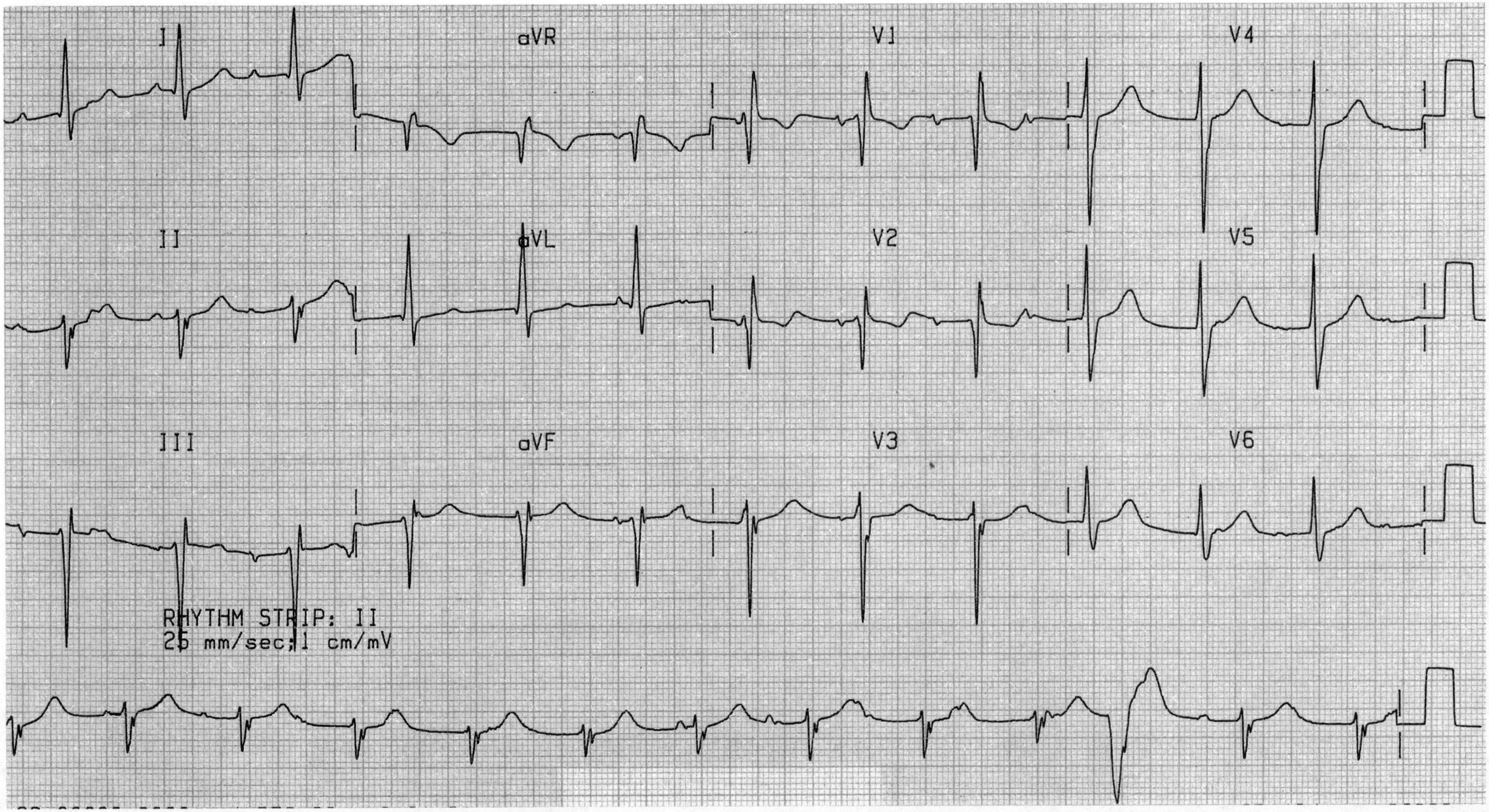

E-19

NARRATIVE INTERPRETATION

Rhythm: **Sinus with complete AV block, accelerated AV junctional rhythm**
Rate: **Atrial rate 88, AV junctional rate 74**
Intervals: **PR –, QRS 0.13, QT 0.40**
Axis: **−45 degrees**

Abnormalities

P waves fail to conduct to ventricles. Axis leftward of −30 degrees. S wave lead III greater than 15. Prolonged QRS with rSR′ and T-wave inversion leads V1–V2. VPC. Alteration and reset of sinus and AV junctional cycle post VPC.

Synthesis

Sinus rhythm with complete AV block. Accelerated AV junctional rhythm. AV dissociation. VPC. Cycle alteration probably secondary to retrograde atrial activation from ventricular depolarization. Left axis deviation. LAFB. RBBB with associated ST-T-wave abnormalities. Probable LVH.

TEST ANSWERS: 1, 23, 26, 47, 53, (55), 64, 70, 72, (78), 104.

Comment: This is a complex ECG. One should first notice there is no constant relationship between the P waves and QRS complex. The P waves "march through," which is characteristic of AV dissociation. An accelerated AV junctional rhythm becomes the dominant pacemaker. The AV junction is not simply an escape focus as the normal intrinsic rate of the AV junction is slower than the current rate of 74 beats per minute; hence, this is an accelerated rhythm. Despite this relatively rapid junctional rhythm, several of the sinus beats would be expected to conduct to the ventricles; therefore, complete AV block is present. Note that following the VPC on the rhythm strip, the next QRS complex has a less-than-compensatory pause, which occurs somewhat earlier than expected. This is usually seen when the dominant rhythm is other than sinus, as the PVC has depolarized the underlying pacemaker in the AV junction. The P wave following the VPC also occurs early, probably secondary to retrograde conduction and a resetting of the sinus cycle. Also remember that with complete RBBB, the first 0.06 s of the complex may be interpreted in a normal fashion. LAFB is present and concomitant LVH is suggested by the increased R- and S-wave voltage in leads aVL and III, respectively.

E-20

Clinical History

A 67-year-old woman with palpitations.

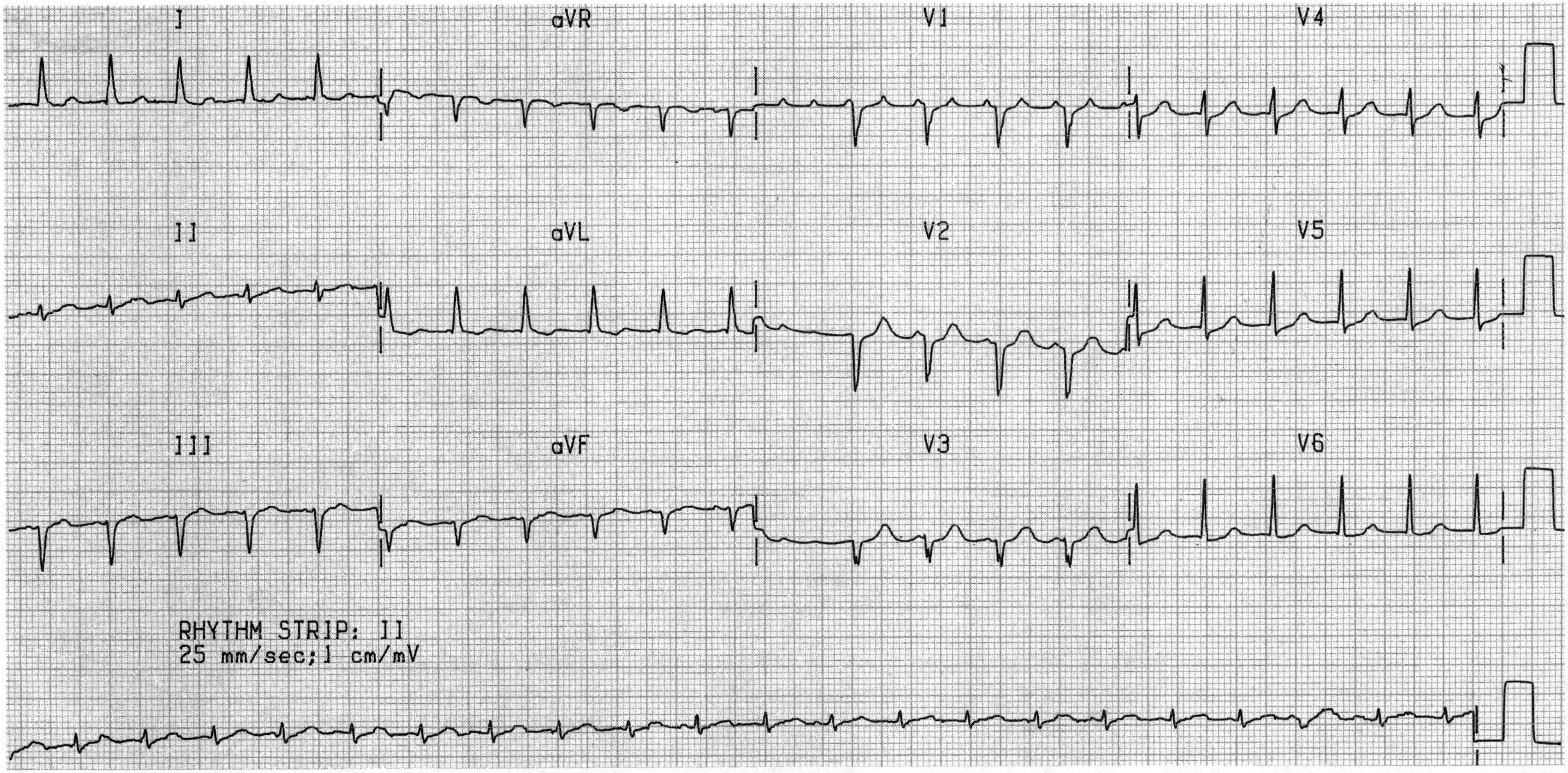

E-20

NARRATIVE INTERPRETATION

Rhythm:	**Atrial tachycardia with variable (predominantly 2:1) AV conduction**
Rate:	**Atrial rate 250, ventricular rate 125**
Intervals:	**PR 0.28, QRS 0.08, QT 0.28**
Axis:	**−30 degrees**

Abnormalities

R-wave amplitude less than 3 mm leads V1–V3. Slight ST depression leads V4–V6. T-wave inversion lead aVL. VPC.

Synthesis

Atrial tachycardia with 2:1 AV conduction and brief period of variable AV conduction. Poor R-wave progression. Nonspecific ST-segment abnormalities. VPC.

TEST ANSWERS: 17, 26, 50, 51, 66, 106.

Comment: On initial examination, the reader might mistakenly interpret this rhythm as sinus tachycardia. However, a brief period of variable AV conduction is evident prior to the first complex of the precordial leads, which demonstrates the P waves of atrial tachycardia. This tracing is difficult to interpret in that the reader might also mistake the rhythm for atrial flutter. Note the isoelectric baseline between the P waves, best seen in lead V1, as well as the absence of true flutter waves. These characteristics help to distinguish this rhythm as atrial tachycardia with 2:1 AV conduction rather than atrial flutter. As is the case with atrial flutter, the AV node conducts in a 2:1 fashion when presented with an atrial rate of 250; therefore, the 2:1 ratio does not actually represent AV block. This is a physiologic property of the AV node. Higher ratios of conduction, however, are not physiologic.

REFERENCES: Chung pp 130, 140. Chou pp 322–324. Friedman p 462.

E-21

Clinical History

A 50-year-old man with dyspnea.

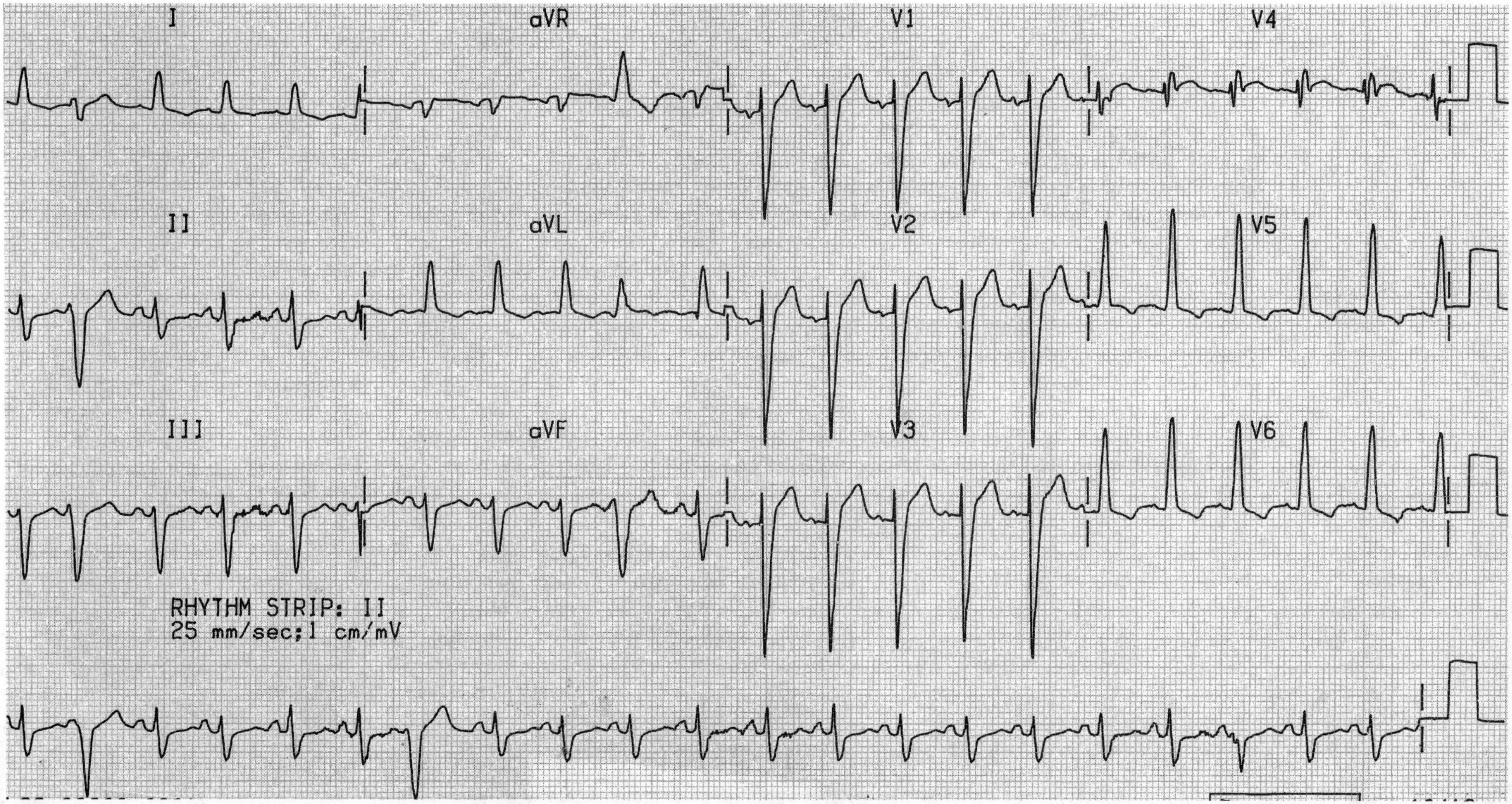

E-21

NARRATIVE INTERPRETATION

Rhythm: **Sinus tachycardia**
Rate: **120**
Intervals: **PR 0.16, QRS 0.10, QT 0.28**
Axis: **−30 degrees**

Abnormalities
Rapid heart rate. VPCs. ST depression leads I, aVL, V5–V6. ST-segment elevation at J point leads V1–V4. T-wave inversion leads I, aVL, V5–V6. SV2 + RV5 greater than 35.

Synthesis
Sinus tachycardia. VPCs. Fusion complex (on rhythm strip). LVH by voltage criteria. Associated ST-T-wave abnormalities. Clinical correlation required to exclude myocardial injury.

TEST ANSWERS: 4, 26, 56, 78, (100), 103.

Comment: This patient had an idiopathic dilated cardiomyopathy with left ventricular dilatation. The ST changes seen in the precordial leads were chronic and secondary to LVH. The different morphologies of the VPCs seen on the rhythm strip are a result of fusion with conduction from the sinus mechanism. Note the fusion complex in the third-from-last beat of the rhythm strip. The relatively short QT interval in this example was most likely related to the effect of digoxin.

E-22

Clinical History

A 77-year-old woman admitted with pneumonia.

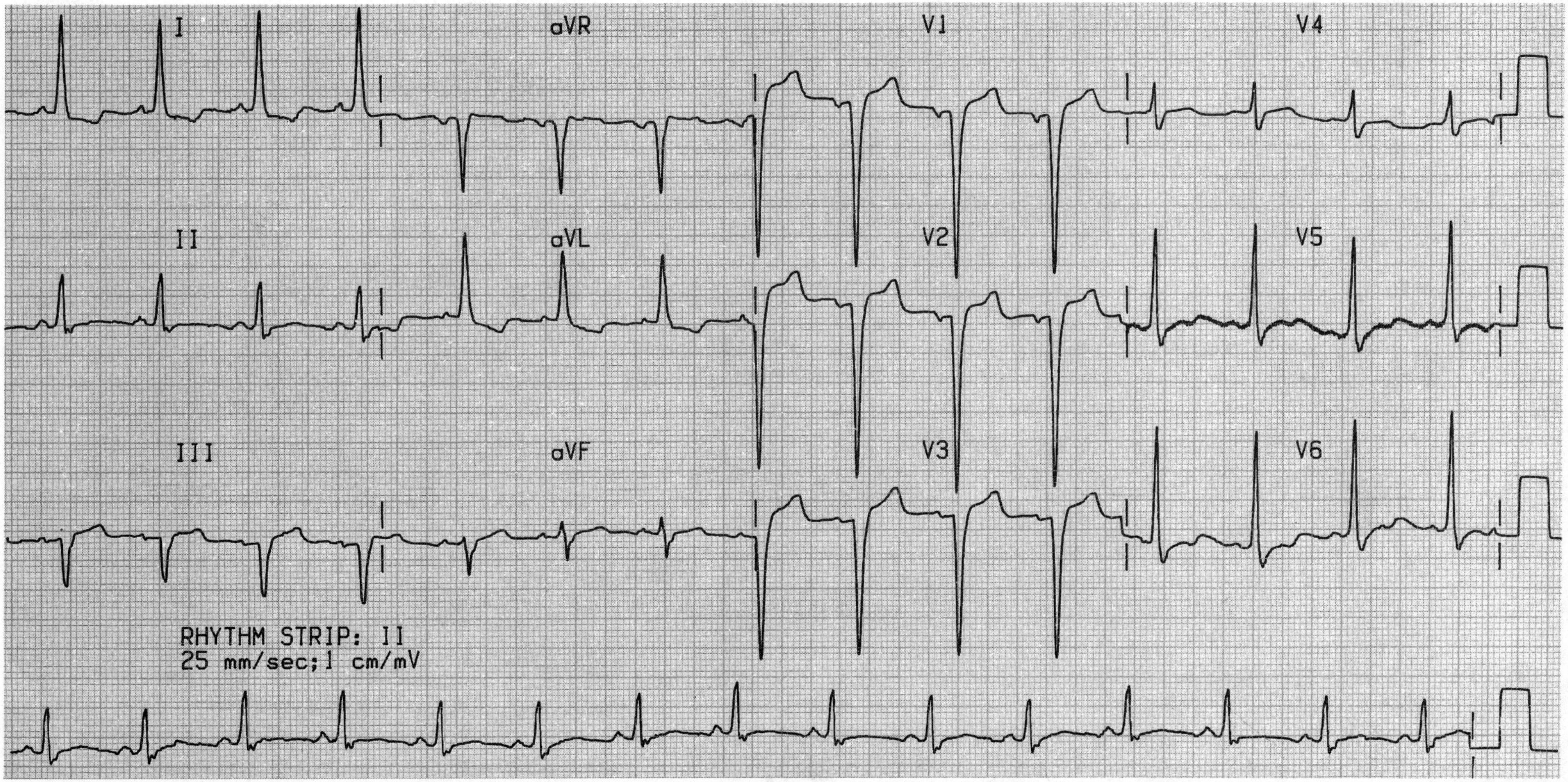

E-22

NARRATIVE INTERPRETATION

Rhythm:	**Sinus**
Rate:	**90**
Intervals:	**PR 0.14, QRS 0.11, QT 0.36**
Axis:	**−15 degrees**

Abnormalities

Abnormal P terminal force V1. SV2 + RV5 greater than 35. ST depression leads I, aVL, V6. T wave inversion leads I, aVL, V6. QS leads V1–V2. "Micro" R wave lead V3. Prolonged QRS duration.

Synthesis

Sinus rhythm. Left atrial abnormality. Left ventricular hypertrophy with associated ST-T-wave abnormalities. Intraventricular conduction delay. Cannot exclude prior anteroseptal myocardial infarction.

TEST ANSWERS: 1, 60, 76, 78, (82), 103.

Comment: Note that a "pseudoinfarction" pattern is present in leads V1–V3. The diagnosis of anteroseptal myocardial infarction is difficult in the presence of LVH. The transitional zone is commonly shifted leftward in patients with LVH and may produce either poor R wave progression, or as in this example, a QS pattern in the right precordial leads. Although an anteroseptal myocardial infarction cannot be excluded, there should be additional supporting evidence with either clinical data or serial electrocardiograms to support this diagnosis.

REFERENCES: Chou p 40. Goldberger I.

E-23

Clinical History

A 79-year-old woman with long-standing COPD.

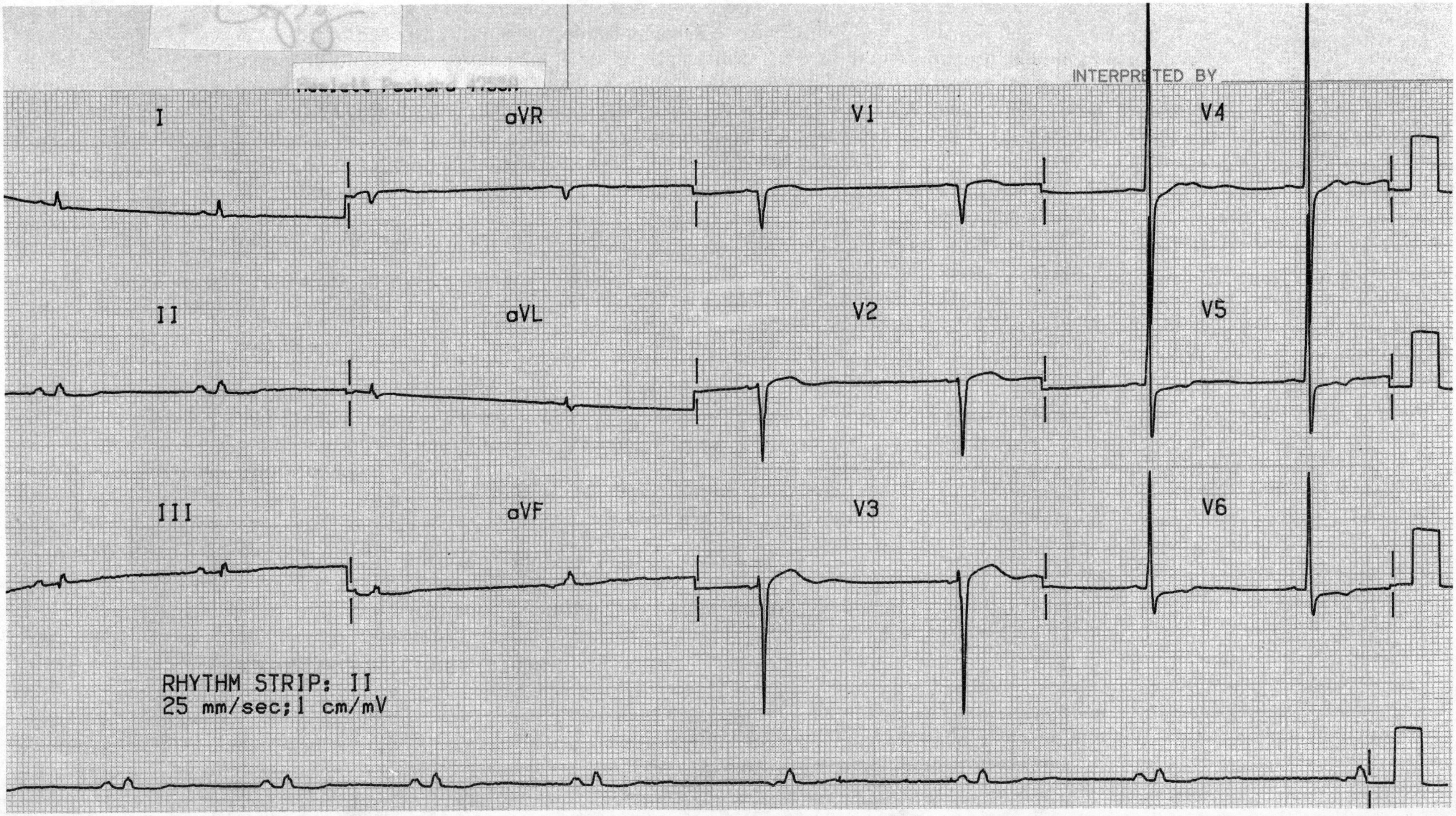

E-23

NARRATIVE INTERPRETATION

Rhythm:	**Sinus bradycardia, sinus pause**
Rate:	**52**
Intervals:	**PR 0.16, QRS 0.08, QT 0.40**
Axis:	**+60 degrees**

Abnormalities
Slow heart rate. Sinus pause with AV junctional escape complexes. Low voltage in limb leads. SV2 + RV5 greater than 35. R wave leads V1–V3 less than 3 mm. ST depression leads II, aVF, V4–V6. Low T-wave voltage in limb leads. T wave biphasic leads V5–V6.

Synthesis
Sinus bradycardia with sinus pause. AV junctional escape complexes. Low voltage in limb leads. Poor R-wave progression. LVH. Associated nonspecific ST-T-wave abnormalities.

TEST ANSWERS: 3, 7, 24, 66, 67, 78, 103.

Comment: This tracing demonstrates sinus bradycardia with a periodic sinus pause and AV junctional escape beats. Note that the intrinsic sinus bradycardic rate is around 52 beats per minute, whereas the AV junctional rate is about 42 beats per minute. Sinus bradycardia with sinus arrhythmia cannot be completely excluded but there is no definite evidence of a gradual prolongation of the PP interval beyond 0.16 s in order to make the diagnosis of sinus arrhythmia. This patient also had the interesting combination of low voltage in the limb leads secondary to chronic pulmonary disease and increased voltage in the precordial leads secondary to long-standing hypertension.

E-24

Clinical History

A 78-year-old woman in the ICU with gastrointestinal bleeding. She has a history of multiple MIs.

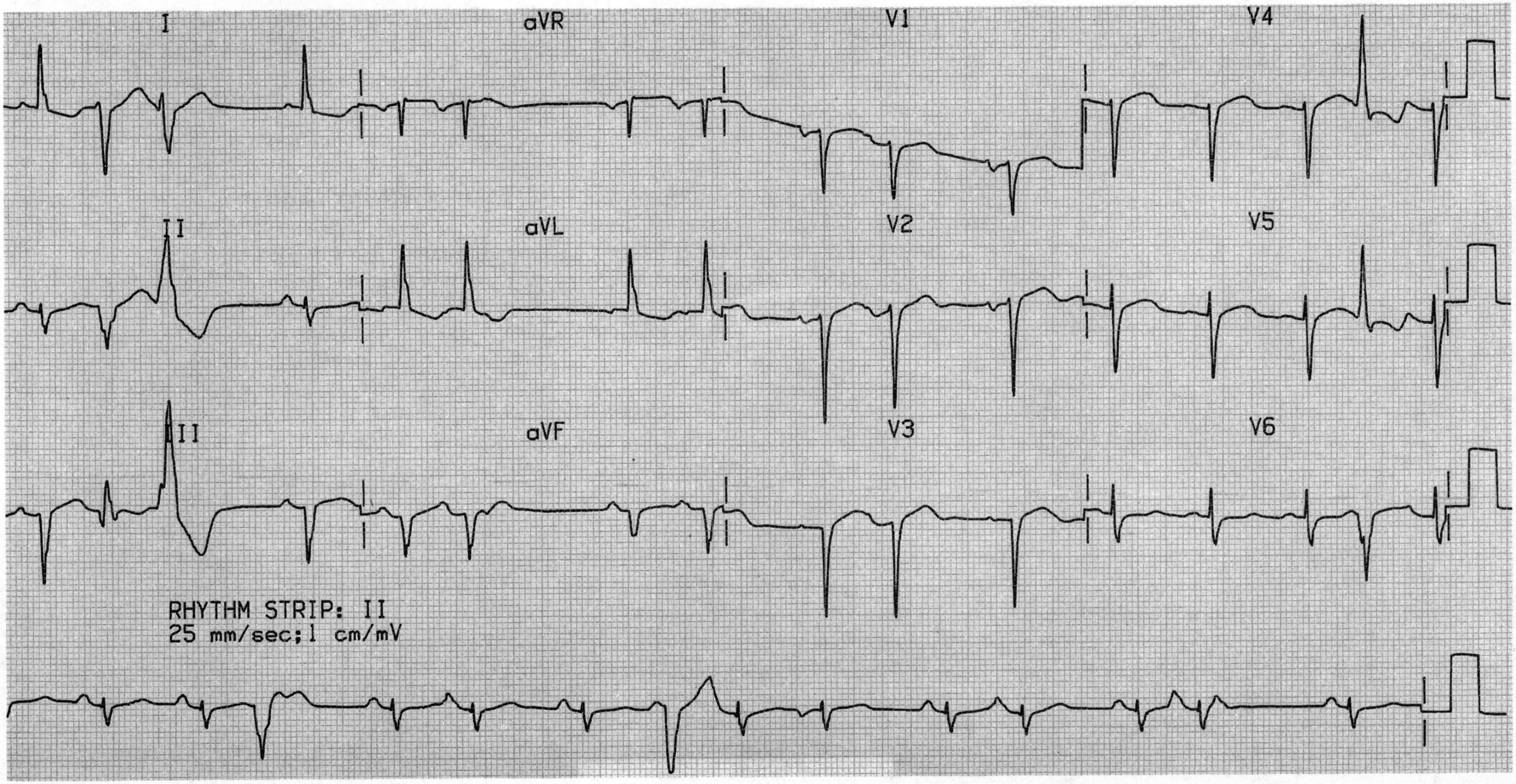

E-24

NARRATIVE INTERPRETATION

Rhythm: **Sinus**
Rate: **87**
Intervals: **PR 0.16, QRS 0.08, QT 0.36**
Axis: **−45 degrees**

Abnormalities

APCs, normally conducted. Nonconducted APC. VPCs. Paired, multiform VPCs. Echo complexes. Axis leftward of −30 degrees. R wave leads V1–V3 less than 3 mm. ST depression leads I, aVL. ST elevation leads III, aVF, V2–V5. T-wave inversion leads I, aVL.

Synthesis

Sinus rhythm. VPCs. Paired, multifocal VPCs. VPC with echo beat and retrograde atrial activation. APCs. Nonconducted APC. Left axis deviation. Left anterior fascicular block. Poor R-wave progression. Probable anterior wall MI of indeterminate age. Nonspecific ST-T-wave abnormalities. Cannot exclude acute myocardial injury.

TEST ANSWERS: 1, 10, 12, 26, 27, 28, 54, 55, 64, 66, 72, (84), (100), 106.

Comment: Note that the basic sinus mechanism is evident in only a few beats in this tracing. The first two complexes of the rhythm strip and the first three complexes in leads V4–V6 demonstrate the native rhythm. Frequent VPCs are noted as well as frequent APCs. The seventh complex of the rhythm strip is a "late" VPC, which occurs just as the P wave is appearing. The T wave of this complex is tall secondary to a retrograde P wave from ventriculoatrial conduction. This retrograde P wave is then conducted back to the ventricles as an echo beat. The negative P wave of the ninth complex of the rhythm strip also suggests one more cycle of retrograde atrial activation with a more prolonged VA interval. A junctional or atrial premature beat is also possible. The sinus mechanism resumes with the next complex. The thirteenth complex of the rhythm strip is a normally conducted APC. A second APC, which is nonconducted, follows immediately afterward.

This example also points out the importance of reviewing prior tracings, if they are available. An anterior wall MI is suggested by the poor (reverse) R-wave progression and ST-T-wave abnormalities. These were unchanged from prior tracings. Acute ST elevation indicative of myocardial injury cannot, however, be excluded on the basis of this single electrocardiogram.

E-25

Clinical History

A 72-year-old woman seen on routine follow-up.

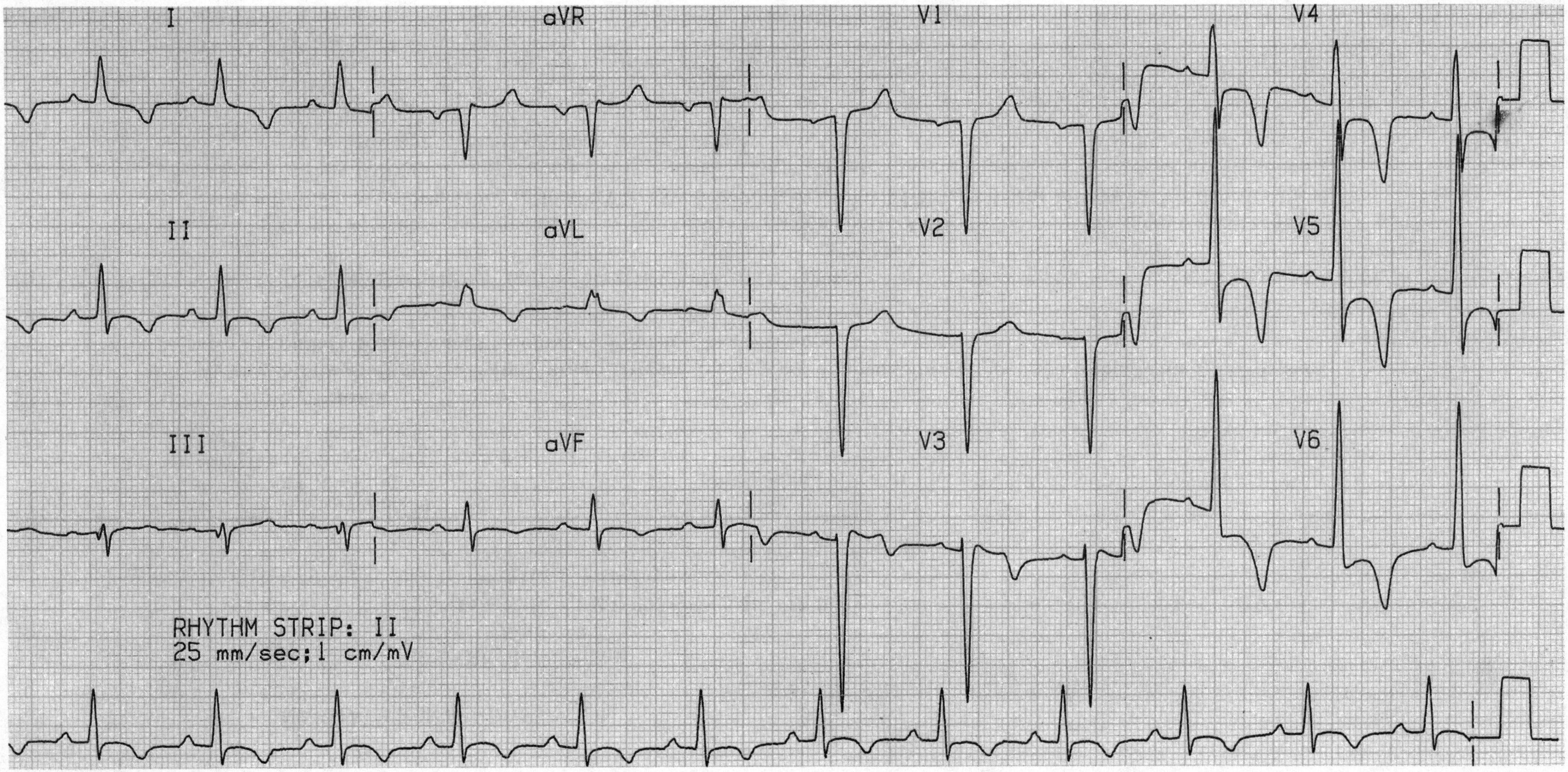

E-25

NARRATIVE INTERPRETATION

Rhythm: **Sinus**
Rate: **74**
Intervals: **PR 0.20, QRS 0.10, QT 0.40**
Axis: **+15 degrees**

Abnormalities

ST depression leads V4–V6. T-wave inversion leads I, II, aVL, aVF, V3–V6. SV2 + RV5 greater than 35. R wave less than 3 mm leads V1–V3.

Synthesis

Sinus rhythm. LVH by voltage criteria. ST-T-wave abnormalities associated either with LVH or secondary to myocardial ischemia. Poor R-wave progression.

TEST ANSWERS: 1, 66, 78, 102, 103.

Comment: This patient has fairly obvious criteria for LVH. At first glance, there appears to be a left bundle branch pattern in lead aVL; however, criteria for LBBB are absent in view of a QRS duration of only 0.10 s. Incomplete LBBB is a consideration, but there is no significant slurring of the R wave in the left precordial leads or delay in the intrinsicoid deflection. There is loss of the septal Q waves in the left precordial leads, a finding in incomplete LBBB and in septal fibrosis. The poor R-wave progression is likely secondary to LVH; however, a prior anteroseptal wall MI cannot be excluded. The ST-T-wave abnormalities appear more pronounced than those normally seen in LVH alone and suggest the diagnosis of coronary heart disease.

REFERENCES: Romanelli. Chou p 81.

E-26

Clinical History

A 38-year-old asymptomatic man.

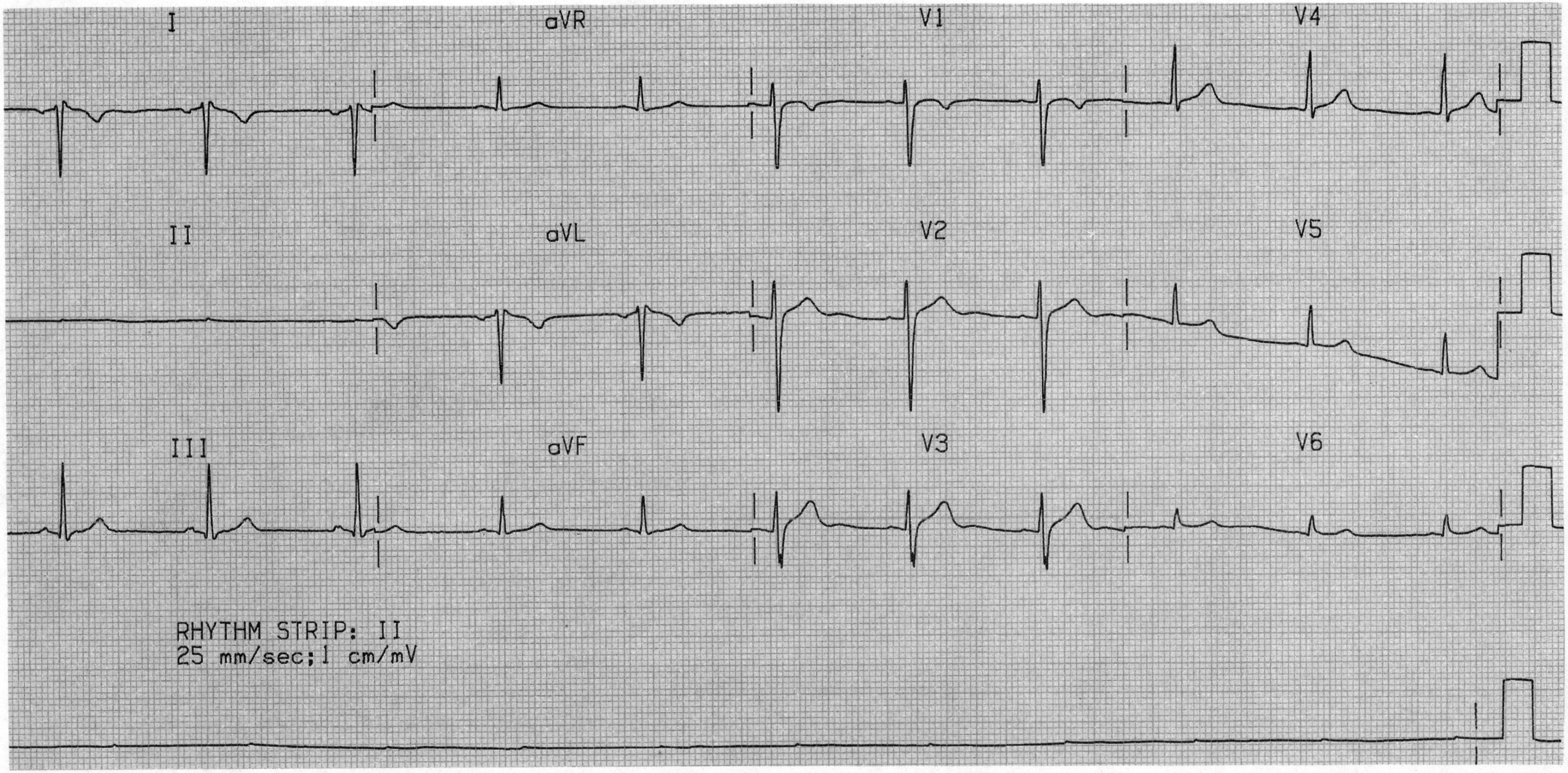

E-26

NARRATIVE INTERPRETATION

Rhythm: **Sinus**
Rate: **61**
Intervals: **PR 0.18, QRS 0.08, QT 0.36**
Axis: **xx degrees**

Abnormalities
Electrode reversal. Tracing uninterpretable.

Synthesis
Sinus rhythm. Right arm and right leg limb electrode reversal.

TEST ANSWERS: 1, 112.

Comment: This tracing demonstrates the characteristic findings of a reversal of the right arm and right leg electrodes. The P wave and QRS complex are negative in leads I and aVL and are positive in lead aVR. Lead II appears as isoelectric because this lead now records the electrical potential between the right and left legs, which is virtually zero. It is important to recognize that apparent asystole in a single lead of the electrocardiogram may be artifactual owing to incorrect electrode placement. More than one monitoring lead is always desirable.

E-27

Clinical History

A 75-year-old man with chronic atrial fibrillation with nausea and dehydration. Medications include digoxin. He is a long-time smoker.

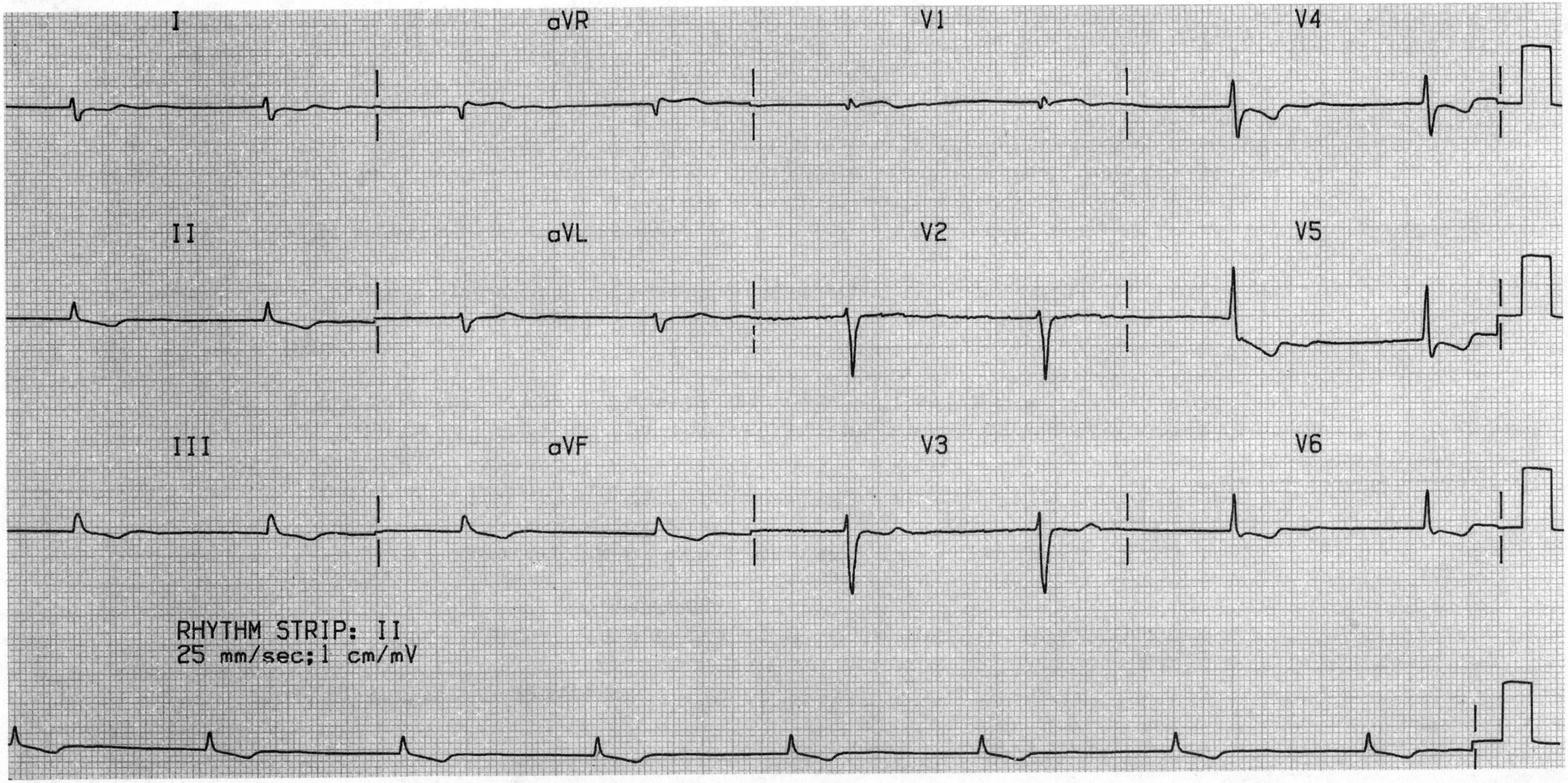

E-27

NARRATIVE INTERPRETATION

Rhythm:	**Atrial fibrillation with complete AV block, AV junctional escape rhythm**
Rate:	**45**
Intervals:	**PR –, QRS 0.08, QT 0.38**
Axis:	**+105 degrees**

Abnormalities

Axis rightward of +90 degrees. Limb-lead voltage less than 6 mm. R wave leads V1–V3 less than 3 mm. ST depression leads I, V3–V6. T-wave inversion leads II, III, aVF, V4–V6.

Synthesis

Atrial fibrillation with complete AV block. AV junctional escape rhythm. Low-voltage limb leads. Right axis deviation. Nonspecific ST-T-wave abnormalities. Poor R-wave progression.

TEST ANSWERS: 20, 22, 47, 65, 66, 67, 106.

Comment: This patient became markedly dehydrated and developed renal insufficiency. As a result, digoxin was accumulated. A "regularized" rhythm in a patient with atrial fibrillation should raise the suspicion of digitalis toxicity. Electronic filtering of an electrocardiogram, present in this electrocardiogram, may occasionally make interpretation more difficult. The presence of "fine" fibrillatory waves is difficult to see but is best observed in lead V2. Confirmation is best made after comparison with prior tracings. Additional points in this electrocardiogram are findings suggestive of chronic pulmonary disease. A mean QRS axis of +105 degrees is unusual in older persons. Low voltage and poor R-wave progression are also characteristic of pulmonary emphysema.

REFERENCES: Fisch. Smith. Chou p 55. Schmock (*Chest* 60:328–334, 1971). Schmock (*Chest* 60:335–340, 1971).

E-28

Clinical History

A 59-year-old asymptomatic man seen in the clinic 1 month following a CCU admission.

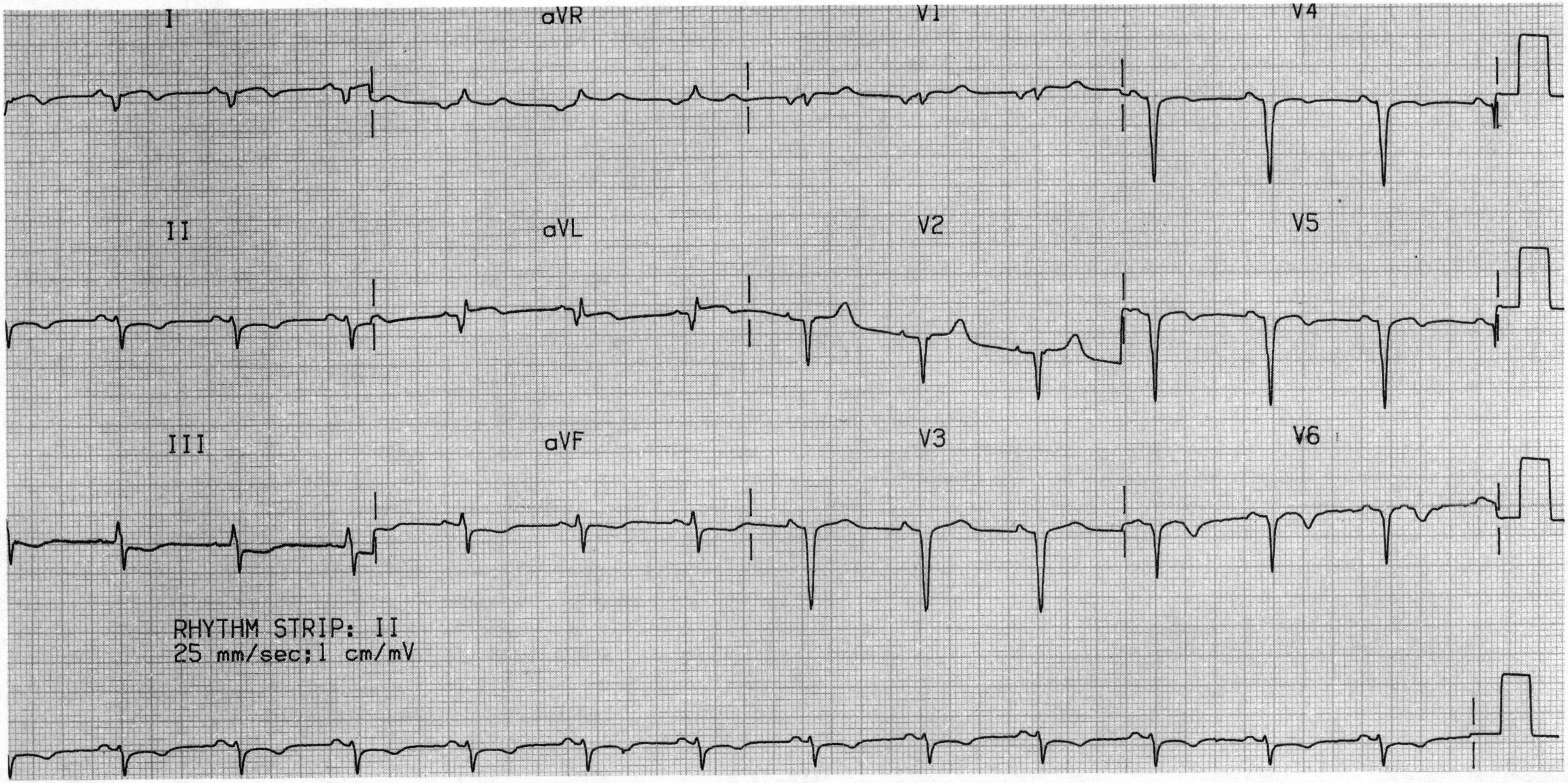

E-28

NARRATIVE INTERPRETATION

Rhythm: **Sinus**
Rate: **76**
Intervals: **PR 0.12, QRS 0.08, QT 0.38**
Axis: **+225 degrees**

Abnormalities

Marked right axis deviation. Q waves leads I, aVL. QS waves leads V2, V6. "Micro" R waves with RS pattern leads V2–V5. ST elevation leads I, aVL, V5–V6. ST depression leads II, III, aVF. T-wave inversion leads I, II, III, aVF, V4–V6. Abnormal P terminal force lead V1.

Synthesis

Sinus rhythm. Right axis deviation. Left anterior fascicular block. Extensive anterior and lateral wall MI. ST-T-wave abnormalities suggesting myocardial ischemia. ST-T-wave abnormalities suggesting aneurysm formation. Left atrial abnormality.

TEST ANSWERS: 1, 60, 65, 72, 88, 90, 95, 102.

Comment: This patient has evidence of extensive myocardial necrosis. There is extensive loss of R forces across the entire precordium with concomitant infarction of the lateral wall. In an asymptomatic person, persistent ST elevation in the lateral leads is evidence of aneurysm formation. In the absence of clinical correlation, one cannot distinguish the ST elevation from that of recent myocardial injury. Lateral wall MI will often produce right axis deviation. The marked axis shift in this example is likely secondary to the left anterior fascicular block combined with lateral and anterior infarction.

REFERENCE: Milliken.

E-29

Clinical History

A 31-year-old man with dyspnea on exertion.

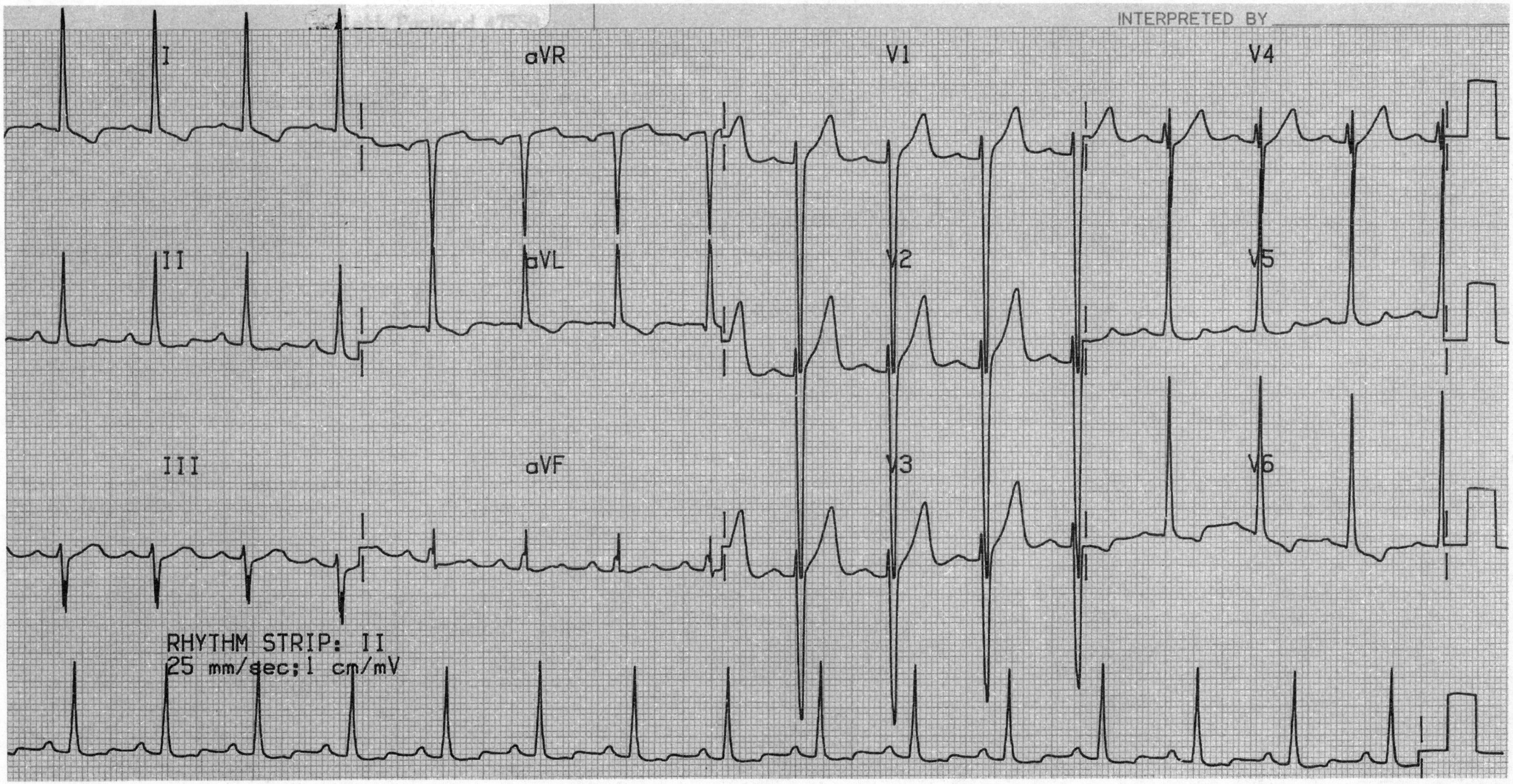

E-29

NARRATIVE INTERPRETATION

Rhythm: **Sinus**
Rate: **90**
Intervals: **PR 0.16, QRS 0.08, QT 0.32**
Axis: **+15 degrees**

Abnormalities

SV2 + RV5 greater than 45. ST depression leads I, II, aVL, aVF, V5–V6. T-wave inversion leads I, aVL, V6. Biphasic T waves leads II, V5.

Synthesis

Sinus rhythm. LVH. Associated ST-T-wave abnormalities.

TEST ANSWERS: 1, 78, 103.

Comment: This patient had LVH on the basis of congenital aortic valve disease with chronic aortic insufficiency. Patients with aortic regurgitation often have massive left ventricular enlargement. The precordial voltage criterion of 45 rather than 35 is used for the diagnosis of LVH because of the patient's age.

REFERENCES: Manning. Walker. Kannel (1987).

E-30

Clinical History

A 28-year-old woman with palpitations seen in the emergency department.

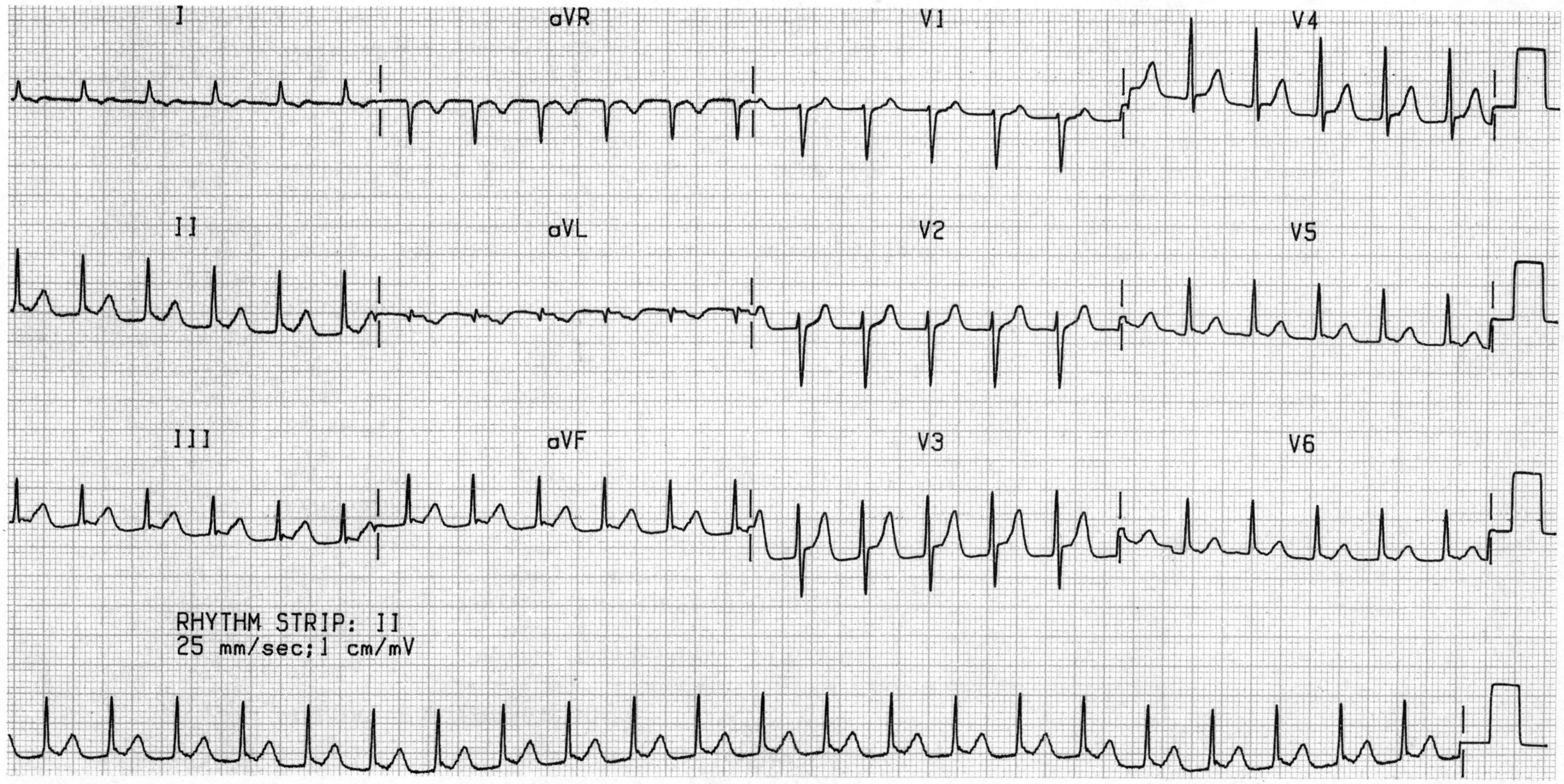

E-30

NARRATIVE INTERPRETATION

Rhythm:	**Supraventricular tachycardia**
Rate:	**135**
Intervals:	**PR –, QRS 0.08, QT 0.28**
Axis:	**+60 degrees**

Abnormalities
Rapid heart rate. ST-segment elevation at J point leads II, III, aVF, V3–V6.

Synthesis
Supraventricular tachycardia. Nonspecific ST-segment abnormalities. Normal variant, J-point elevation.

TEST ANSWERS: 18, 96, 106.

Comment: This tracing may represent an orthodromic AV reciprocating tachycardia that involves the AV node as the antegrade limb and an AV nodal bypass tract as the retrograde limb. This is the second most common mechanism of supraventricular tachycardia (second only to AV nodal reentrant tachycardia). A clue for involvement of an accessory pathway in the retrograde limb of the reentry circuit is a P wave seen after the QRS complex. With careful examination, an inverted P wave may be seen in lead I, with a suggestion of this in leads II, III, and aVF as well.

REFERENCE: Manolis.

E-31

Clinical History

A 63-year-old man with chest discomfort.

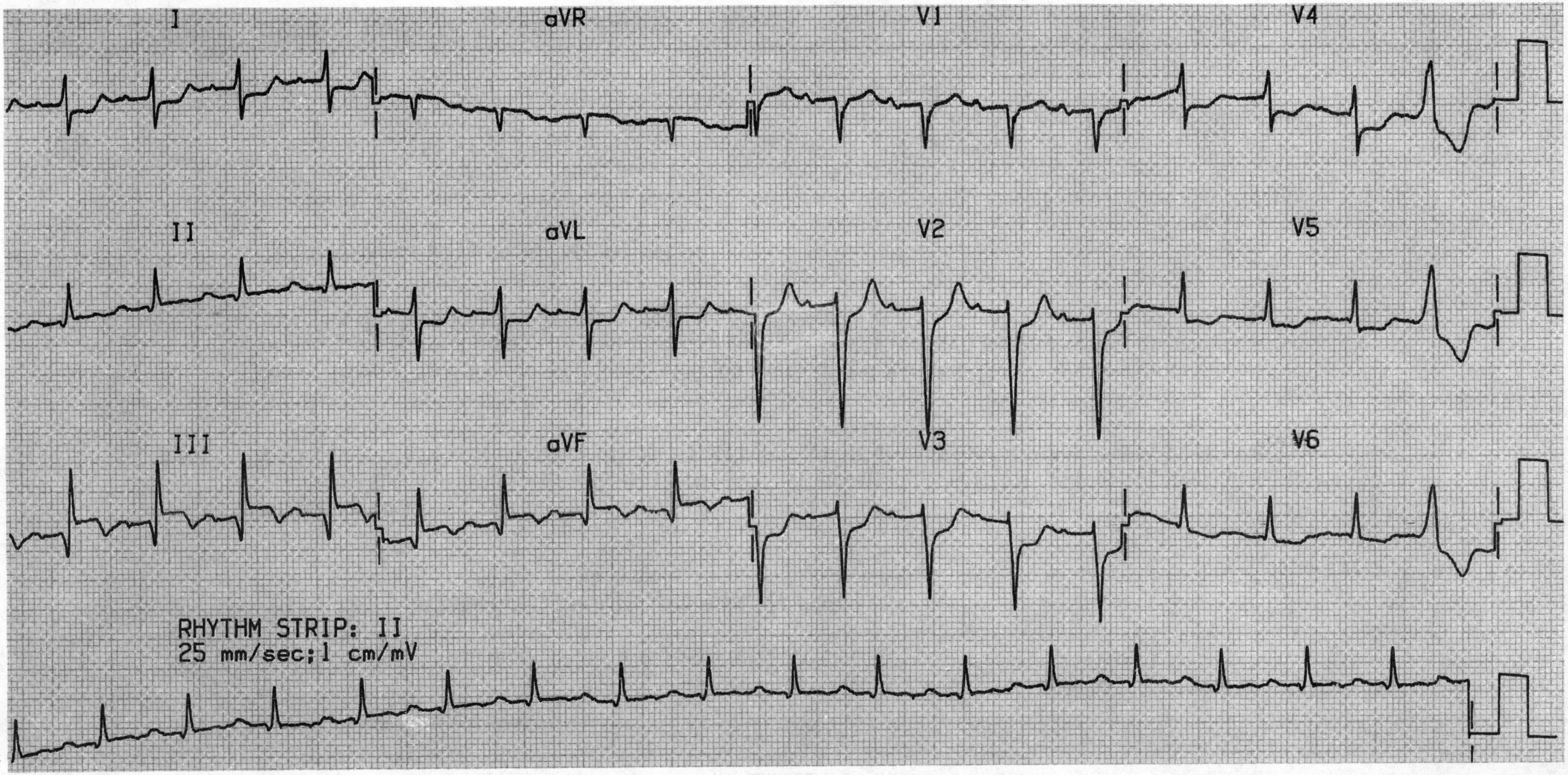

E-31

NARRATIVE INTERPRETATION

Rhythm: **Sinus with first-degree AV block**
Rate: **100**
Intervals: **PR 0.24, QRS 0.08, QT 0.34**
Axis: **+90 degrees**

Abnormalities

Prolonged PR interval. Q waves leads II, III, aVF. ST elevation leads II, III, aVF. ST depression leads I, aVL, V2–V6. T-wave inversion leads III, aVF, V4–V6. R wave leads V1–V3 less than 3 mm. VPC.

Synthesis

Sinus rhythm. First-degree AV block. VPC. Inferior wall MI with ST-T-wave abnormalities suggestive of acute myocardial injury. ST abnormalities in leads I, aVL, V2–V6 suggestive of either myocardial ischemia or reciprocal changes. Poor R-wave progression.

TEST ANSWERS: 1, 26, 42, 66, 91, 100, 101.

Comment: It is quite controversial whether or not the anterior ST-segment depression seen in patients with acute inferior MI represents additional myocardial ischemia or is simply a reciprocal electrical phenomenon. The ST depression in leads V2 and V3 should also raise the suspicion of posterior infarction; however, there is no supporting ST depression in lead V1. Posterior infarction is also unlikely in view of the very small, narrow R waves in the right precordial leads.

REFERENCES: Shah. Croft. Schweitzer (1990).

E-32

Clinical History

A 68-year-old woman admitted to the CCU for dyspnea.

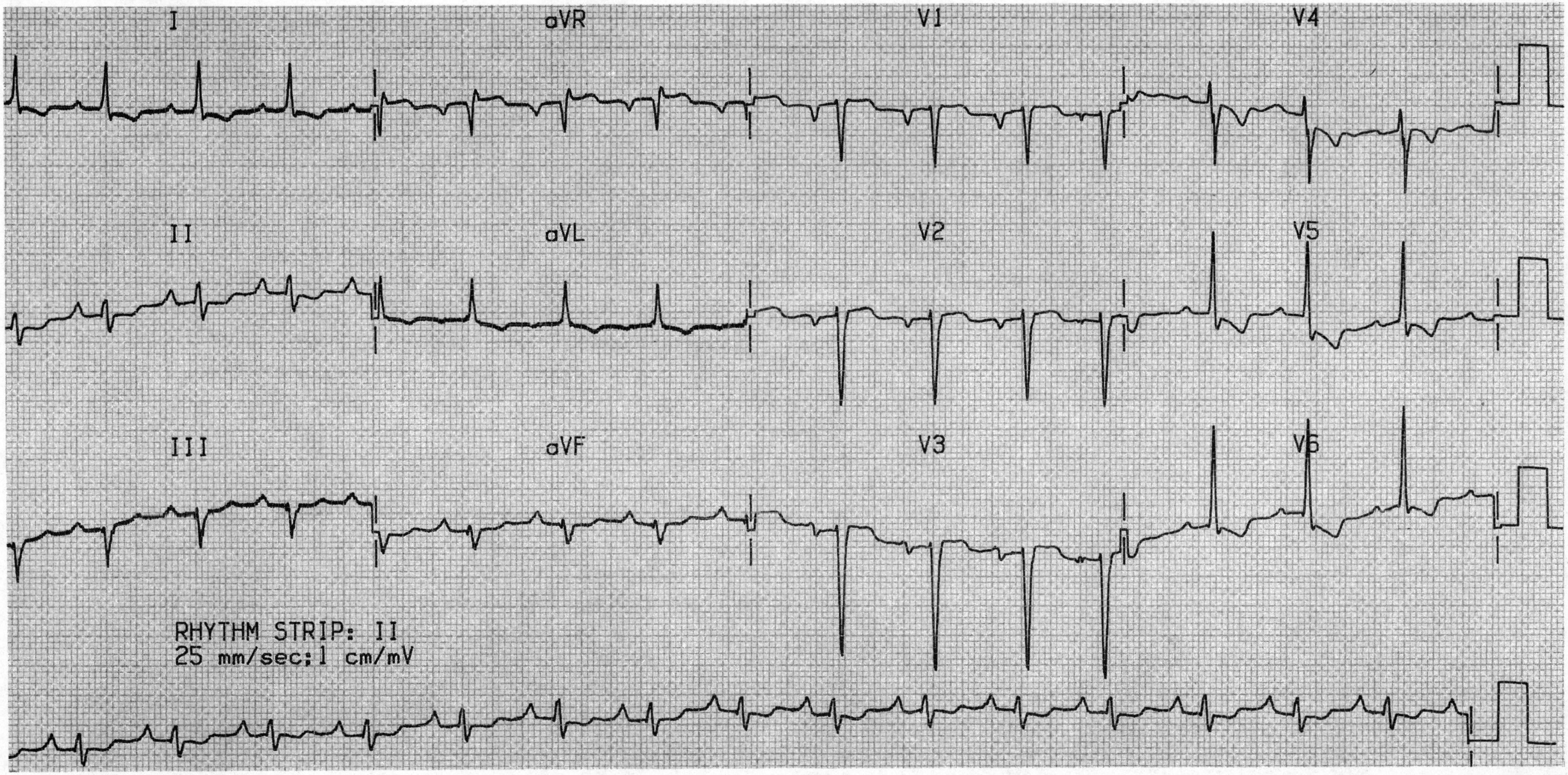

E-32

NARRATIVE INTERPRETATION

Rhythm: **Sinus**
Rate: **96**
Intervals: **PR 0.20, QRS 0.08, QT 0.30**
Axis: **−30 degrees**

Abnormalities

Abnormal P terminal force lead V1. ST depression leads I, II, aVL,aVF, V5, V6. T-wave inversion leads I, aVL, V4–V6. Biphasic T waves leads II, aVF, V2, V3. R-wave voltage less than 3 mm leads V1–V3. APC.

Synthesis

Sinus rhythm. APC. Left atrial abnormality. Nonspecific ST-T-wave abnormalities. Poor R-wave progression.

TEST ANSWERS: 1, 10, 60, 66, 106.

Comment: At first glance the reader might suspect that LVH is evident; however, voltage criteria are not met in either the limb or precordial leads. The ST-T-wave abnormalities are also nonspecific. This patient did have mild cardiomegaly secondary to long-standing mitral insufficiency. Left atrial abnormality is easily appreciated in lead V1. The reader is cautioned not to overlook the APC (fourth complex of the right precordial leads).

REFERENCES: Surawicz. Romhilt (1968). Romhilt (1969).

E-33

Clinical History

An 80-year-old man admitted to the ICU.

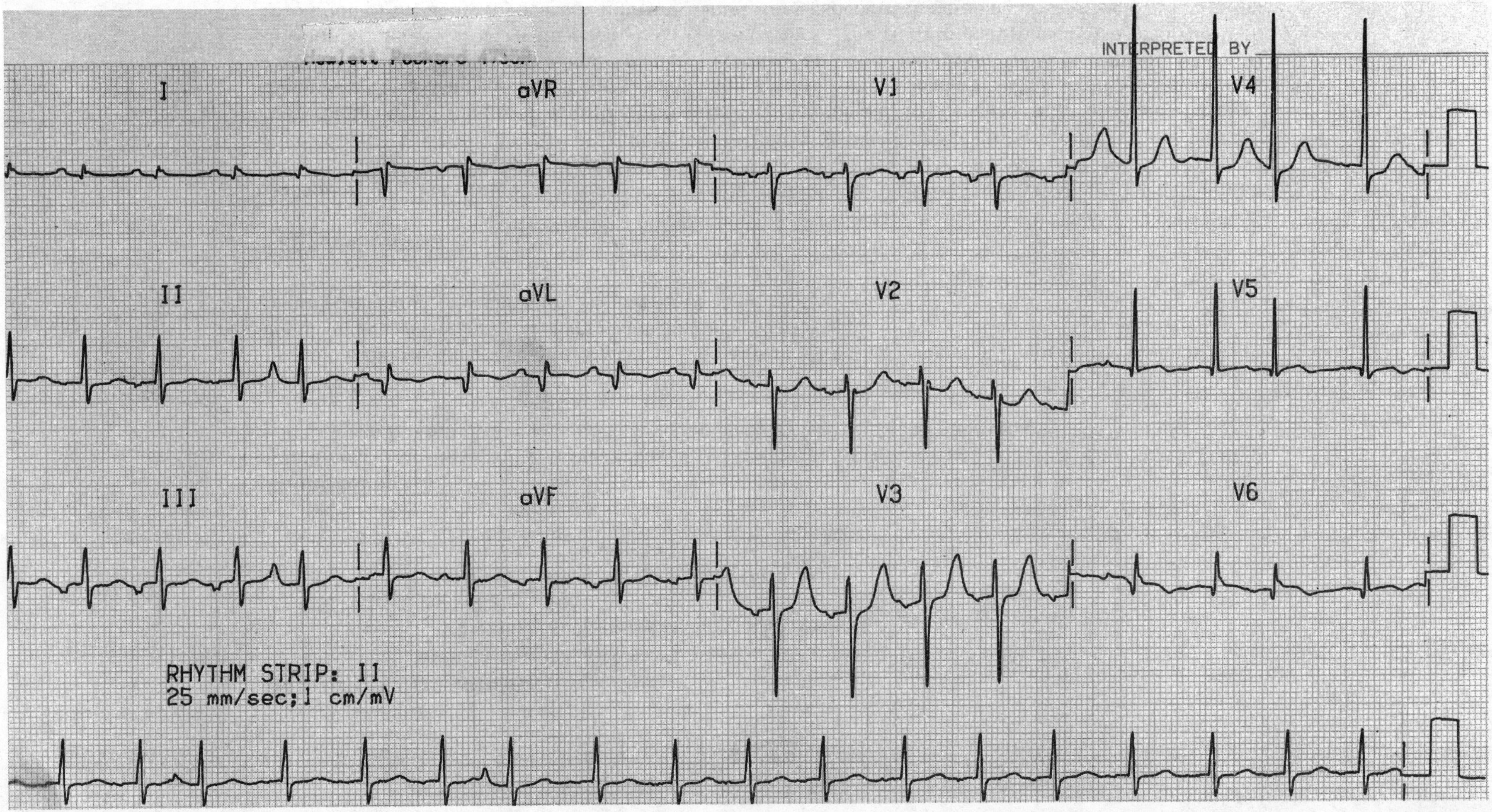

E-33

NARRATIVE INTERPRETATION

Rhythm: **Accelerated ectopic atrial rhythm**
Rate: **105**
Intervals: **PR 0.16, QRS 0.08, QT 0.36**
Axis: **+60 degrees**

Abnormalities

Rapid heart rate. Inverted P waves leads II, III, aVF. PR elevation leads II, III, aVF. APCs. Small Q waves leads I, V6. Q wave aVL. ST elevation leads aVL, V5–V6. ST depression leads V2–V4.

Synthesis

Ectopic atrial rhythm, accelerated. APCs. Lateral wall MI with ST-segment abnormalities suggestive of acute myocardial injury. ST depression in leads V2–V4 suggestive of either myocardial ischemia or reciprocal change. PR elevation suggestive of atrial injury.

TEST ANSWERS: 9, 10, (23), 89, 100, 101.

Comment: This is a difficult tracing to interpret for a number of reasons. The rhythm may be accelerated AV junctional with antegrade block, which thus allows for a normal PR interval, or it may represent an accelerated ectopic atrial focus. By definition, the rate of an accelerated ectopic atrial rhythm is greater than 100 beats per minute. It is difficult to diagnose a lateral wall MI because of the absence of a clear diagnostic Q wave in lead I to accompany the abnormal Q wave in lead aVL. The slight ST elevation in leads aVL and V6 requires some comment regarding an acute infarction. This patient did go on to develop a lateral wall MI with positive CPK isoenzymes. The rhythm disturbance also resolved with resolution of the acute myocardial injury. An interesting aspect of this tracing is the PR elevation in the inferior limb leads, which suggests atrial injury. Atrial arrhythmias often accompany atrial infarction.

REFERENCES: Chou p 318. Friedman p 134.

E-34

Clinical History

A 70-year-old woman seen in the emergency department for nausea. She is prescribed digoxin and diuretics for congestive heart failure.

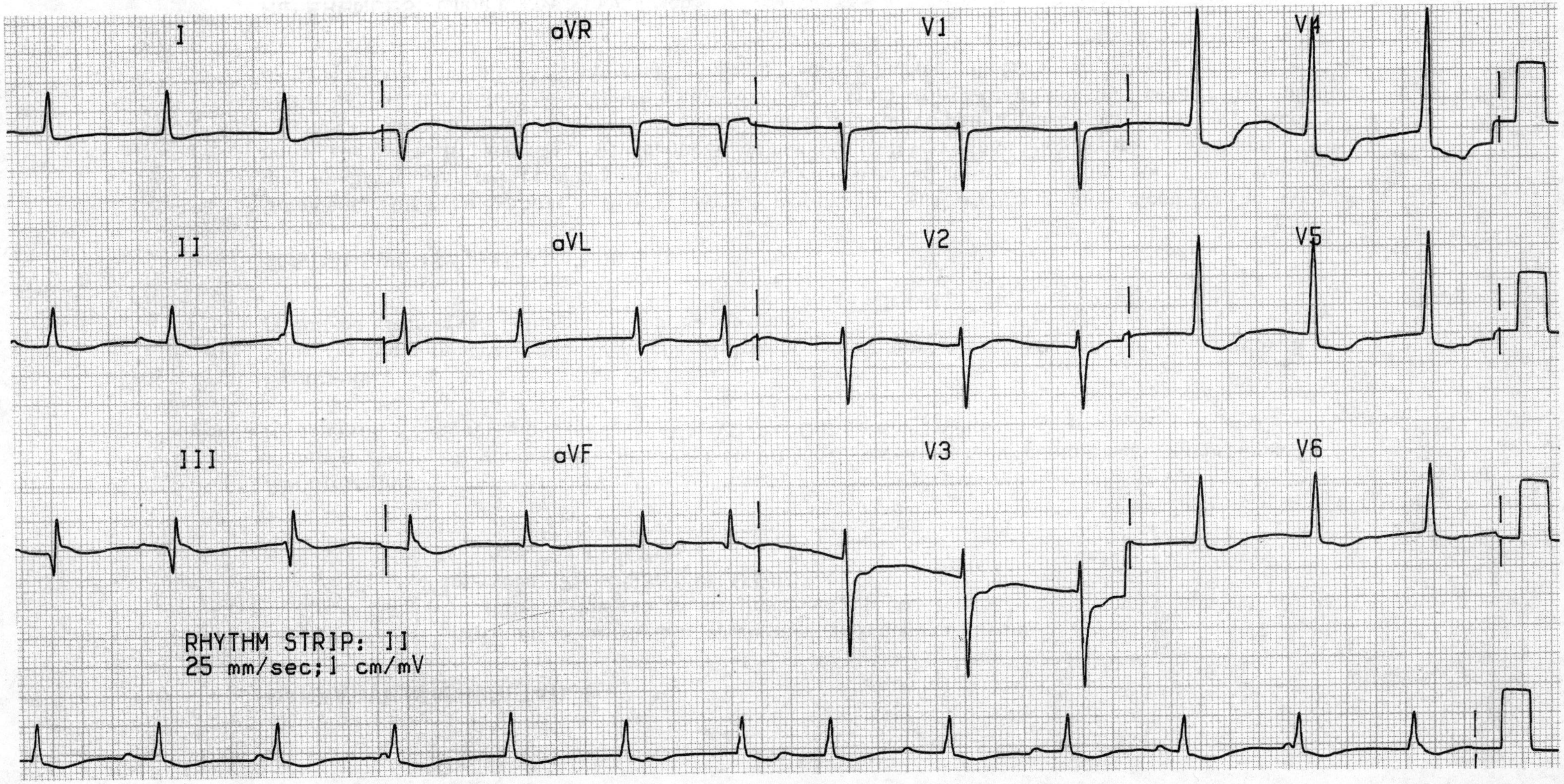

E-34

NARRATIVE INTERPRETATION

Rhythm:	**Sinus rhythm, accelerated AV junctional rhythm**
Rate:	**Sinus rate 68, AV junctional rate 74**
Intervals:	**PR –, QRS 0.08, QT 0.38**
Axis:	**+45 degrees**

Abnormalities

Failure of P waves to conduct to ventricles. Isorhythmic dissociation. Sinus capture beat with prolonged PR interval. ST depression leads I, II, aVF, V2–V6. Diffuse low T voltage.

Synthesis

Sinus rhythm with accelerated AV junctional rhythm. Isorhythmic AV dissociation. Sinus capture with prolonged PR interval. Diffuse ST-T-wave abnormalities.

TEST ANSWERS: 1, 23, 53, 57, 106.

Comment: This is an example of two supraventricular mechanisms' occurring simultaneously. The AV junction has accelerated secondary to digitalis toxicity and usurped control of the normally slower sinus node. The two heart rates are nearly identical and manifest as P waves and QRS complexes that appear together but are unrelated. Although AV dissociation is present, complete heart block is not, as proved by the ventricular capture beat (eighth complex on the rhythm strip). Additional signs of the effects of digitalis are the generalized ST-segment depression and low T-wave voltage.

REFERENCES: Chou p 459. Saner. Fisch.

E-35

Clinical History

An 81-year-old asymptomatic man.

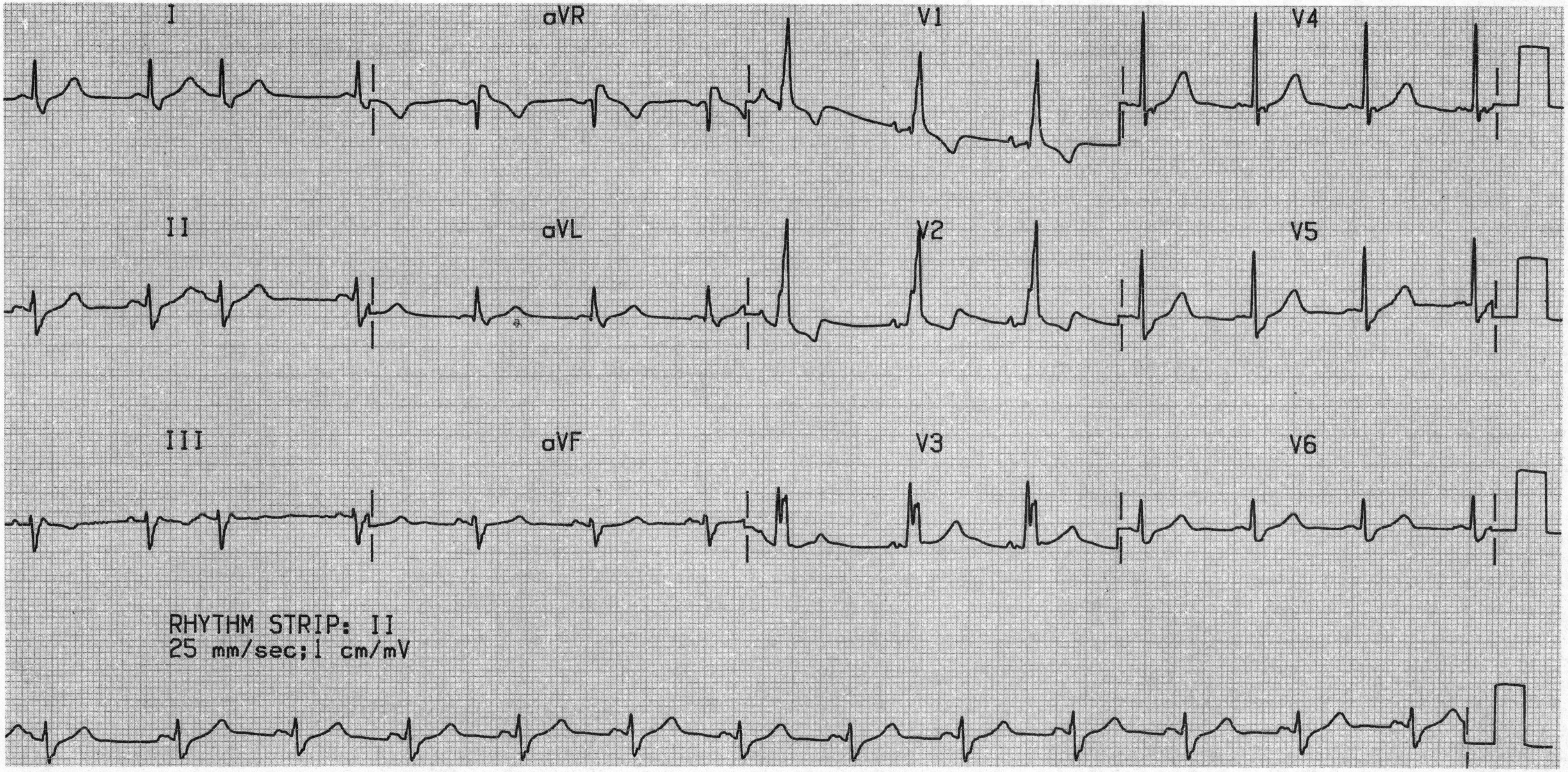

E-35

NARRATIVE INTERPRETATION

Rhythm: **Sinus**
Rate: **80**
Intervals: **PR 0.12, QRS 0.12, QT 0.36**
Axis: **−45 degrees**

Abnormalities

APC. Axis leftward of −30 degrees. Broad QRS with rsR′ leads V1–V3 and T-wave inversion leads V1–V2.

Synthesis

Sinus rhythm. APC. RBBB. Associated ST-T-wave abnormalities. Left axis deviation. Left anterior fascicular block.

TEST ANSWERS: 1, 10, 64, 70, 72, 104.

Comment: This tracing is from an asymptomatic patient with "bifascicular block." Although patients with bifascicular block have an excess mortality over patients without such findings, the causes of death are related to underlying cardiac disease and not to advanced heart block. Accordingly, prophylactic permanent pacing is not indicated in asymptomatic patients. Note that the PR interval is at the lower limits of normal but does not have characteristics that suggest an ectopic or AV junctional focus.

REFERENCE: McAnulty.

E-36

Clinical History

A 90-year-old asymptomatic man.

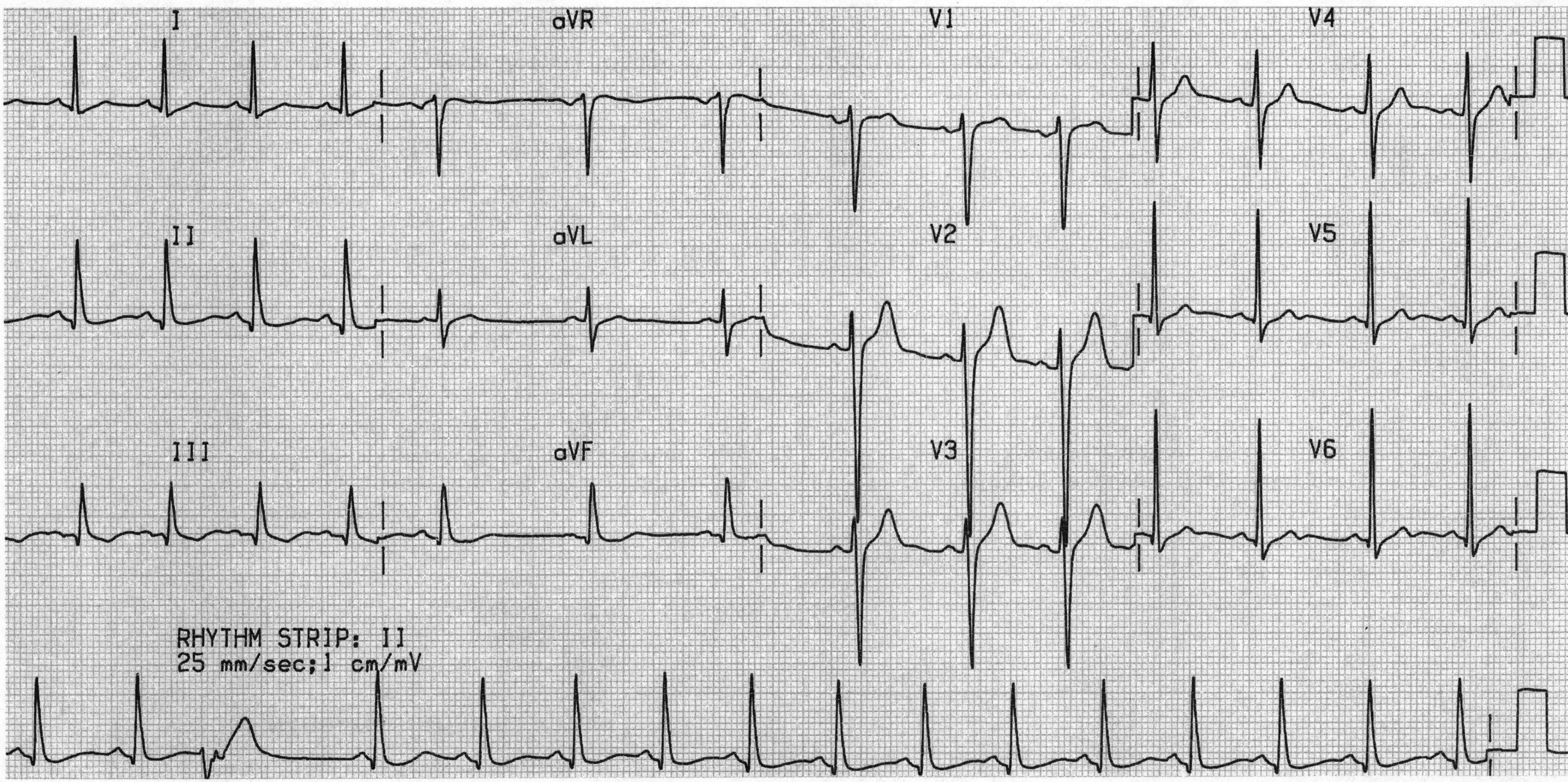

E-36

NARRATIVE INTERPRETATION

Rhythm: **Sinus**
Rate: **100**
Intervals: **PR 0.16, QRS 0.08, QT 0.36**
Axis: **+60 degrees**

Abnormalities

VPC on rhythm strip with prolonged postectopic pause. Complex following pause with short PR interval. Sinus pause with temporary abrupt change in sinus rate. Slight ST depression lead aVF. SV2 + RV5 greater than 35.

Synthesis

Sinus rhythm. Sinus pause probably secondary to SA block. VPC with prolonged postectopic interval and probable junctional escape complex. LVH. Associated ST-segment abnormality.

TEST ANSWERS: 1, 7, (8), 24, 26, 78, 103.

Comment: The patient's sinus rhythm is seen to pause abruptly after the fifth complex in the limb leads. The interval between the next three slower beats is not identical and is not a multiple of the intrinsic sinus rate, which thus excludes a diagnosis of 2:1 second-degree SA block. First-degree SA block is the likely mechanism of these pauses, although this cannot be confirmed on the surface electrocardiogram. Note also the prolonged postectopic interval after the VPC on the rhythm strip. The following P wave occurs later than expected and demonstrates a short PR interval. This is probably a junctional or "low" atrial escape beat.

E-37

Clinical History

An 88-year-old man with a history of a diastolic murmur.

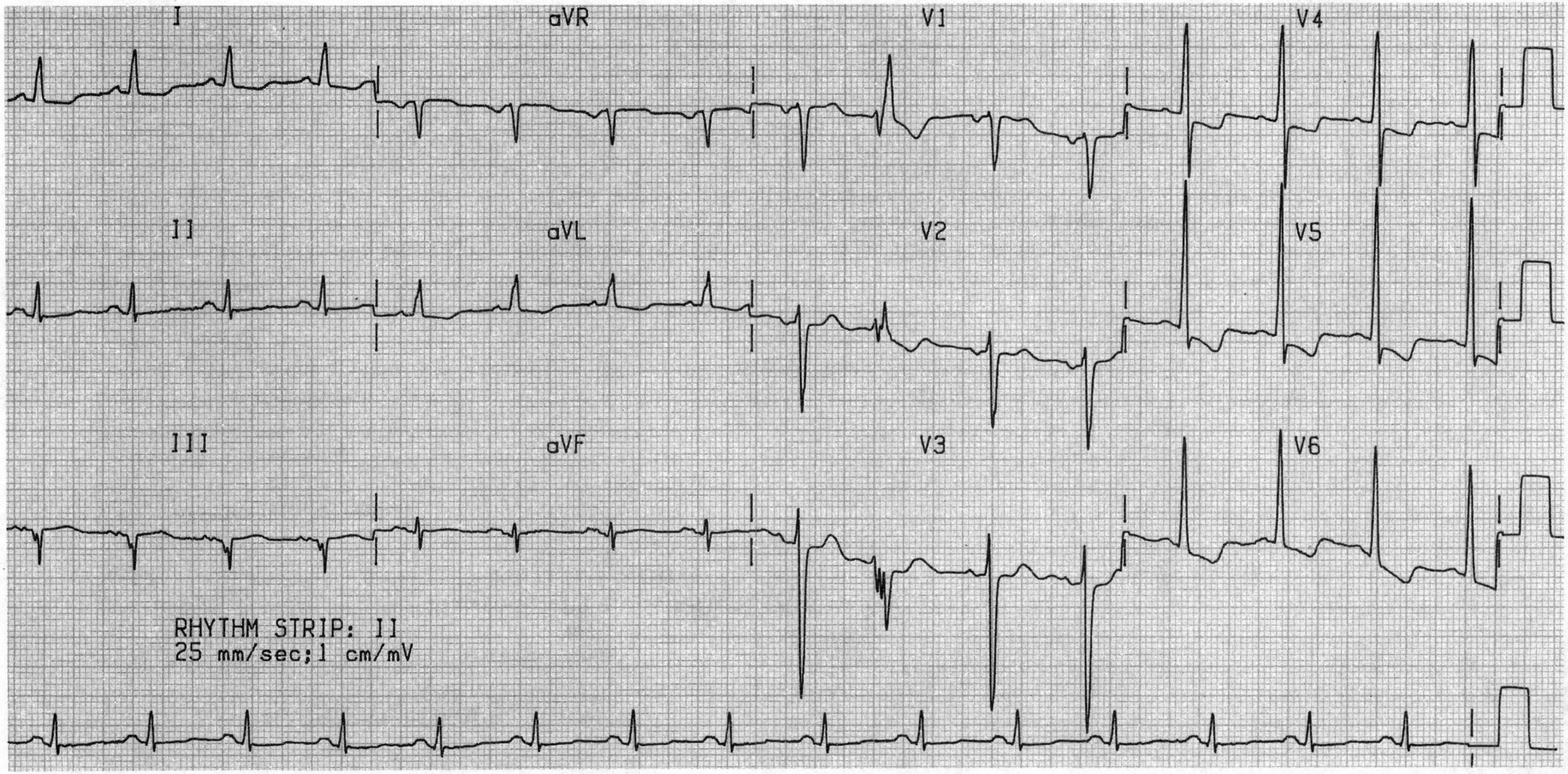

E-37

NARRATIVE INTERPRETATION

Rhythm: Sinus
Rate: 90
Intervals: PR 0.16, QRS 0.08, QT 0.34
Axis: − 15 degrees

Abnormalities

ST depression leads I, aVL, V4–V6. T-wave inversion leads I, aVL, V4–V6. SV2 + RV5 greater than 35. VPC.

Synthesis

Sinus rhythm. VPC. LVH by voltage criteria with associated ST-T-wave abnormalities.

TEST ANSWERS: 1, 26, 78, 103.

Comment: This patient has characteristic findings for LVH. There is increased precordial voltage and ST depression with an asymmetrically inverted T wave. The ST- and T-wave abnormalities have been called the left ventricular "strain" pattern. It is interesting to note that despite obvious criteria for LVH in the precordial leads the QRS voltage in the limb leads is quite low. This is due to the fact that the major forces of the QRS vector are perpendicular to the frontal plane. The LVH was secondary to chronic aortic insufficiency. The relatively short QT interval was secondary to treatment with digoxin.

E-38

Clinical History

A 35-year-old man seen in the emergency department.

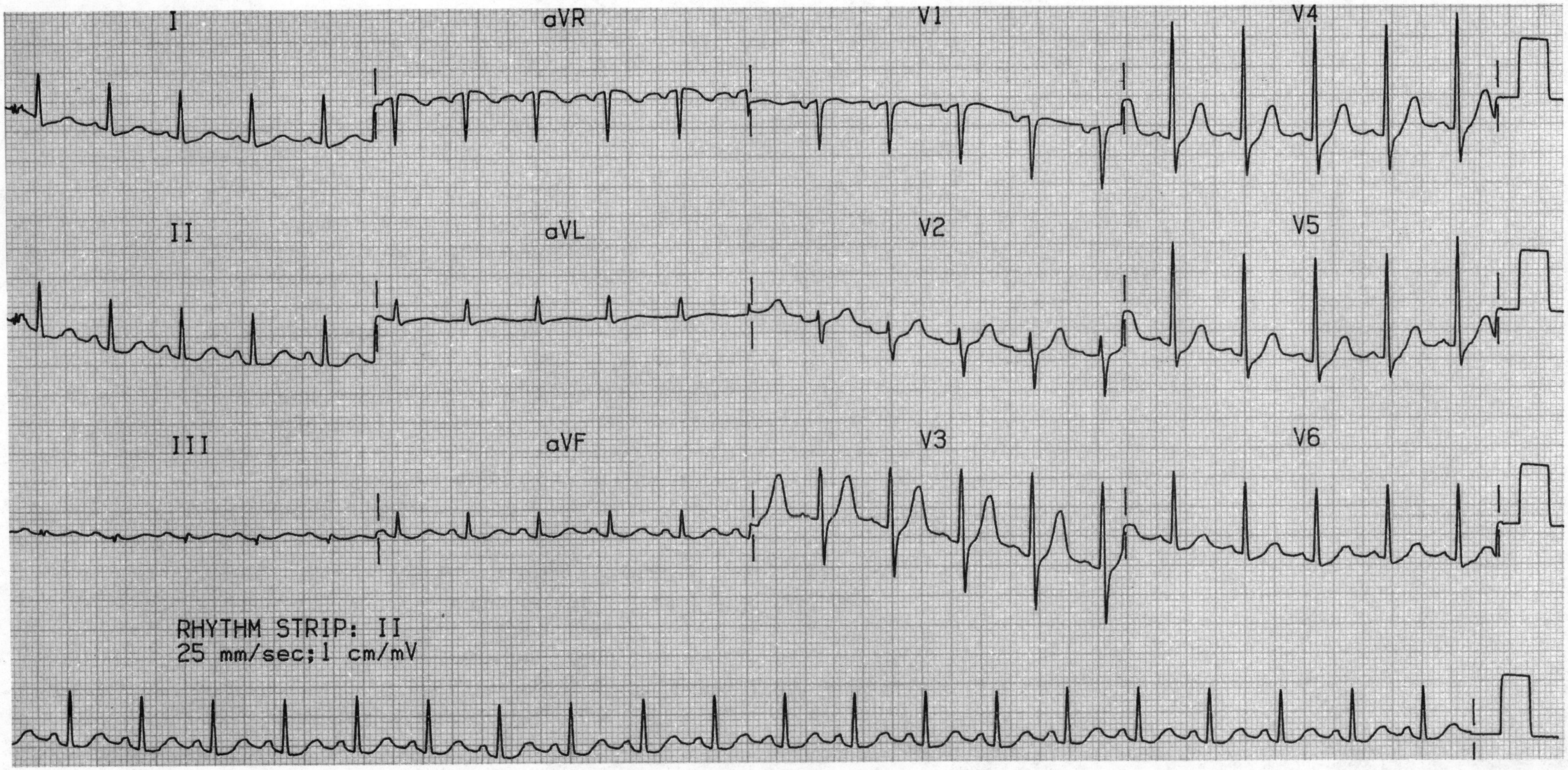

E-38

NARRATIVE INTERPRETATION

Rhythm:	**Sinus tachycardia**
Rate:	**126**
Intervals:	**PR 0.14, QRS 0.06, QT 0.30**
Axis:	**+30 degrees**

Abnormalities
Rapid heart rate. Slight ST depression leads I, II, aVF, V4–V6.

Synthesis
Sinus tachycardia. Nonspecific ST-segment abnormalities.

TEST ANSWERS: 4, 106.

Comment: The only significant abnormality of this electrocardiogram is the rapid heart rate. The minor, nonspecific ST abnormalities are likely associated with the sinus tachycardia and are not indicative of underlying cardiac disease. Remember that sinus tachycardia at rest is generally secondary to some other medical condition. Therapy should be directed to the primary disorder, not to the tachycardia itself. Conditions that frequently result in sinus tachycardia include hypotension, hypovolemia, hypoxia, fever, pain, and anxiety. Endocrine disorders such as hyperthyroidism or pheochromocytoma may also present with unexplained sinus tachycardia.

E-39

Clinical History

A 75-year-old man with mild "indigestion."

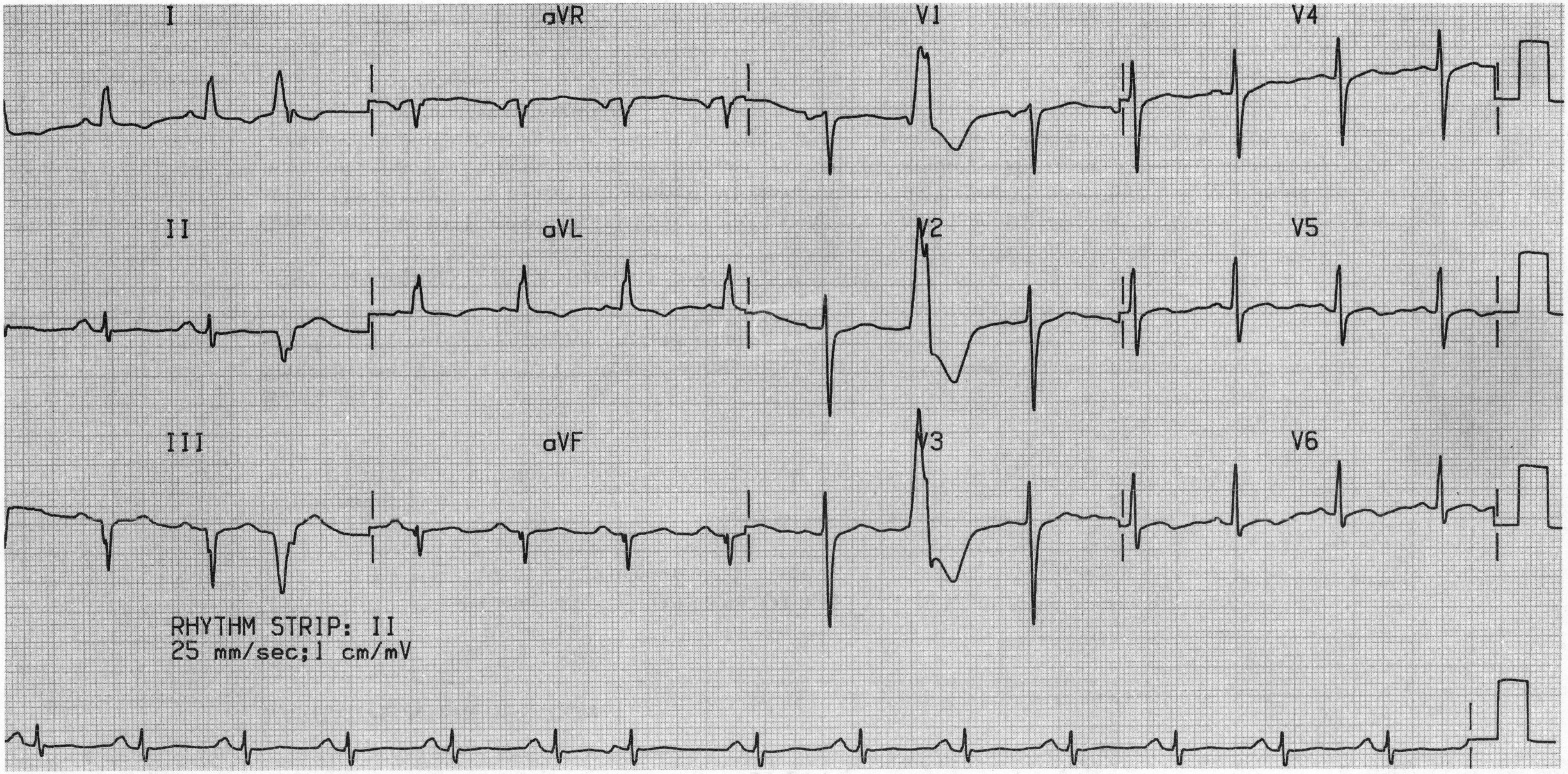

E-39

NARRATIVE INTERPRETATION

Rhythm:	**Sinus**
Rate:	**86**
Intervals:	**PR 0.19, QRS 0.08, QT 0.36**
Axis:	**−30 degrees**

Abnormalities

Slight ST elevation with downward concavity (coved) leads V5–V6. T-wave inversion leads I, aVL, V6. VPC. APC.

Synthesis

Sinus rhythm. VPC. APC. ST-T-wave abnormalities in leads V5–V6 suggesting myocardial injury. Nonspecific ST-T-wave abnormalities in leads I and aVL.

TEST ANSWERS: 1, 10, 26, 100, (102), 106.

Comment: The ST-T-wave abnormalities in this example are nondiagnostic but are somewhat worrisome. The "coved," or concave downward, ST elevation in leads V5 and V6 may represent myocardial injury and appear a bit more significant than just "nonspecific" findings. The reader is also reminded to carefully check the rhythm strip on each tracing. The VPC is easily seen; however, the APC might be overlooked by the casual interpreter.

E-40

Clinical History

A 62-year-old woman in the CCU.

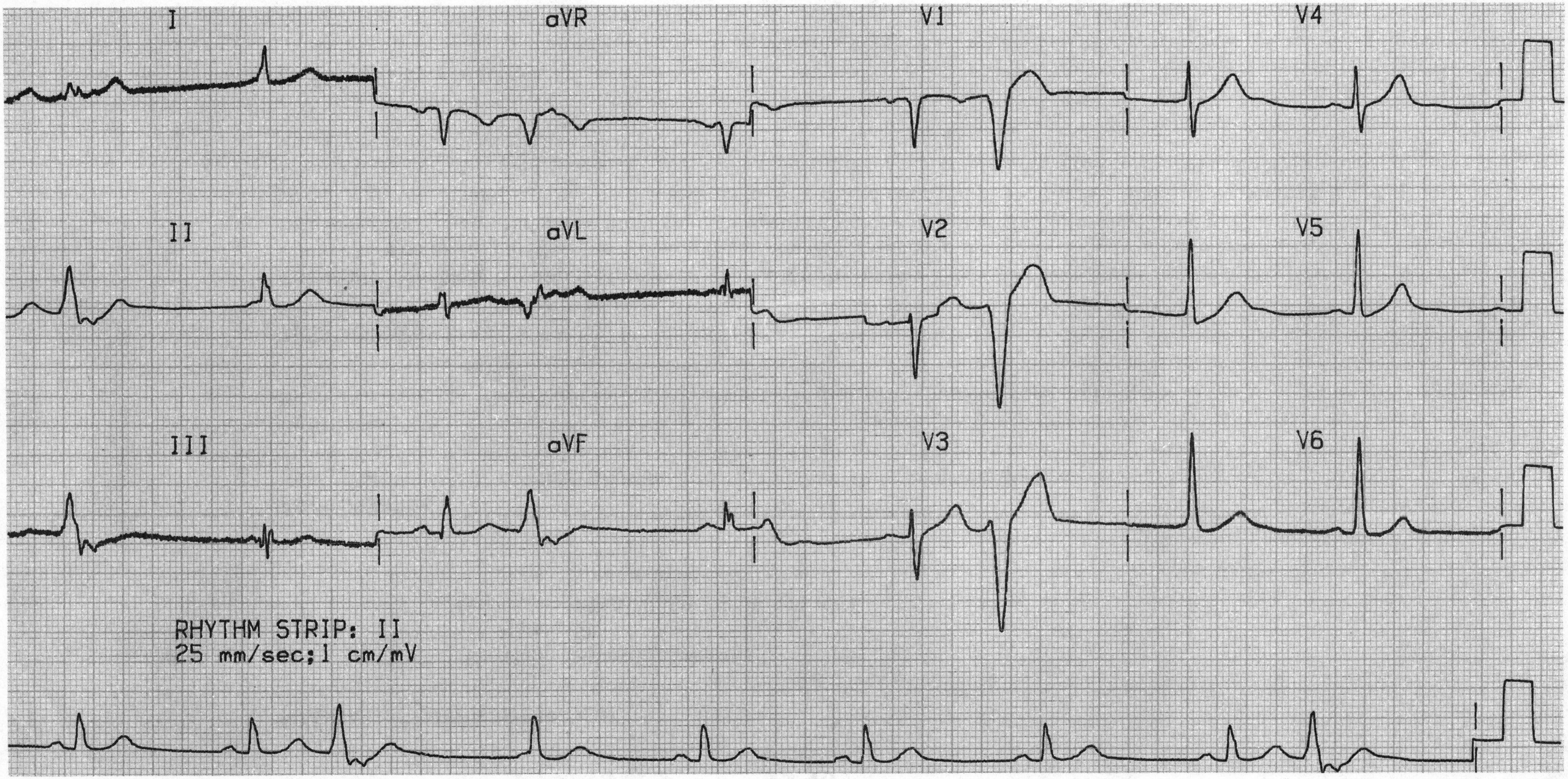

E-40

NARRATIVE INTERPRETATION

Rhythm: **Sinus bradycardia**
Rate: **50**
Intervals: **PR 0.20, QRS 0.08, QT 0.42**
Axis: **Unable to be determined**

Abnormalities

Slow heart rate. VPCs with retrograde atrial activation. Junctional escape complexes.

Synthesis

Sinus bradycardia. VPCs with retrograde atrial activation. Junctional escape complexes.

TEST ANSWERS: 3, 24, 26, 55.

Comment: The basic rhythm is sinus bradycardia interrupted by VPCs. On close inspection, an inverted P wave can be appreciated in the ST segment of the VPC. Because the sinus node is depolarized earlier than its normal cycle, the subsequent sinus depolarization occurs somewhat later than expected. As can be seen in this example, this may allow for a subsidiary pacemaker in the AV junction to emerge. Because the intrinsic rate of the AV junction is slower than the normal sinus rate, the sinus node can quickly regain control in the following complex.

REFERENCE: Chung p 354.

References

JOURNALS

Akhtar M, Shenasa M, Jazayeri M, et al: Wide QRS complex tachycardia. *Ann Intern Med* 109:905–912, 1988.

Alpert JS: "Conduction disturbances: Temporary and permanent pacing in patients with acute myocardial infarction." In Gersh BJ, Rahimtoola SH (eds): *Acute Myocardial Infarction*. New York, Elsevier, 1991, pp 249–258.

Alpert MA, Munuswamy K: Electrocardiographic diagnosis of left atrial enlargement. *Arch Intern Med* 149:1161–1165, 1989.

Bar FW, Brugada P, Dassen WRM, et al: Prognostic value of Q waves, R/S ratio, loss of R wave voltage, ST-T segment abnormalities, electrical axis, low voltage and notching: Correlation of electrocardiogram and left ventriculogram. *J Am Coll Cardiol* 4:17–27, 1984.

Bar FW, Brugada P, Dassen WRM, Wellens HJJ: Differential diagnosis of tachycardia with narrow QRS complex (shorter than .12 second). *Am J Cardiol* 54:555–560, 1984.

Barold SS, Linhart JW, Hildner FJ, et al: Incomplete left bundle branch block. *Circulation* 38:702–710, 1968.

Barrett PA, Peter CT, Swan HJC, et al: The frequency and prognostic significance of electrocardiographic abnormalities in clinically normal individuals. *Prog Cardiovasc Dis* 23:299–319, 1981.

Belardinelli L, Linden JH, Berne RM: The cardiac effects of adenosine. *Prog Cardiovasc Dis* 32:73–97, 1989.

Benchimol A, Desser KB: "The electrovectorcardiographic diagnosis of posterior wall myocardial infarction." In Fisch C (ed): *Complex Electrocardiography I*. Philadelphia, Davis, 1973, pp 184–197.

Berger PB, Ruocco NA Jr, Ryan TJ, et al: Incidence and prognostic implications of heart block complicating inferior myocardial infarction treated with thrombolytic therapy: Results from TIMI II. *J Am Coll Cardiol* 20:533–540, 1992.

Berk WA: ECG findings in nonpenetrating chest trauma: A review. *J Emerg Med* 5:209–215, 1987.

Blackman NS, Kuskin L: Inverted T waves in the precordial electrocardiogram of normal adolescents. *Am Heart J* 67:304–312, 1964.

Brugada P, Brugada J, Mont L, et al: A new approach to the differential diagnosis of a regular tachycardia with a wide QRS complex. *Circulation* 83: 1649–1659, 1991.

Bush HS, Ferguson JJ III, Angelini P, Willerson JT: Twelve-lead electrocardiographic evaluation of ischemia during percutaneous transluminal coronary angioplasty and its correlation with acute reocclusion. *Am Heart J* 121:1591–1599, 1991.

Casale PN, Devereux RB, Kligfield P, et al: Electrocardiographic detection of left ventricular hypertrophy: Development and prospective validation of improved criteria. *J Am Coll Cardiol* 6:572–580, 1985.

Chaitman BR: Posterior myocardial infarction revisited. *J Am Coll Cardiol* 12:1167–1168, 1988.

Cox J, Krajden M: Cardiovascular manifestations of Lyme disease. *Am Heart J* 122:1449–1455, 1991.

Crenshaw JH, Mirvis DM, El-Zeky F, et al: Interactive effects of ST-T wave abnormalities on survival of patients with coronary artery disease. *J Am Coll Cardiol* 18:413–420, 1991.

Croft CH, Woodward W, Nicod P, et al: Clinical implications of anterior S-T segment depression in patients with acute inferior myocardial infarction. *Am J Cardiol* 50:428–436, 1982.

DePace NL, Colby J, Hakki A, et al: Poor R wave progression in the precordial leads: Clinical implications for the diagnosis of myocardial infarction. *J Am Coll Cardiol* 2:1073–1079, 1983.

de Zwaan C, Bar FWHM, Wellens HJJ: Characteristic electrocardiographic pattern indicating a critical stenosis high in left anterior descending coronary artery in patients admitted because of impending myocardial infarction. *Am Heart J* 103:730–737, 1982.

Dunsmore LD, LoPointe MA, Dunsmore RA: Radiation-induced coronary artery disease. *J Am Coll Cardiol* 8:239–244, 1986.

Eisenstein I, Samnarco ME, Madrid WL, Selvester RH: Electrocardiographic and vectorcardiographic diagnosis of posterior wall myocardial infarction. *Chest* 88:409–416, 1985.

Farnham DJ, Shah PM: Left anterior hemiblock simulating anteroseptal myocardial infarction. *Am Heart J* 92:363–367, 1976.

Fass AE, Zimmerman FH: "Electrocardiographic abnormalities associated with cerebrovascular accidents." In Weintraub MI, Fass AE (eds): *Heart and Brain: Interactions of Cardiac and Neurologic Disease*. Santa Ana, California, PMA Publishing, 1991, pp 163–170.

Feigl D, Ashkenazy J, Kishon Y: Early and late atrioventricular block in acute inferior myocardial infarction. *J Am Coll Cardiol* 4:35–38, 1984.

Ferguson DW, Pandian N, Kioschos JM, et al: Angiographic evidence that reciprocal ST-segment depression during acute myocardial infarction does not indicate remote ischemia: Analysis of 23 patients. *Am J Cardiol* 53:55–62, 1984.

Fisch C, Knoebel SB: Digitalis cardiotoxicity. *J Am Coll Cardiol* 5:91A–98A, 1985.

Fisher ML, Mugmon MA, Carliner NH, et al: Left anterior fascicular block: Electrocardiographic criteria for its recognition in the presence of inferior myocardial infarction. *Am J Cardiol* 44:845–849, 1979.

Flowers NC: Left bundle branch block: A continuously evolving concept. *J Am Coll Cardiol* 9:684–697, 1987.

Fuchs RM, Aschuff SC, Grunwald L, et al: Electrocardiographic localization of coronary artery narrowings: Studies during myocardial ischemia and infarction in patients with one-vessel disease. *Circulation* 66:1168–1176, 1982.

Garson A Jr: Stepwise approach to the unknown pacemaker ECG. *Am Heart J* 119:924–941, 1990.

Gertsch M, Theler A, Foglia E: Electrocardiographic detection of left ventricular hypertrophy in the presence of left anterior fascicular block. *Am J Cardiol* 61:1098–1101, 1988.

Gintzon LE, Laks MM: The differential diagnosis of acute pericarditis from the normal variant: New electrocardiographic criteria. *Circulation* 65: 1004–1009, 1982.

Goldberger AL: ECG simulators of myocardial infarction. Part I: Pathophysiology and differential diagnosis of pseudo-infarct Q wave patterns. *PACE* 5:106–119, 1982.

Goldberger AL: ECG simulators of myocardial infarction. Part II: Pathophysiology and differential diagnosis of pseudo-infarct ST-T wave patterns. *PACE* 5:414–430, 1982.

Green M, Heddle B, Dassen W, et al: Value of QRS alternation in determining the site of origin of narrow QRS supraventricular tachycardia. *Circulation* 68:368–373, 1983.

Gulamhusein S, Yee R, Ko PT, Klein GJ: Electrocardiographic criteria for differentiating aberrancy and ventricular extrasystole in chronic atrial fibrillation: Validation by intracardiac recordings. *J Electrocardiol* 18:41–50, 1985.

Haft JI: "Clinical implications of atrioventricular and intraventricular conduction abnormalities. II. Acute myocardial infarction." In Rios JC (ed): *Clinical Electrocardiographic Correlations*. Philadelphia, Davis, 1977, pp. 65–78.

Haines DE, Raabe DS, Gundel WD, Wackers FJT: Anatomic and prognostic significance of new T-wave inversion in unstable angina. *Am J Cardiol* 52:14–18, 1983.

Hands ME, Cook EF, Stone PH, et al: Electrocardiographic diagnosis of myocardial infarction in the presence of complete left bundle branch block. *Am Heart J* 116:23–31, 1988.

Haraphongse M, Tanomsup S, Jugdutt BI: Inferior ST segment depression during acute anterior myocardial infarction: Clinical and angiographic correlations. *J Am Coll Cardiol* 4:467–476, 1984.

Hart GJ, Barrett PA, Barnaby PF, et al: Diagnosis of old anterior myocardial infarction in emphysema with poor R wave progression in anterior chest leads. *Br Heart J* 45:523–526, 1981.

Hazen MS, Marwick TH, Underwood DA: Diagnostic accuracy of the resting electrocardiogram in detection and estimation of left atrial enlargement: An echocardiographic correlation in 551 patients. *Am Heart J* 122:823–828, 1991.

Hecht HH, Kossmann CE, Childers RW, et al: Atrioventricular and intraventricular conduction: Revised nomenclature and concepts. *Am J Cardiol* 31:232–244, 1973.

Hindman MC, Wagner GS, JaRo M, et al: The clinical significance of bundle branch block complicating acute myocardial infarction. I. Clinical characteristics, hospital mortality, and one-year follow-up. *Circulation* 58:679–688, 1978.

Hindman MC, Wagner GS, JaRo M, et al: The clinical significance of bundle branch block complicating acute myocardial infarction. II. Indications for temporary and permanent pacemaker insertion. *Circulation* 58:689–699, 1978.

Horowitz LN: Electrophysiologic evaluation of patients with preexcitation syndromes. *Cardiol Clin* 4:447–457, 1986.

Howard RL, Dunn M: Left axis deviation with left bundle branch block. *Am J Noninvas Cardiol* 1:98–101, 1987.

Huey BL, Beller GA, Kaiser DL, Gibson RS: A comprehensive analysis of myocardial infarction due to left circumflex artery occlusion: Comparison with infarction due to right coronary artery and left anterior descending artery occlusion. *J Am Coll Cardiol* 12:1156–1166, 1988.

James KB, Obarski TP, Underwood DA: Electrocardiographic criteria for anterior myocardial infarction. *Cleve Clin J Med* 57:618–621, 1990.

Joy M, Trump DW: Significance of minor ST segment and T wave changes in the resting electrocardiogram of asymptomatic subjects. *Br Heart J* 45:48–55, 1981.

Kafka H, Burggraf GW, Milliken JA: Electrocardiographic diagnosis of left ventricular hypertrophy in the presence of left bundle branch block: An echocardiographic study. *Am J Cardiol* 55:103–106, 1985.

Kalbfleisch SJ, El-Atassi R, Calkins H, et al: Differentiation of paroxysmal narrow QRS complex tachycardias using the 12-lead electrocardiogram. *J Am Coll Cardiol* 21:85–89, 1993.

Kannel WB, Abbott RD, Savage DD, McNamara PM: Epidemiologic features of chronic atrial fibrillation: The Framingham study. *N Engl J Med* 306:1018–1022, 1982.

Kannel WB, Dannenberg AL, Levy D: Population implications of electrocardiographic left ventricular hypertrophy. *Am J Cardiol* 60:851–931, 1987.

Kastor JA: Multifocal atrial tachycardia. *New Engl J Med* 322:1713–1717, 1990.

Kastor JA, Yurchak PM: Recognition of digitalis intoxication in the presence of atrial fibrillation. *Ann Intern Med* 67:1045–1054, 1967.

Keefe DL, Miura D, Somberg JC: Supraventricular tachyarrhythmias: Their evaluation and therapy. *Am Heart J* 111:1150–1161, 1986.

Kilcoyne MM, Davis AL, Ferrer MI: A dynamic electrocardiographic concept useful in the diagnosis of cor pulmonale. *Circulation* 42:903–924, 1970.

Kindwall KE, Brown J, Josephson ME: Electrocardiographic criteria for ventricular tachycardia in wide complex left bundle branch block morphology tachycardias. *Am J Cardiol* 61:1279–1283, 1988.

Kishida H, Cole JS, Surawicz B: Negative U wave: A highly specific but poorly understood sign of heart disease. *Am J Cardiol* 49:2030–2036, 1982.

Klein GJ, Yee R, Sharma AD: Longitudinal electrophysiologic assessment of asymptomatic patients with the Wolff-Parkinson-White electrocardiographic pattern. *N Engl J Med* 320:1229–1233, 1989.

Klein RC, Vera Z, DeMaria JA, Mason DT: Electrocardiographic diagnosis of left ventricular hypertrophy in the presence of left bundle branch block. *Am Heart J* 108:502–506, 1984.

Koskinen P, Kupari M, Leinonen H, Luomanmaki K: Alcohol and new onset atrial fibrillation: A case-control study. *Br Heart J* 57:468–473, 1987.

Krahn AD, Manfreda J, Tate RB, et al: The natural history of electrocardiographic preexcitation in men. *Ann Intern Med* 116:456–460, 1992.

Kremers MS, Black WH, Wells PJ, Solodnya M: Effect of preexisting bundle branch block on the electrocardiographic diagnosis of ventricular tachycardia. *Am J Cardiol* 62:1208–1212, 1988.

REFERENCES

Kremers MS, Miller JM, Josephson ME: Electrical alternans in wide complex tachycardias. *Am J Cardiol* 56:305–308, 1985.

Langendorf R, Cohen H, Gozo EG Jr: Observations on second degree atrioventricular block, including new criteria for the differential diagnosis between type I and type II block. *Am J Cardiol* 29:111–119, 1972.

Lepeschkin E: The U wave of the electrocardiogram. *Mod Concepts Cardiovasc Dis* 38:39–45, 1969.

Liao Y, Emidy LA, Dyer A, et al: Characteristics and prognosis of incomplete right bundle branch block: An epidemiologic study. *J Am Coll Cardiol* 7:492–499, 1986.

Lopez-Sendon J, Coma-Canella I, Alcasena S, et al: Electrocardiographic findings in acute right ventricular infarction: Sensitivity and specificity of electrocardiographic alterations in right precordial leads V4R, V3R, V1, V2 and V3. *J Am Coll Cardiol* 6:1273–1279, 1985.

Louridas G, Patakas D, Angomachalelis N: Concomitant presence of left anterior hemiblock and inferior myocardial infarction: Electrocardiographic recognition of each entity. *J Electrocardiol* 14:365–370, 1981.

Macdonald RC, O'Neill CD, Ledingham IM: Myocardial contusion in blunt chest trauma. *Intensive Care Med* 7:265–268, 1981.

Mangiardi LM, Bonamini R, Conte M, et al: Bedside evaluation of atrioventricular block with narrow QRS complexes: Usefulness of carotic sinus massage and atropine administration. *Am J Cardiol* 49:1136–1145, 1982.

Manning GW, Smiley JR: QRS voltage criteria for left ventricular hypertrophy in a normal male population. *Circulation* 29:224–230, 1964.

Manolis AS, Estes AM: Supraventricular tachycardia: Mechanism and therapy. *Arch Intern Med* 147: 1706–1716, 1987.

Marriott HJL, Sandler IA: Criteria, old and new, for differentiating between ectopic ventricular beats and aberrant ventricular conduction in the presence of atrial fibrillation. *Prog Cardiovasc Dis* 9:18–28, 1966.

McAnulty JH, Rahimtoola SH, Murphy E, et al: Natural history of "high risk" bundle branch block. *N Engl J Med* 307:137–143, 1982.

Milliken JA: Isolated and complicated left anterior fascicular block: A review of suggested electrocardiographic criteria. *J Electrocardiol* 16:199–212, 1983.

Mirvis DM: Physiologic basis for anterior ST segment depression in patients with acute inferior wall myocardial infarction. *Am Heart J* 116:1308–1322, 1988.

Mymin D, Matewson FAL, Tate RB, Manfreda J: The natural history of primary first-degree atrioventricular heart block. *N Engl J Med* 315:1183–1187, 1986.

Nestico PF, Hakki A-Hamid, Iskandrian AS, Anderson GJ: Electrocardiographic diagnosis of posterior myocardial infarction revisted: A new approach using a multivariate discriminant analysis and thallium-201 myocardial scintigraphy. *J Electrocardiol* 19:33–40, 1986.

Nicod P, Gilpin E, Dittrich H, et al: Long-term outcome in patients with inferior myocardial infarction and complete atrioventricular block. *J Am Coll Cardiol* 12:589–594, 1988.

Parisi AF, Beckmann CH, Lancaster MC: The spectrum of ST segment elevation in the electrocardiograms of healthy adult men. *J Electrocardiol* 4:137–144, 1971.

Perloff JK: The recognition of strictly posterior myocardial infarction by conventional scalar electrocardiography. *Circulation* 30:706–718, 1964.

Perloff JK, Roberts NK, Cabeen WR Jr: Left axis deviation: A reassessment. *Circulation* 60:12–21, 1979.

Pritchett ELC: Management of atrial fibrillation. *N Engl J Med* 326:1264–1271, 1992.

Reddy GV, Schamroth L: The localization of bypass tracts in the Wolff-Parkinson-White syndrome from the surface electrocardiogram. *Am Heart J* 113:984–993, 1987.

Robalino BD, Whitlow PL, Underwood DA, Salcedo EE: Electrocardiographic manifestations of right ventricular infarction. *Am Heart J* 118:138–144, 1989.

Romanelli R, Willis WH Jr, Mitchell WA, Boucek RJ: Coronary arteriograms and myocardial scintigrams in the electrocardiographic syndrome of septal fibrosis. *Am Heart J* 100:617–621, 1980.

Romhilt DW, Bove KE, Norris RJ, et al: A critical appraisal of the electrocardiographic criteria for the diagnosis of left ventricular hypertrophy. *Circulation* 40:185–195, 1969.

Romhilt DW, Estes EH: A point score system for the ECG diagnosis of left ventricular hypertrophy. *Am Heart J* 75:752–758, 1968.

Rosenbaum MB, Yesuron J, Lazzaari JO, Elizari MV: Left anterior hemiblock obscuring the diagnosis of right bundle branch block. *Circulation* 48:298–303, 1973.

Rubin DA, Nieminski RN, Monteferrante JC, et al: Ventricular arrhythmias after coronary artery bypass graft surgery: Incidence, risk factors and long-term prognosis. *J Am Coll Cardiol* 6:307–310, 1985.

Rubin DA, Sorbera C, Nikitin P, et al: Prospective evaluation of heart block complicating early Lyme disease. *PACE* 15:252–255, 1992.

Saner HE, Lange HW, Pierach CA, Aeppli DM: Relation between serum digoxin concentration and the electrocardiogram. *Clin Cardiol* 11:752–756, 1988.

Schaeffer JW, Pryor R: Pseudo left axis deviation and the S1S2S3 syndrome in chronic airway obstruction. *Chest* 4:453–455, 1977.

Schamroth L, Bradlow BA: Incomplete left bundle branch block. *Br Heart J* 26:285–288, 1964.

Schmock CL, Mitchell RS, Pomerantz B, et al: The electrocardiogram in emphysema with and without chronic airways obstruction. *Chest* 60:328–334, 1971.

Schmock CL, Mitchell RS, Pomerantz B, et al: The electrocardiogram in chronic airways obstruction. *Chest* 60:335–340, 1971.

Schneider JF, Thomas HE, Kreger BE, et al: Newly acquired left bundle branch block. *Ann Intern Med* 90:303–310, 1979.

Schneider JF, Thomas HE, Kreger BE, et al: Newly acquired right bundle branch block. *Ann Intern Med* 92:37–44, 1980.

Schweitzer P: The electrocardiographic diagnosis of acute myocardial infarction in the thrombolytic era. *Am Heart J* 119:642–654, 1990.

Schweitzer P: The values and limitations of the QT interval in clinical practice. *Am Heart J* 124: 1121–1126, 1992.

Selvester RH, Rubin HB: New criteria for the electrocardiographic diagnosis of emphysema and cor pulmonale. *Am Heart J* 69:437–447, 1965.

Shah PK: "New insights into the electrocardiogram of acute myocardial infarction." In Gersh BJ, Rahimtoola SH (eds): *Acute Myocardial Infarction*. New York, Elsevier, 1991, pp 128–143.

Simonson E, Cady LD, Woodbury M: The normal Q-T interval. *Am Heart J* 63:747–753, 1962.

Smith TW, Antman EM, Friedman PL, et al: Digitalis glycosides: Mechanisms and manifestations of toxicity. *Prog Cardiovasc Dis* 27:21–56, 1984.

Spodick DH: Differential characteristics of the electrocardiogram in early repolarization and acute pericarditis. *N Engl J Med* 295:523–526, 1976.

Spodick DH: Left axis deviation and left anterior fascicular block. *Am J Cardiol* 61:869–870, 1987.

Steinman RT, Herrera C, Schuger CD, Lehmann MH: Wide QRS tachycardia in the conscious adult. *JAMA* 261:1013–1016, 1989.

Stewart RB, Bardy GH, Greene HL: Wide complex tachycardia: Misdiagnosis and outcome after emergent therapy. *Ann Intern Med* 104:766–771, 1986.

Stratmann HG, Kennedy HL: Torsades de pointes associated with drugs and toxins: Recognition and management. *Am Heart J* 113:1470–1482, 1987.

Surawicz B: Electrocardiographic diagnosis of chamber enlargement. *J Am Coll Cardiol* 8:711–724, 1986.

Tchou P, Young P, Mahmud R, et al: Useful clinical criteria for the diagnosis of ventricular tachycardia. *Am J Med* 84:53–56, 1988.

Tenzer ML: The spectrum of myocardial contusion: A review. *J Trauma* 25:620–627, 1985.

Thomas JL, Dickstein RA, Parker FB Jr, et al: Prognostic significance of the development of left bundle conduction defects following aortic valve replacement. *J Thorac Cardiovasc Surg* 84:382–386, 1982.

Timmis GC, Gangadharan V, Ramos RG, Gordon S: Reassessment of Q waves in left bundle branch block. *J Electrocardiol* 9:109–114, 1976.

Tuzcu EM, Emre A, Goormastic M, et al: Incidence and prognostic significance of intraventricular conduction abnormalities after coronary bypass surgery. *J Am Coll Cardiol* 16:607–610, 1990.

Vandenberg BF, Romhilt DW: Electrocardiographic diagnosis of left ventricular hypertrophy in the presence of bundle branch block. *Am Heart J* 122:818–822, 1991.

Wackers FJT: The diagnosis of myocardial infarction in the presence of left bundle branch block. *Cardiol Clin* 5:393–401, 1987.

Waldo AL: "Atrial flutter." In Horowitz LN (ed): *Current Management of Arrhythmias*. Philadelphia, Decker, 1991, pp 58–63.

Walker CHM, Rose RL: Importance of age, sex and body habitus in the diagnosis of left ventricular hypertrophy from the precordial electrocardiogram in childhood and adolescence. *Pediatrics* 28:705–711, 1961.

Wanner WR, Schaal SF, Bashore TM, et al: Repolarization variant vs acute pericarditis. *Chest* 83: 180–184, 1983.

Warner RA, Hill NE, Mookherjee S, Smulyan H: Electrocardiographic criteria for the diagnosis of combined inferior myocardial infarction and left anterior hemiblock. *Am Heart J* 51:718–722, 1983.

Warner RA, Hill NE, Mookherjee S, Smulyan H: Improved electrocardiographic criteria for the diagnosis of left anterior hemiblock. *Am J Cardiol* 51:723–726, 1983.

Warner RA, Hill NE, Sheehe PR, et al: Improved electrocardiographic criteria for the diagnosis of inferior myocardial infarction. *Circulation* 66:422–428, 1982.

Warner RA, Reger M, Hill NE, et al: Electrocardiographic criteria for the diagnosis of anterior myocardial infarction: Importance of the duration of precordial R waves. *Am J Cardiol* 52:690–692, 1983.

Wellens HJJ, Barr FWHM, Lie KI: The value of the electrocardiogram in the differential diagnosis of a tachycardia with a widened QRS complex. *Am J Med* 84:27–33, 1978.

Wexelman W, Lichstein E, Cunningham JN, et al: Etiology and clinical significance of new fascicular conduction defects following coronary bypass surgery. *Am Heart J* 111:923–927, 1986.

Willems JL, Robles de Medina EO, Bernard R, et al: Criteria for intraventricular conduction disturbances and pre-excitation. *J Am Coll Cardiol* 5:1261–1275, 1985.

Witham AC: "VCG patterns of myocardial scarring in the absence of diagnostic Q waves." In Schlant RC, Jurst JW (eds): *Advances in Electrocardiography*. New York: Grune & Stratton, 1972, pp 349–365.

Zehender M, Meinertz T, Keul J, Just H: ECG variants and cardiac arrhythmias in athletes: Clinical relevance and prognostic importance. *Am Heart J* 119:1378–1391, 1990.

Zema MJ: Electrocardiographic tall R waves in the right precordial leads. *J Electrocardiol* 23:147–156, 1990.

Zema MJ, Kligfield P: Electrocardiographic poor R wave progression. I: Correlation with the Frank vectorcardiogram. *J Electrocardiol* 12:3–10, 1979.

Zema MJ, Kligfield P: Electrocardiographic poor R wave progression. II: Correlation with angiography. *J Electrocardiol* 12:11–15, 1979.

Zema MJ, Luminais SK, Chiaramida S, et al: Electrocardiographic poor R wave progression. III: The normal variant. *J Electrocardiol* 13:135–142, 1980.

Zema MJ, Kligfield P: ECG poor R wave progression. *Arch Intern Med* 142:1145–1148, 1982.

Zema MJ, Kligfield P: Electrocardiographic tall R waves in the right precordial leads: Vectorcardiographic and electrocardiographic distinction of posterior myocardial infarction from prominent anterior forces in normal subjects. *J Electrocardiol* 17:129–138, 1984.

Zimmerman FH, Gustafson GM, Kemp HG Jr: Recurrent myocardial infarction associated with cocaine abuse in a young man with normal coronary arteries: Evidence of coronary artery spasm culminating in thrombosis. *J Am Coll Cardiol* 9:964–968, 1987.

Zipes DP: Second degree atrioventricular block. *Circulation* 60:465–472, 1979.

BOOKS

Chou TC: *Electrocardiography in Clinical Practice,* 3d ed. Philadelphia, Saunders, 1991.

Chung EK: *Principles of Cardiac Arrhythmias,* 4th ed. Baltimore, William & Wilkins, 1989.

Cooksey JD, Dunn M, Massie E: *Clinical Vectorcardiography and Electrocardiography,* 2d ed. Chicago, Year Book Medical Publishers, 1977.

Falk RH, Podrid PJ (eds): *Atrial Fibrillation: Mechanisms and Management*. New York, Raven, 1992.

Friedman HH: *Diagnostic Electrocardiography and Vectorcardiography,* 3d ed. New York, McGraw-Hill, 1985.

Horowitz LN: *Current Management of Arrhythmias*. Philadelphia, Decker, 1991.

Marriott HJL: *Practical Electrocardiography,* 8th ed. Baltimore, William & Wilkins, 1988.

Marriott HJL, Conover MH: *Advanced Concepts in Arrhythmias*. St. Louis, Mosby, 1983.

Schamroth L: *The Disorders of Cardiac Rhythm*. Philadelphia, Davis, 1971.

Schlant RC, Hurst JW (eds): *Advances in Electrocardiography*. New York, Grune & Stratton, 1972.

Index for Electrocardiographic Diagnoses

89. Lateral or high lateral, acute or recent C-13, D-5, E-9, E-33
90. Lateral, old or of indeterminate age E-28
91. Inferior or diaphragmatic, acute or recent A-3, A-28, B-16, B-35, B-38, C-8, C-10, C-16, C-22, C-30, C-36, C-37, D-21, D-32, E-13, E-31
92. Inferior or diaphragmatic, old or of indeterminate age A-20, A-25, A-37, B-10, B-18, C-3, C-28, D-11, D-24
93. Posterior, acute or recent B-18, C-10, C-30, E-13
94. Posterior, old or of indeterminate age A-17, B-38, C-11, C-18, C-29
95. Suggestive of ventricular aneurysm A-20, A-25, C-28, E-10, E-28

IX. ST-, T-, U-WAVE ABNORMALITIES

96. Normal variant, isolated J-point elevation (early repolarization pattern) B-2, C-3, C-5, E-30
97. Isolated J-point depression
98. Normal variant, RSR′ pattern lead V1 A-21
99. Normal variant, persistent juvenile T-wave pattern A-8
100. ST- and/or T-wave abnormalities suggesting acute or recent myocardial injury A-3, A-19, A-28, A-32, A-40, B-16, B-19, B-27, B-35, B-38, B-40, C-4, C-8, C-10, C-13, C-15, C-16, C-22, C-30, C-36, C-37, D-5, D-19, D-21, D-31, D-32, E-4, E-13, E-31, E-33, E-39
101. ST- and/or T-wave abnormalities in the setting of acute myocardial injury suggesting either reciprocal change or myocardial ischemia A-3, A-28, B-35, C-8, C-10, C-13, C-22, C-30, D-31, D-32, E-4, E-9, E-31, E-33
102. ST- and/or T-wave abnormalities in the absence of acute myocardial injury suggesting myocardial ischemia B-23, D-27, D-39, E-25, E-28
103. ST- and/or T-wave abnormalities associated with ventricular hypertrophy A-2, A-13, A-22, A-30, A-36, A-37, A-39, B-11, B-12, B-13, B-22, B-24, B-25, B-32, B-34, B-37, C-2, C-12, C-16, C-21, C-31, C-32, C-38, D-1, D-4, D-13, D-33, D-34, D-35, D-37, D-38, E-5, E-7, E-16, E-21, E-22, E-23, E-25, E-29, E-36, E-37
104. ST- and/or T-wave abnormalities associated with ventricular conduction abnormality A-11, A-23, A-31, A-37, B-1, B-4, B-7, B-10, B-17, B-20, B-25, B-26, B-40, C-8, C-9, C-19, C-23, C-37, C-39, D-7, D-11, D-12, D-24, D-26, D-28, D-29, D-30, E-1, E-2, E-14, E-19, E-35
105. ST- and/or T-wave abnormalities suggesting early, acute pericarditis B-3, C-35
106. Nonspecific ST- and/or T-wave abnormalities A-4, A-5, A-7, A-9, A-17, A-24, A-27, A-29, A-35, A-38, B-7, B-28, B-31, B-33, B-36, B-39, B-40, C-1, C-3, C-5, C-6, C-7, C-15, C-18, C-20, C-26, C-27, C-28, C-34, D-2, D-3, D-9, D-10, D-14, D-15, D-20, D-25, D-36, E-3, E-6, E-10, E-12, E-15, E-20, E-27, E-30, E-32, E-34, E-38, E-39
107. Postextrasystolic T-wave abnormality
108. Peaked T waves A-4
109. Prolonged QT interval for heart rate (QTc) A-4, A-39, B-33, C-28, C-34, D-10, D-17, D-27, D-35, E-4, E-16
110. Prominent U waves B-28, B-37, D-4, D-34
111. Inverted U waves B-37

X. GENERAL FEATURES

112. Incorrect electrode placement B-31, E-26
113. Artifact secondary to tremor B-37